Best Wishes—

John B. [illegible], M.D.

Vascular Surgery

Vascular Surgery

Edited by
John B. Chang, M.D.
Director
Long Island Vascular Clinic
Roslyn, New York

MEDICAL & SCIENTIFIC BOOKS
A DIVISION OF SPECTRUM PUBLICATIONS, INC.
NEW YORK

SPECTRUM PUBLICATIONS, INC.
175-20 Wexford Terrace
Jamaica, NY 11432

Library of Congress Cataloging in Publication Data
Main entry under title:

Vascular surgery.

Based on the International Vascular Symposium, "Vascular Surgery–1983," held in New York City in the spring of 1983.
Includes bibliographies and index.
1. Blood-vessels–Surgery–Congresses. I. Chang, John B. II. International Vascular Symposium, "Vascular Surgery–1983" (1983: New York, N.Y.)
[DNLM: 1. Vascular Surgery–congresses. WG 170 V3312]
RD598.5.V373 1985 617′.413 85-2319
ISBN 0-89335-232-2

Printed in the United States of America

Dedication

This book is dedicated
to my lifetime friend and cherished wife,
Lucy Chang, M.D.

Contributors

Hon. Seymour Boyers Former Associate Justice, Appellate Division, Second Department; Former Presiding Justice, Medical Malpractice Panel, Supreme Court, Queens County, New York

John B. Chang, M.D. Director, Long Island Vascular Clinic and Long Island Vascular Laboratory, Roslyn, New York; Attending Surgeon, Long Island Jewish-Hillside Medical Center, New Hyde Park, New York; Assistant Professor of Clinical Surgery, Health Sciences Center, State University of New York at Stony Brook

Denton A. Cooley, M.D. Surgeon-in-Chief, Texas Heart Institute, Houston; Clinical Professor of Surgery, University of Texas Medical School, Houston

Charles T. Dotter, M.D. Chairman, Department of Radiology, Oregon Hospital and Clinic, Portland; Professor of Radiology, University of Oregon Health Sciences Center School of Medicine, Portland

Alfred R. Ernst, M.D. Chief of Vascular Surgery, Mary Immaculate Hospital, Jamaica, New York; Clinical Instructor of Surgery, State University of New York, Downstate Medical Center College of Medicine, Brooklyn

Moshe Haimov, M.D. Co-Chief, Vascular Surgical Service, Department of Surgery, Mt. Sinai Hospital, New York, New York; Associate Clinical Professor of Surgery, Mt. Sinai School of Medicine of the City University of New York

Larry H. Hollier, M.D. Consultant in Vascular Surgery, Mayo Clinic; Assistant Professor of Surgery, Mayo Medical School, Rochester, Minnesota

Anthony M. Imparato, M.D. Professor of Surgery, New York University School of Medicine, New York

Eric P. Lofgren, M.D. Consultant in Surgery, Mayo Clinic; Associate Professor of Surgery, Mayo Medical School, Rochester, Minnesota

Edward Meilman, M.D. Director Emeritus, Department of Medicine, Long Island Jewish-Hillside Medical Center, New Hyde Park, New York; Professor of Medicine, Health Sciences Center, State University of New York at Stony Brook

Marshall J. Orloff, M.D. Chairman and Professor, Department of Surgery, University of California School of Medicine, San Diego

Malcolm O. Perry, M.D. Chief Vascular Surgeon, Division of Vascular Surgery, Department of Surgery, New York Hospital-Cornell Medical Center; Professor of Surgery, Cornell University Medical College, New York, New York

George J. Reul, Jr., M.D. Associate Surgeon, Texas Children's Hospital, St. Luke's Hospital, and Texas Heart Institute; Associate Clinical Professor of Surgery, University of Texas Medical School at Houston

Harry Schanzer, M.D. Director, Vascular Laboratory and Transplantation Laboratory, Mt. Sinai Hospital, New York, New York; Associate Professor of Surgery, Mt. Sinai School of Medicine of the City University of New York

Ernst Schneider, M.D. Department of Angiology, Medical Polyclinic, Universitätsspital, Zurich, Switzerland

D. E. Strandness, Jr., M.D. Professor, Department of Surgery, University of Washington School of Medicine, Seattle

D. Emerick Szilagyi, M.D. Consultant, Vascular Surgery, Henry Ford Hospital, Detroit, Michigan; Clinical Professor of Surgery, The University of Michigan Medical School, Ann Arbor

Marko Turina, M.D. Professor of Surgery, Chirurgische Klinik, Universitätsspital, Zurich, Switzerland

Ronald Virag, M.D. Centre d'Etudes et de Recherches de l'Impuissance, Paris, France

Preface

This publication is based on the International Vascular Symposium, "Vascular Surgery—1983," which took place in New York City in the spring of 1983. The book presents the current state of the art of vascular surgery to physicians and surgeons who deal with vascular disease problems. The reader will have a handbook of up-to-date clinical and laboratory information applicable to patient care, with a current review of selected surgical problems and management, all from the most outstanding surgeons and physicians in the field today. It is my sincere hope that the reader will find this book both valuable and thought-provoking, and an incentive for further research and sharing of knowledge.

I appreciate the encouragement given to this conference by Robert K. Match, M.D., President of Long Island Jewish-Hillside Medical Center and Professor of Community and Preventive Medicine, School of Medicine, State University of New York at Stony Brook, and the strong support and guidance given to me throughout the convention by Leslie Wise, M.D., Chairman, Department of Surgery, Long Island Jewish-Hillside Medical Center and Professor of Surgery, School of Medicine, State University of New York at Stony Brook. My thanks also go to Ms. Ann Boehme, Continuing Education Coordinator at the Medical Center, who helped to make the Vascular Symposium so successful, and to the entire staff of the Long Island Vascular Clinic and of the Long Island Vascular Laboratory for their great efforts in making the Symposium a wonderful reality. I would also like to thank Ms. Barbara Messner for the excellent editing of the manuscripts.

My particular thanks go to the Hon. Seymour Boyers, a distinguished judge and my dear friend, who has contributed greatly to lessen the unnecessary stress on our profession from malpractice problems. His lecture at our convention was extremely well received. My sincere appreciation goes to all the guest speakers at the Symposium, and to our special luncheon speaker, Mr. H. H. G. Eastcott of London.

My deepest gratitude goes to my dear wife, Lucy, without whose untiring endeavors in my behalf, my professional life would not be so fulfilling.

As future symposia evolve, we hope to add to the knowledge of those dedicated surgeons and doctors who care for patients in the fields of vascular surgery and medicine. It is also my hope that this educational project will give guidelines and direction to interns and residents, who give me great challenges and for whom I have great compassion. I am grateful to the patients whom I have been privileged to attend. They are my major source of inspiration for understanding, love, and commitment beyond the complexities of vascular surgery. I hope this book will be a milestone in our ever-growing interest in teaching and patient care at our institutions, and that the information contained herein can be shared with our many colleagues throughout the world.

John B. Chang, M.D., F.A.C.S.

Contents

CHAPTER 8
Transluminal Angioplasty

CHAPTER 9
Arteriosclerotic Peripheral Vascular Disease

CHAPTER 10
Venous Problems

Vascular Surgery

1

Noninvasive Vascular Studies

1
Noninvasive Vascular Studies of Extracranial Vascular System and Current Concepts

D. E. Strandness, Jr.

The methods available to assess the extracranial arterial system can be classified into two major groups. The indirect tests are those which sense changes in pressure and flow at some point removed from the carotid bifurcation. These include periorbital Doppler and oculoplethysmography. Both of these methods are useful only in situations in which the pressure and flow across the bifurcation have been reduced either by high grade stenoses or total occlusions. Thus, they will not be of value for the detection of those lesions which do not reduce pressure and flow. Another disadvantage of these indirect methods is that once positive, they will not change back and thus cannot be used to detect further progression of an existing lesion.

Because of the need to assess both the anatomy and physiology of the carotid bifurcation, direct ultrasonic methods have been developed. While there is some disagreement concerning the relative worth of anatomic visualization (B-mode) versus the role of spectral analysis of velocity signals by Doppler, all of the

Incidence of Coma-Death (Long-Term Follow-Up)

	Patients	C-D	Percent
Group I (unilateral C.E.)	146	3	2.0%
Group II (unilateral C.E.—contralateral ICA occlusion)	45	3	6.6%
Group III (bilateral C.E.)	86	1	1.2%

Late Strokes

Carotid territory	26
Coma-death	7
Total	33

Carotid Artery Surgery
Long-Term Follow-Up (1970–1975)

298 patients → 13 died
↓
285 survived → 8 lost
↓
277 followed (97.2%)

277 Patients followed 4–9 years

80 deaths	27.0%
33 strokes	11.9%

Perioperative Stroke

Contralateral carotid artery status	Operations	Strokes	Percent
70% Stenosis	665	12	1.8%
70–99% Stenosis	165	3	1.8%
Totally occluded	103	8	7.8%
Totals	933	23	

Carotid Complications by Symptoms (Amaurosis Fugax Only)

Stroke	1.4%
Death	1.4%

Myocardial Infarction after Carotid Endarterectomy (683 Patients)

Myocardial infarction	2.3%
Death from M.I.	0.7%

Correlation of Heart Disease and Postoperative M.I.

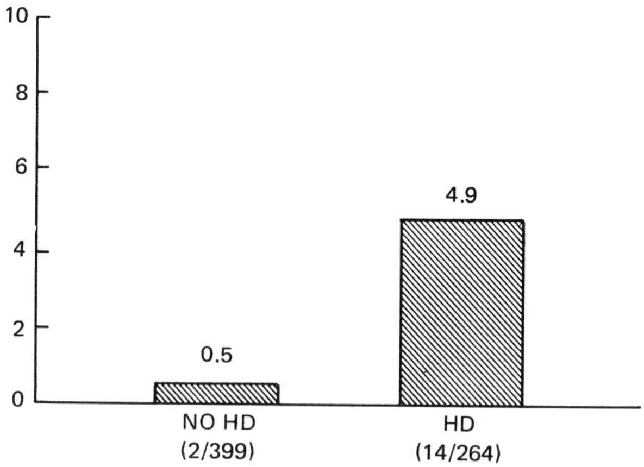

BIBLIOGRAPHY

Blaisdell FW, Clauss RH, Goldberg AF, Johnson AL, Imparato AM, Ransohoff J. Joint study of cerebrovascular disease—a review of surgical considerations. JAMA 209:1889, 1969.

Eastcott HHG, Bickering GW, Rob C. Reconstruction of internal carotid artery in a patient with intermittent attacks of hemiplegia. Lancet 1954(2):994–996.

Ehrenfeld WK, Royt WF, Wylie EJ. Embolization and transient blindness from carotid atheroma. Surgical considerations. Arch Surg 93:787–794, 1966.

Fisher M. Occlusion of the internal carotid artery. Arch Neurol Psychiat 72: 187–204, 1954.

Hass WK, Clauss RH, Goldberg AF, Johnson AL, Imparato AM, Ransohoff J. Special problems associated with surgical and thrombolytic treatment of strokes. Arch Surg 92:27, 1966.

Hutchinson EC, Yates PO. The cervical portion of the vertebral artery, a clinico-pathological study. Brain 79:319–331, 1956.

Imparato AM. Carotid predominance: the major and minor carotid artery in surgical reconstructions. In WK Hass (ed.), Current Concepts in Cerebrovascular Disease. Stroke 9:15–18, 1974.

Imparato AM, Bracco A, Kim GE, Bergmann L. The hypoglossal nerve in carotid arterial reconstructions. Stroke 3:576, 1972.

Imparato AM, Riles TS, Kim GE. Cervical vertebral angioplasty for brain stem ischemia: 16 years experience. Surg Gynec Obstet, submitted for publication.

Larsen GP Jr, Ehrenfeld WK, Wade JG, Wylie EJ. Jugular venous oxygen saturation as an index of adequacy of cerebral oxygenation. Surg 62:31–39, 1967.

McDowell FH, Potes J, Groch S. The natural history of internal carotid and vertebral-basilar artery occlusion. Neurology 11:153–157, 1961.

Millikan CH. The pathogenesis of transient focal cerebral ischemia. Circulation 32:438–450, 1965.

Ransohoff J. Surgery for extracranial cerebrovascular insufficiency. In J Ransohoff (ed.), Modern Technics in Surgery, pp 14–38. Mount Kisco, NY, Futura, 1980.

Riles TS, Kopelman I, Imparato AM. Myocardial infarction following carotid endartectomy: a review of 683 operations. Surg 85:249–251, 1979.

Riles TS, Imparato AM, Kopelman I. Carotid artery stenosis with contralateral internal carotid occlusions: long term results in 52 patients. Surg 87: 363, 1980.

Riles TS, Imparato AM, Mintzer R. Comparison of results of bilateral and unilateral carotid endartectomy five years after surgery. Stroke 12:124, 1981 (abstract).

Spielberger S, Turndorf H, Culliford A, Imparato AM. Hand-held toy squeaker during carotid endartectomy in the awake patient. Arch Surg 114:103, 1979.

Thompson JE. Complication of carotid endarterectomy and their prevention. (Invited commentary by AM Imparato) World J Surg 3:155–165, 1979.

Thompson JE, Austin DJ, Patman RD. Endartectomy of the totally occluded carotid artery for stroke: results in 100 operations. Arch Surg 95:791–801, 1967.

Wells BA, Keats AS, Cooley DA. Increased tolerance to cerebral ischemia produced by general anesthesia during temporary carotid occlusion. Surg 54:216–223, 1963.

4
Carotid Artery Disease: Pathogenesis and Management

Larry H. Hollier

In the United States, stroke remains one of the major causes of death and carries an increasing incidence with advancing age. Cerebral infarction accounts for almost 80 percent of strokes, with subarachnoid hemorrhage and intracerebral hemorrhage causing less than 20 percent [1,2]. About three-fourths of patients with ischemic strokes have occlusive lesions at a surgically accessible site, and about 40 percent have the offending lesion confined to the extracranial arteries [3].

This relatively high degree of accessibility encourages one to look very closely at the development and consequences of these lesions, since timely intervention may allow the prevention of stroke. To better delineate the problems and the rationale of treatment, a thorough understanding of the pathogenesis of stroke and the clinical manifestations of cerebrovascular disease is necessary.

PATHOGENESIS

Because of mechanical and rheologic factors, the carotid bulb and bifurcation are particularly prone to the development of atherosclerotic plaque. One can postulate that the turbulent flow in this area may damage the endothelium, which then may precipitate the cycle of platelet adhesion, release of platelet-derived growth factor, proliferation of subendothelial smooth muscle cells and the increasing deposition of lipoprotein into these cells, resulting in the atherosclerotic plaque. As the plaque grows larger, the foam cells eventually disintegrate, resulting in the accumulation of cholesterol crystals in the plaque. The continued growth of the plaque may occlude the lumen of the carotid artery, or the endothelium of the plaque may break down, discharging the cholesterol and other atherosclerotic debris into the arterial blood stream. The ulcerated plaque is then even more thrombogenic and platelets may alternately accumulate and be washed off to occlude small distal vessels [4]. Thus the production of symptoms may result from one or a combination of three factors: the enlarging stenotic plaque which decreases or completely occludes blood flow, the rupture of the plaque with embolism of atherosclerotic material, or the embolism of platelet aggregates from an endothelial ulceration.

CLINICAL CLASSIFICATION

To better discuss clinical presentations and the associated risk factors, it is helpful to classify cerebrovascular ischemic disease into clinical syndromes. The usual categories are: frank stroke and reversible ischemic neurologic deficit (RIND), amaurosis fugax, transient ischemic attack (TIA), chronic cerebral ischemia, and asymptomatic bruits.

Frank stroke is defined as the sudden onset of the neurologic deficit, persisting for more than 24 hours, which is caused by reduced or absent blood flow in the cerebral vessels. *RIND* is a subcategory of stroke wherein the neurologic deficit generally clears entirely within a week or so of the time of onset. A frank stroke implies a destruction of neuronal tissue that is irreversible. However, in stroke there is generally a surrounding zone of damaged but viable neurons that may recover with time. As a result, many patients will show dramatic recovery of function after a period of time [5,6]. Although surgical intervention in cases of frank stroke will not change the neurologic deficit, one may prevent recurrent cerebral infarction, which occurs in about one-fourth of patients without treatment [5,7]. It is also important to note that transient ischemic attacks frequently occur prior to ischemic stroke, and 50 percent of the infarctions occur within the first year after the onset of TIAs, with 21 percent of strokes occurring within the 30 days following the first TIA [2,5,7].

Chronic cerebral ischemia denotes a syndrome wherein total cerebral blood flow is reduced to the extent that there results generalized impairment in thought processes, memory or motor functions [6,8,9]. This is a relatively rare syndrome, generally without focal neurologic deficit, and should not be confused with those patients who have senility or chronic cerebral atrophy. Chronic cerebral ischemia implies severe stenosis or occlusion of both carotid and both vertebral arteries with such resultant decrease in blood flow that cerebral function is compromised. Restoration of flow through just one vessel is generally enough to completely reverse the clinical picture and return function to normal.

Amaurosis fugax is a transient loss of vision in one eye due to reduction or interruption of blood flow to the retina. This is usually due to embolization of platelet aggregates or cholesterol debris to the retina from a more proximal carotid lesion. The implications of amaurosis fugax are the same as for transient ischemic attacks [6,8].

A *transient ischemic attack* (TIA) is, by definition, a localized ischemic neurologic deficit that may last minutes to hours, but is completely resolved within 24 hours. Although many mechanisms for transient ischemic attacks have been postulated [10,11], most symptoms are related to sudden severe reduction in blood flow through the carotid artery or, most commonly, to microemboli arising from ulcerated carotid plaques [10–15]. In 1961, Hollenhorst described bright orange retinal plaques in the eyegrounds of patients with amaurosis fugax, TIAs, or ipsilateral strokes [12]. He postulated then that these plaques represented cholesterol crystals that had embolized from ulcerating carotid lesions. He also described dull, white, nonrefractile emboli in the retinal vessels. Other investigators subsequently demonstrated that the orange plaques do represent cholesterol crystals and that the dull white emboli represent aggregates of platelets.

Asymptomatic bruits are audible findings in the neck caused by turbulent flow and are included in the classification since they are suggestive of a carotid artery lesion. Atherosclerotic lesions generally do not cause enough turbulence to produce a bruit until they occlude at least 50 percent of the lumen. Bruits may disappear when a high-grade stenosis restricts flow to such a degree that the turbulence is not great enough to cause audible vibrations. The importance of asymptomatic bruits relates entirely to their implied causal relationship to transient ischemic attacks and strokes. However, there are no definitive studies that adequately define these risks. Javid [16] in 1970 found progressive worsening of carotid bifurcation plaques in 62 percent of patients in a retrospective study. In a 10-year followup of 102 patients with asymptomatic bruits, Thompson and associates [17] found 27 percent developed TIAs and 19 percent had frank strokes without antecedent symptoms. Levin [18] and Humphries [19] suggested that patients with asymptomatic bruits had up to a 17 percent risk of developing TIAs, but only a small risk of frank stroke as the initial presenting event. However, many patients in the latter two studies had previously undergone carotid endarterectomy on the opposite carotid. That may provide a protective factor, since patent intracranial collaterals could provide adequate cerebral blood flow and pressures and thus lessen the risk of ischemic or embolic strokes.

Obviously, many other studies can be found to support or reject the supposition that carotid bruits represent harbingers of TIA and stroke. Perhaps, however, one needs to be more precise in discussing carotid bifurcation plaques and specify whether these lesions are hemodynamically significant. Busuttil and associates [20] used oculopneumoplethysmography (OPPG) to identify those patients who had pressure and flow-reducing carotid lesions, and noted that 6.6 percent developed strokes, while no strokes occurred in the OPPG-negative patients. This would suggest that carotid atherosclerotic plaques that become hemodynamically significant may pose an increased risk for stroke.

DIAGNOSIS

Noninvasive vascular laboratory procedures have now become commonplace for the evaluation of suspected carotid artery disease. Various techniques either assess the carotid bifurcation directly (phonoangiography, spectral analysis of flow, Doppler ultrasonic scanning, and real-time B-scan imaging [21-27]), or indirectly suggest the presence or absence of occlusive disease by assessing the hemodynamics of the carotid vessels (ophthalmodynamometry, thermography, oculophethysmography, oculopneumoplethysmography, and directional Doppler flow studies [12,28-36]). These techniques are not mutually exclusive and, in fact, when used in combination, may increase the sensitivity and specificity of the overall evaluation. In general, however, most noninvasive techniques can reliably detect those patients with complete occlusion or severe stenosis of one or both carotid arteries; nonstenotic ulcerative lesions and stenoses of less than 50 percent are detected with less accuracy and poor reliability. Regardless of noninvasive tests, one must remember that symptoms may occur with minimal demonstrable carotid disease, and yet severe carotid stenosis may never cause symptoms [21]. Therefore, patients with classic hemispheric transient ischemic attacks will generally need angiography, regardless of any noninvasive findings, but a positive finding on a noninvasive test does not, in itself, dictate the need of further diagnositc or therapeutic intervention in an otherwise asymptomatic patient.

In our experience, oculopneumoplethysmography (OPPG) is useful in evaluating asymptomatic bruits, since it helps to identify those patients with hemodynamically significant lesions. This may be useful information in some clinical situations, as suggested by Busuttil [20].

A simplified diagnostic approach to patients with asymptomatic cervical bruits or suspected carotid occlusive disease is shown diagrammatically in Figure 1.

Angiography remains the "gold standard" against which all noninvasive tests are measured and generally provides the definitive information that must be utilized when one contemplates carotid endarterectomy. However, even angiography may provide inaccurate interpretation if radiographic techniques are inadequate [37,38]. Biplane angiography with good radiographic techniques of penetration and definition is important to be able to adequately evaluate the question of ulcerative lesions, as well as stenotic plaques.

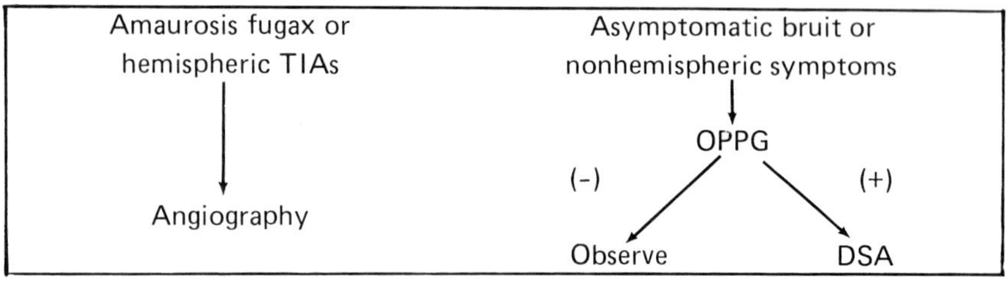

Figure 1. Diagnostic approach.

More recently, the advent of digital subtraction angiography (DSA) has provided a safer technique for visualizing the carotid and intracranial circulation [39]. The morbidity is exceedingly low and the angiographic resolution approaches 1 mm. Therefore, in most cases this provides an adequate and safe technique for screening patients with suspected cerebrovascular occlusive disease. However, it should be emphasized that, in patients with hemispheric transient ischemic attacks, the DSA may occasionally miss a small nonstenotic ulcerative plaque that is the source of microemboli. Conventional angiography is somewhat more accurate in this regard.

TREATMENT

For patients with transient ischemic attacks or amaurosis fugax, carotid endarterectomy appears to be the treatment of choice [40–43], because without treatment 40–50 percent of these patients develop strokes. With appropriate attention to detail, surgical treatment should be accomplished with an operative stroke rate and mortality rate of less than 2 percent each. Anatomic patency of the carotid can generally be attained in over 98 percent of cases and late patency should be in the range of 95 percent. Recurrent symptomatic stenosis remains very low and long-term relief of symptoms should exceed 90 percent [41].

Some patients may simply be unacceptable candidates for carotid endarterectomy because of overwhelming medical problems. In such situations anticoagulant therapy can reduce the incidence of TIA and stroke, although these patients are prone to possible hemorrhagic complications including intracerebral hemorrhage [9].

Recently, much attention has been directed toward the use of antiplatelet drugs for the management of patients with amaurosis fugax or TIA. In 1977 Fields et al [44], reported a controlled trial of aspirin in patients with cerebral ischemia. This multi-institutional study in patients with TIA or amaurosis fugax suggested that aspirin reduced the incidence of symptoms when compared with patients who received placebos. However, this study was severely flawed in that patients were not randomized until *after* some had been selected for surgical treatment. Furthermore, in the aspirin-vs-placebo groups there was no statistical difference in regard to stroke, retinal infarction and death.

A second randomized trial of antiplatelet agents was reported in 1978 by the Canadian Cooperative Study Group [45]. In this study (in which, unfortunately, angiography was not routinely performed), aspirin again appeared to reduce the incidence of TIAs in males, but it did not sufficiently establish that aspirin prevented strokes.

Because of the antiplatelet activity, it appears realistic to expect that aspirin can decrease the incidence of TIAs and amaurosis fugax as caused by platelet-aggregate emboli arising from ulcerated plaques. However, the natural maturation of an atherosclerotic plaque and its ultimate ulceration and embolization of cholesterol debris will not be affected by aspirin. Thus, one should expect a continuing incidence of stroke despite therapy.

It is our feeling that patients presenting with amaurosis fugax, or TIAs, after thorough medical and neurologic evaluation, should have four-vessel biplane angiography, including the aortic arch and intracranial vessels. Stenotic or ulcerative lesions in the carotid vessels appropriate to the symptoms (i.e., ipsilateral in amaurosis fugax and contralateral in TIAs) should undergo carotid endarterectomy without undue delay. If no specific vascular lesion is found, persistent transient ischemic attacks should warrant further workup to identify other possible causes of TIAs. If no other source is found, aspirin and Persantin may reduce the frequency of symptoms.

Surgical treatment is generally not indicated for complete occlusions of the internal carotid or for acute strokes. Attempts at carotid endarterectomy for acute strokes carry a risk of mortality approaching 40 percent. The immediate goal of therapy should be to provide medical support for the multiple systems indirectly affected by the neurologic deficit. If the patient recovers significant function over a period of time, one might consider angiography if recurrent symptoms develop.

Patients who have relatively minor strokes with early recovery should be considered for carotid endarterectomy after they have completely stabilized. If computerized tomography demonstrates a small area of cerebral infarction, both angiography and surgery should be delayed until the blood-brain barrier is restored, generally in about six weeks [46].

As mentioned previously, true chronic cerebral ischemia is rare, but is often dramatically benefited by carotid endarterectomy. Patients who fit the clinical syndrome, who have abnormal EEGs compatible with reduced blood flow, and who otherwise would be good surgical risks, should be evaluated by non-invasive testing. If these tests suggest bilaterally occlusive disease, digital subtraction angiography would be indicated. Severe stenoses would potentially be an indication for carotid endarterectomy. Patients with total occlusion of one

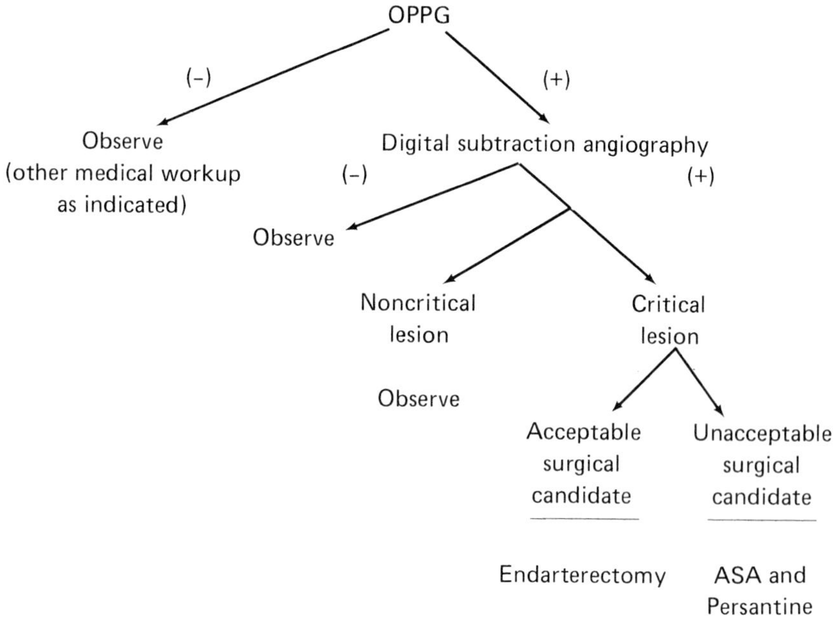

Figure 2. Therapeutic approach. Asymptomatic bruit or nonhemispheric symptoms.

internal carotid artery and stenosis of the other should have surgery only on the stenotic vessel. Patients who have complete occlusion of both internal carotid arteries may be considered candidates for possible extracranial-intracranial bypass by neurosurgery.

The question of surgical intervention for patients with asymptomatic stenotic lesions of the carotid bifurcation is more difficult to answer. Patients who are poor surgical risks should not be considered candidates for surgery if they are truly asymptomatic. Also, patients with no signs of other peripheral vascular occlusive disease and who might, therefore, be considered at relatively lower risk of developing progressive carotid disease, especially if they are elderly, should generally not be subjected to carotid endarterectomy, nor should patients with only mildly stenotic nonhemodynamically significant lesions. On the other hand, patients who have evidence of generalized atherosclerosis but are acceptable surgical risks from a cardiac standpoint and who have hemodynamically significant lesions might be potentially benefited by carotid endarterectomy. This is particularly true in patients with bilateral stenoses, stenoses on the side of the dominant hemisphere, and stenoses with extensive ulcerations or near-total occlusion. It is vitally important to remember, however, that surgical intervention in these patients will be acceptable only if the individual surgeon consistently maintains an exceedingly low mortality and stroke rate in such patients.

A schematic approach to patients with asymptomatic lesions or nonhemispheric TIAs is presented in Figure 2. Patients who are acceptable surgical risks and who have positive OPGs (hemodynamically significant lesions) are subjected to digital subtraction angiography. If worrisome lesions are found, carotid endarterectomy may be considered or, if correctable risk factors exist, may be delayed until a more appropriate time.

TECHNIQUE OF CAROTID ENDARTERECTOMY

Attention to every detail is of utmost importance in carotid endarterectomy. Every effort must be made to minimize the risk of stroke as a result of blood pressure fluctuations, embolization, cerebral ischemia, postoperative occlusion and intracranial hemorrhage.

Anesthetic management is an important consideration in carotid endarterectomy. We prefer general endotracheal anesthesia for this procedure, as it assures the most reliable method of precise ventilatory control and reliable oxygenation, while increasing the tolerance of the brain to ischemia during endarterectomy by reducing the cerebral metabolic demands for oxygen. It is preferable to maintain carbon dioxide tension at normal levels and to keep the systemic blood pressure only slightly above the patient's usual blood pressure. Anesthetic monitoring includes continuous measurement of arterial pressure via an intraarterial line.

Various techniques of cerebral protection during carotid endarterectomy have been recommended [47-57]. The techniques that currently seem most reliable are routine shunting in all cases, selective shunting based on stump pressures measured from the internal carotid artery after occlusion, and selective shunting based on routine EEG monitoring. In the hands of an experienced surgeon, all appear to be equally reliable when one is completely familiar with the technique used. Although we prefer selective shunting based on EEG monitoring, routine shunting is the safest if facilities for monitoring are not available.

After appropriate prepping and draping, a vertical incision is made along the anterior border of the sternocleidomastoid and the carotid sheath is exposed. The facial vein is divided and doubly ligated, allowing the internal jugular vein to be retracted laterally; then the hypoglossal nerve can readily be identified and preserved without injury. The artery and vein to the sternocleidomastoid muscle loop over the hypoglossal nerve and tether it down. These small vessels can be ligated and divided, freeing the hypoglossal nerve for high exposure of the internal carotid artery. The area of the carotid sinus at the carotid bifurcation is carefully infiltrated with 1% Xylocaine to avoid fluctuation in blood pressure and pulse rate. Exceedingly gentle dissection is mandatory throughout the procedure to avoid embolization. Vessel loops are placed around the superior thyroid, external carotid and internal carotid arteries and an umbilical tape and rubber tourniquet are placed around the common carotid artery. After intravenous heparin is given, flow is occluded in the carotid vessels and an incision is made in the common carotid artery and extended up into the internal carotid artery. This incision is continued beyond the level of the uppermost extent of the atherosclerotic plaque. If a shunt is to be used, it is now inserted into the internal carotid artery above the plaque. The proximal end of the shunt is then inserted into the common carotid artery and flow is reinstituted through the shunt. The plaque is removed by careful endarterectomy of the carotid vessels. If the intima of the internal carotid artery does not feather out to a smooth endpoint, the intima is sharply divided distal to the plaque and tacked down with interrupted sutures of 7–0 Prolene. The upper end of the internal carotid arterotomy is extended for about 1 cm beyond the site of the intimal edge and the arteriotomy is generally closed with a reversed saphenous vein patch harvested from the leg. Just prior to completion of the patch closure, flow in the carotid vessels is again interrupted and the shunt is removed. The closure is completed and flow is again restored through the carotid vessels. Two small Penrose drains are brought out from the lower aspect of the wound and the platysma and skin are closed in layers. The heparin is generally not reversed. The drains are removed after 24 hours.

Customarily, we give aspirin, 10 gr twice a day, starting immediately after surgery, with the first dose given rectally while the patient is in the recovery room. Close monitoring of blood pressure is essential and every attempt is made to maintain systolic pressure in the range of 120–160 mm Hg. If the patient becomes hypertensive, a nitroprusside drip is cautiously instituted. If hypotension is evident, additional fluid is given; if this does not restore adequate pressure, a slow infusion of dilute Neosynephrine® is started and carefully controlled.

With meticulous attention to detail, wound complications are unusual and postoperative discomfort is minimal. In patients requiring bilateral endarterectomy, we generally delay the second procedure for about 7 days, to decrease potential problems from laryngeal edema, cerebral edema or difficulty with deglutition.

For adequate continuing assessment of our surgical results, we routinely obtain postoperative OPPG and digital subtraction angiography on all patients after carotid endarterectomy. Patients are generally discharged 3–5 days after surgery.

SUMMARY

Atherosclerotic occlusive cerebrovascular disease remains prevalent in the aging population. Although noninvasive vascular studies are able to identify carotid lesions with increasing accuracy, careful judgment is required to identify those patients whose clinical situation justifies surgical intervention.

Since it is readily accepted that amaurosis fugax and transient ischemic attacks predict the increased likelihood of stroke, these patients should clearly receive treatment. Good-risk patients with accessible lesions should generally undergo carotid endarterectomy. If surgery is not feasible, anticoagulant therapy is acceptable, though less desirable. Aspirin and Persantine, or other antiplatelet agents, have not at this time proven to be effective in reducing the risk of stroke in these patients and thus cannot be recommended without qualification.

The true natural history of asymptomatic atherosclerotic lesions is not fully known at this time. It is probable that, in many patients, there is no great risk of stroke without antecedent warning TIAs. However, it also seems probable that patients with diffuse atherosclerotic occlusive disease are more likely to have progression of carotid lesions and thus be at greater risk of sudden stroke. In carefully selected patients, carotid endarterectomy may be beneficial in reducing this risk, especially in patients with hemodynamically significant lesions.

APPENDIX

Carotid Occlusive Disease (Natural History)

No change	38%
Increase in stenosis	62%

>25%/year 34%

Transient Cerebral Ischemia (Natural History)

Author	Cases	Strokes	Follow-Up (months)
Fisher 1958	23	8-35%	0
Baker 1968	73	17-23%	41
Stekart 1963	160	51-32%	60
Whisnant 1971	140	43-31%	180
Acheson 1971	151	94-62%	96

TIAs

Microemboli	80%
Internal carotid stenosis	15%

8–15% have strokes per year
51% of strokes occur in first year after TIA
20–50% of strokes occur within first month

Ischemic Stroke Prognosis

Recurrent cerebrovascular event		38%
TIA	20%	
CVA	26%	
Mortality with recurrent CVA		62%

Carotid Endarterectomy TIA–145 Cases)

Mortality	1.5%
Major morbidity	1.0%
Minor morbidity	1.0%
Transient neurologic dysfunction	2.0%

Carotid Artery Stenosis (Hemodynamic Significance and Clinical Course)

	OPPG (+)	OPPG (-)
Total late stroke	16.2%	2.2%
Asymptomatic late stroke	6.6%	0%
Late stroke after carotid endarterectomy		1.9%

Asymptomatic Carotid Bruits (10 Year Follow-Up—102 Patients)

Asymptomatic	54%
TIAs	27%
Frank stroke	19%

Asymptomatic Bruits
(Population Study—Evans County, Georgia)

Bruits in asymptomatic patients >45 y/o		4.4%
Risk of stroke (6 year)		13.9%
Men	27.8%	
Women	9.3%	
(stroke often nonspecific)		
Risk of stroke without bruit		3.4%

Asymptomatic Carotid Stenosis
(12 Year Follow-Up—168 Patients)

Asymptomatic	82%
TIAs	17%
Frank stroke	0.6%

Asymptomatic Carotid Stenosis
(20 Year Follow-Up—147 Patients)

Asymptomatic	88%
TIAs	12%
Frank stroke	0%

REFERENCES

1. Eisenberg H, Morrison JT, Sullivan P, et al. Cerebrovascular accidents: Incidence and survival rates in a defined population, Middlesex County, Connecticut. JAMA 189:883–888, 1964.
2. Whisnant JP, Matsumoto N, Elveback LR. Transient cerebral ischemic attacks in a community: Rochester, Minnesota, 1955–1969. Mayo Clin Proc 48:194–198, 1973.
3. Bauer R, Meyer J, Fields W, et al. Joint study of extracranial arterial occlusion: III. Progress report of controlled study of long-term survival in patients with and without operation. JAMA 208:509–518, 1969.
4. Kotte BA, Ravi Suffiah MP. Pathogenesis of atherosclerosis. Mayo Clin Proc 53:35–48, 1978.
5. Baker R, Schwartz W, Ramseyer J. Prognosis among survivors of ischemic stroke. Neurology 18:933–941, 1968.

6. Thompson JE. Surgery for Cerebrovascular Insufficiency: Stroke. Springfield, IL, Charles C Thomas, 1968.
7. Matsumoto N, Whisnant J, Kurland L, et al. Natural history of stroke in Rochester, Minnesota, 1955 through 1969: An extention of a previous study, 1945 through 1954. Stroke 4:20–29, 1973.
8. Thompson J, Austin D, Patman R. Carotid endarterectomy for cerebrovascular insufficiency: Long-term results in 592 patients followed up to 13 years. Ann Surg 172:663–679, 1970.
9. Millikan C, McDowell F. Treatment of transient ischemic attacks. Stroke 9:299–308, 1978.
10. Moore W, Hall A. Carotid artery back pressure: A test of cerebral tolerance to temporary carotid occlusion. Arch Surg 99:702–710, 1969.
11. Kollarits C, Lubow M, Hissong S. Retinal strokes: Incidence of carotid atheromata. JAMA 222:1273–1275, 1972.
12. Hollenhorst R. Significance of bright plaques in the retinal arterioles. JAMA 178:23–29, 1961.
13. Pessin M, Hinton R, Davis K, et al. Mechanisms of acute carotid stroke. Ann Neurol 6:245–252, 1974.
14. Hertzer N, Beven E, Benjamin S. Ultramicroscope ulcerations and thrombi of the carotid bifurcation. Arch Surg 112:1394–1402, 1977.
15. Crawford E, DeBakey M, Blaisdell F, et al. Hemodynamic alterations in patients with cerebral arterial insufficiency before and after operation. Surg 48:76–94, 1960.
16. Javid H, Ostermiller W, Hengesh J, et al. Natural history of carotid bifurcation atheroma. Surg 67:80–86, 1970.
17. Thompson J, Patman R, Persson A. Management of asymptomatic carotid bruits. Amer Surg 42:77–80, 1976.
18. Levin S, Sondheimer F, Levin J. The contralateral diseased but asymptomatic carotid artery: To operate or not? An update. Amer Surg 140:203–205, 1980.
19. Humphries A, Young J, Santelli P, et al. Unoperated, asymptomatic significant internal carotid artery stenosis: A review of 182 instances. Surg 80: 695–698, 1976.
20. Busuttil R, Baker J, Davidson R, Machelder H. Carotid artery stenosis: hemodynamic significance and clinical course. JAMA 245:1438–1441, 1981.
21. Sandok B. Non-invasive techniques for diagnosis of carotid artery disease. Stroke 9:427–428, 1978.
22. Kartchner M, McRae L. Auscultation for carotid bruits in cerebrovascular insufficiency. JAMA 210:494–497, 1969.
23. Duncan G, Gruber J, Dewey C, et al. Evaluation of carotid stenosis by phonoangiography. New Engl J Med 293:1124–1128, 1975.
24. Reid J, Spencer M. Ultrasonic Doppler technique for imaging blood vessels. Science 176:1235–1236, 1972.
25. Thomas G, Spencer M, Jones T, et al. Non-invasive carotid bifurcation mapping: Its relation to surgery. Amer J Surg 128:168–174, 1974.

26. Blackwell E, Merory J, Toole J, et al. Doppler ultrasound scanning of the carotid bifurcation. Arch Neurol 34:145–148, 1977.
27. Hokanson D, Mazersky D, Sumner D, et al. Ultrasonic arteriography: A non-invasive method of arterial visualization. Radiology 102:435–436, 1972.
28. Best M, Keyes M, Plechatz G, et al. Graphic analysis of the ocular pulse in carotid occlusion. Arch Ophthal 85:315–319, 1971.
29. Capistrant T, Gumnit R. Detecting carotid occlusive disease by thermography. Stroke 4:57–64, 1973.
30. Shapiro H, Ng L, Mishkin M, Reivich M. Direct thermometry, ophthalmodynamometry, auscultation and palpation in extracranial cerebrovascular disease: an evaluation of rapid diagnostic methods. Stroke 1:205–217, 1970.
31. Kartchner M, McRae L, Morrison F. Non-invasive detection and evaluation of carotid occlusive disease. Arch Surg 106:528–535, 1973.
32. Gee W, Aller D, Wylie E. Non-invasive diagnosis of carotid occlusion by ocluar pneumoplethysmography. Stroke 7:18–21, 1971.
33. Lye C, Sumner D, Strandness D Jr. The accuracy of the supraorbital Doppler examination in the diagnosis of hemodynamically significant carotid occlusive disease. Surg 79:42–45, 1976.
34. Machleder H, Barker W. Non-invasive methods for evaluation of extracranial cerebrovascular disease: A comparison. Arch Surg 112:944–946, 1977.
35. Moore M, Bean B, Burtau R, et al. The use of ophthalmosonometry in the diagnosis of carotid artery stenosis. Surg 82:107–115, 1977.
36. Kartchner M, McRae L, Crain V, et al. Oculophethysmography: An adjunct to arteriography in the diagnosis of extracranial carotid occlusive disease. Amer J Surg 132:728–732, 1976.
37. Croft R, Ellam L, Harrison M. Accuracy of carotid angiography in the assessment of atheroma of the internal carotid artery. Lancet 1980 (1): 997–999.
38. Kerber C, Cromwell L, Drayer B, et al. Cerebral ischemia: Current angiographic techniques, complications and safety. Amer J Roent 130:1097–1103, 1978.
39. Chilcote W, Modic M, Pavlicek W, et al. Digital subtraction angiography of the carotid arteries: A comparative study in 100 patients. Radiology 139: 287–295, 1981.
40. Fields W, Maslenokov V, Meyer J, et al. Joint study of extracranial arterial occlusion: V. Progress report of prognosis following surgery or nonsurgical treatment for transient ischemic attacks and cervical carotid artery lesions. JAMA 211:1993–2003, 1970.
41. Thompson J, Talkington C. Carotid endarterectomy. Ann Surg 184:1–15, 1976.
42. DeWeese J, Rob C, Satran R, et al. Results of carotid endarterectomies for transient ischemic attacks—five years later. Ann Surg 178:258–264, 1973.
43. Riles T, Imparato A, Kapelman L. Carotid artery stenosis with contralateral internal carotid occlusion: long-term results in 54 patients. Surg 81:363–368, 1980.

44. Fields W, Lemak N, Frankowski R, et al. Controlled trial of aspirin in cerebral ischemia. Stroke 8:301–315, 1977.
45. The Canadian Cooperative Study Group. A randomized trial of aspirin in threatened stroke. New Engl J Med 299:53–59, 1978.
46. Cohen A, Verden T, Blaisdell F, et al. Blood-brain barrier as a guide to surgical revascularization. Amer J Surg 116:158–163, 1968.
47. Hays R, Levinson S, Wylie E. Intraoperative measurements of carotid back pressure as a guide to operative management for carotid endarterectomy. Surg 72:953–960, 1972.
48. Hobson R, Wright C, Sublett J, et al. Carotid artery back pressure and endarterectomy under regional anesthesia. Arch Surg 109:682–687, 1974.
49. Howe J, Kindt G. Cerebral protection during carotid endarterectomy. Stroke 5:340–343, 1974.
50. Hughes R, Bustos M, Byrne J. Internal carotid artery pressures: A guide for use of shunt during carotid repair. Arch Surg 109:494–495, 1974.
51. Moore W, Yee J, Hall A. Collateral cerebral blood pressure: A index of tolerance to temporary carotid occlusion. Arch Surg 106:520–523, 1973.
52. Rich N, Hobson R. Carotid endarterectomy under regional anesthesia. Amer J Surg 41:253–259, 1975.
53. Sundt T, Sharbrough F, Anderson R, et al. Cerebral blood flow measurements and electroencephalograms during carotid endarterectomy. J Neurosurg 41:310–320, 1974.
54. Young J, Humphries A, Beven E, et al. Carotid endarterectomy without a shunt. Arch Surg 99:293–297, 1969.
55. Alexander S, Lassen N. Cerebral circulatory response to acute brain disease: Implications for anesthetic practice. Anesthesiology 32:60–68, 1970.
56. Ehrenfeld W, Hamilton F, Larson C, et al. Effect of CO_2 and systemic hypertension on downstream cerebral arterial pressure during carotid endarterectomy surgery. Surg 67:87–96, 1970.
57. Sundt T, Sharbrough F, Piepgras D, et al. Correlation of cerebral blood flow and electroencephalographic changes during carotid endarterectomy: With results of surgery and hemodynamics of cerebral ischemia. Mayo Clin Proc 56:553–543, 1981.

5
Extracranial Revascularization

John B. Chang

Since the first carotid endarterectomy was done nearly three decades ago, it has been shown repeatedly that the most frequent cause of symptoms of cerebral vascular insufficiency is atheromatous disease of the carotid bifurcation [1]. Atherosclerotic occlusive disease of the great vessels arising from the aortic arch was described by Broadbent [2] in 1875 and Chiari [3] in 1906. Operations performed for atherosclerotic occlusive disease of the carotid bifurcation by Strully et al [4], Eastcott [5], and Cooley [6] have made it possible to restore the cerebral vascular circulation to normal. Because of the systemic disorder arising from atherosclerosis, patients with carotid or vertebral artery disease are likely to have, therefore, occlusive disease in other circulations, the most important of which is the coronary circulation [7,8].

Cerebral protection during carotid endarterectomy includes two different approaches, as indicated in Figure 1. The efficacy of any method of cerebral protection is difficult to determine, since it can be measured ultimately only by the incidence of new neurological deficit appearing postoperatively. There are general factors affecting the incidence of postoperative neurological deficit (Figure 2). Riles et al [9] indicated the use of metaraminol for increasing stump pressures responsible for the high incidence of postoperative myocardial infarction in patients with preexisting heart disease, and recommended increased use of a shunt rather than vasopressors (Table 1A). Ennix et al [8] reported decreased mortality on patients with preoperative angina treated by coronary artery bypass before, or at the same time of, carotid endarterectomy (Table 1B, Group III). Because of unknown incidence of postoperative stroke from ischemia or carotid cross-clamping alone, the uncertain benefits of any method of cerebral protection, and the well-known mortality rate of postoperative myocardial infarction, it would seem wise to avoid any method of cerebral protection which might increase the likelihood of perioperative myocardial infarction, such as inducing hypertension in patients with symptomatic coronary artery disease [10].

Coronary artery disease is the most common cause of early and postoperative death following carotid endarterectomy [11]. In a series of patients followed for more than five years after carotid endarterectomy performed for transient ischemic attacks, DeWeese and associates [12] found late mortality rate of 27% for patients who had no clinical indication of coronary artery disease

INCREASING TOLERANCE TO ISCHEMIA

GENERAL ANESTHESIA
•
HYPERCARBIA
•
HYPOCARBIA
•
INDUCED HYPERTENSION
•
HYPOTHERMIA
•
THIOPENTAL

DIAGNOSIS OF ISCHEMIA: INDICATION FOR SHUNT

LOCAL ANESTHESIA
•
JUGULAR VENOUS O_2 SATURATION
•
STUMP PRESSURE O_2 TENSION
•
EEG
•
REGIONAL CEREBRAL BLOOD FLOW

Figure 1. Protection of the brain during carotid endarterectomy. From Keats [10].

at the time of operation, and 56% for those with suspected coronary artery disease. Thompson and associates [13] found that myocardial infarction caused 52% of late death, and stroke only in 16% of late death in a series of 592 patients followed as long as thirteen years after carotid endarterectomy. Indication for carotid endarterectomy in a Cleveland Clinic study showed focal transient cerebral ischemia in 35%, asymptomatic carotid stenosis in 25%, previous completed stroke 15%, vertebral basilar syndrome 15%, two of more factors,

PATIENTS WITH PRIOR STROKE
◊
PATIENTS WITH CONTRALATERAL CAROTID OCCLUSION
◊
EXTENT OF COLLATERAL CIRCULATION AND DURATION OF CLAMPING
◊
EXPERIENCE OF SURGEON AND/OR INSTITUTION

Figure 2. Factors affecting incidence of postoperative neurological deficits.

Table 1A. Myocardial Infarction Following Carotid Endarterectomy

	No heart disease	Heart disease[a]
Number of patients	288	203
Postoperative myocardial infarction	0.7% No Aramine 2.0% With Aramine 8.1%	6.9%
Death from myocardial infarction	0%	2.5%

Riles et al, 1979
[a]Angina, congestive heart failure, arrhythmias, previous myocardial infarction.

10%. Carotid endarterectomy was performed preceding another peripheral vascular procedure in 15%, and preceding myocardial revascularization in 15%. Myocardial revascularization at the time carotid endarterectomy was performed was shown in 1% of their series (Table 18) [11]. In their series, the causes of late mortality among 325 operative survivors from one to eleven years after surgery revealed myocardial infarction in 18%, stroke in 8%, malignant neoplasm in 5%, congestive heart failure in 3%, and pulmonary embolism in 1%. The remainder consisted of other problems.

Considering the ominous implications of coronary artery disease in patients with intracranial cerebral vascular disease, routine coronary angiography has been recommended for all patients who are to undergo carotid endarterectomy at the Cleveland Clinic since 1978. Although late follow-up information is not

Table 1B. Coronary Artery Disease in 1238 Patients Who Underwent Carotid Endarterectomy (1967–1977)

	I	II	III[a]
Coronary artery disease symptoms (angina)	0	+	+
Number of patients	1026	77	135
Unstable angina	0	22%	28%
Previous myocardial infarction	18%	55%	50%
Myocardial infarction	1.0%	13%	2.6%
Cardiac/cerebral deaths	2/10	11/3	1/1
In-hospital mortality	1.5%	18.2%	3.0%

Forty-two percent of all deaths were from myocardial infarction

From Ennix et al [8]. Reprinted by permission of *Stroke*.
[a]Prior or simultaneous coronary artery bypass.

yet clearly available for patients whose management presently is determined with the use of routine coronary angiography, their report describes a history of a control group with which such patients will eventually be compared, in an effort to define those patients for whom survey coronary angiography and, if indicated, myocardial revascularization, will be advisable for safe, carotid reconstruction and improved late survival rate.

In Mayo Clinic series, the following were the major considerations in determining the patient's surgical risk [14]:

1. *Medical Risk Factors*: The presence of symptomatic coronary artery disease (angina pectoris) or myocardial infarction within six months before the date of surgery; severe hypertension (blood pressure more than 180/110 mmHg); chronic obstructive lung disease; physiological age more than 70 years; or severe obesity.
2. *Neurological Risk Factors*: Progressing neurological deficit; a deficit less than 24 hours old before surgery; frequent daily transient ischemic attacks; or symptoms of generalized, in contrast to focal, cerebral ischemia.
3. *Angiographically Determined Risks*: Coexisting stenosis of the internal carotid artery, the siphon area; extensive involvement of the vessel to be operated upon, with plaque extending more than 3 cm. distally in the internal carotid artery or 5 cm. proximally in the common carotid artery; bifurcation of the carotid artery at the level of second cervical vertebra in conjunction with a short or thick neck; occlusion of the opposite internal carotid artery; evidence of a short thrombus extending from the ulcerative lesion or small vessel occlusions from the multiple emboli; and slowed intracranial circulation time on angiography. The degree of stenosis, per se, was not considered a risk factor.

On the basis of the above-noted general risk factors, the patients were graded as follows:

Grade 1: Neurologically stable (no neurological risk factors) with no major medical or angiographically determined risk and with unilateral or bilateral ulcerative-stenotic disease.

Grade 2: Neurologically stable with no major medical risks but with significant angiographically determined risk.

Grade 3: Neurologically stable with major medical risks with or without significant angiographically determined risk.

Grade 4: Major neurological risk with or without associated major medically or angiographically determined risk. The angiograms

Table 2A. Results of Carotid Endarterectomy[a] (Neurologic Function)

			New deficit		Mortality etiology		
Grade of risk	Procedures	Normal unchanged or improved	Major	Minor	Intracerebral hemorrhage	Myocardial infarction	Other complications
1	398	394 (4)	0	4	0	0	0
2	237	233 (4)	2	2	0	0	0
3	310	297 (4)	5	3	0	6	1
4	200	180 (7)	5	4	5	2	2
Total	1,145	1,104 (19)	12	13	5	8	3

From Sundt et al [14].
Numbers in parentheses are patients with transient neurologic dysfunction (transient ischemic attacks, seizures, migraine variants).
[a]Overall, mortality was 1.5%. Major morbidity was 1% and minor morbidity was 1%.

in this group frequently showed both slower flow and multiple small vessel occlusions.

These analyses gave the information on Table 2A.

Antiplatelet drugs have become a prime mode of therapy in ischemic cerebral vascular disease. Aspirin is foremost among the medications used. The current use is based on the result of double-blind studies comparing aspirin to placebo in patients with TIAs [17]. A U.S. medical study and a Canadian study revealed significant differences in favor of aspirin for the combination endpoint of cerebral infarct, TIA and death. The Heidelberg study favored aspirin for ischemic events in patients with internal carotid artery TIAs. The beneficial effect of aspirin in cerebral vascular disease presumably arises from inhibition of platelet aggregation. Aspirin inhibits cyclo-oxygenase in platelets by acetylation and thus halts the formation of thromboxine A_2, an important cause of platelet aggregation, from arachidonic acid metabolites (Figure 3) [18]. It is the balance between thromboxane and prostacyclin that is thought to regulate intraarterial platelet aggregation, thrombus formation and perhaps the subsequent smooth muscle formation in atherosclerotic plaque [18, 19]. Computer assisted EEG analysis, for monitoring brain function during

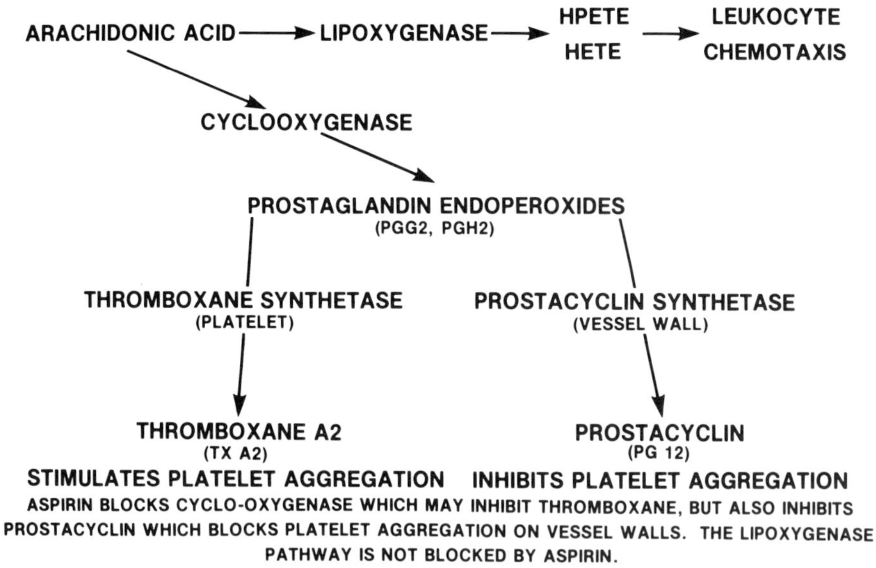

Figure 3. Pathways of arachidonic acid metabolism in the biosynthesis of prostacyclin, thromboxane, and eicosatetraeonic (HPETE, HETE) acids.

administration of anesthesia and operation, may prove valuable even for relatively low-risk procedures. Observations made by Grundy et al [20] can assist in the development of effective monitors by defining patterns of intraoperative EEG changes associated with postoperative neurological deficit. According to Lees and Hertzer at the Cleveland Clinic [21], the introduction of normocarbic general anesthesia and routine intraoperative carotid shunting has been associated with highly significant improvement in the incidence of postoperative stroke for patients with preoperative TIA ($p < 0.01$), and for those with subtotal stenosis of the contralateral internal carotid artery ($p < 0.02$). Though absolute conclusions concerning the value of routine shunting are compromised by differences in anesthetic management, during this consecutive period of study, data tended to support the contention that routine carotid shunting is associated with minimal risk for iatrogenic stroke during carotid endarterectomy. The role of routine carotid shunting in the prevention of intraoperative stroke will continue to be controversial, however, because of conflicting results which continue to be presented by dependable observers. Identical postoperative neurological complication rate of 3.2% has been reported by Thompson et al [22] using routine carotid shunting, and by Ott et al [23] using no shunting whatsoever. These differences are difficult, if not impossible, to reconcile other than by conceding that such results should be the goal of every surgeon performing carotid endarterectomy, and must be obtained if each patient is to receive the full benefit of carotid reconstruction.

The incidence of bilateral operations in the Cleveland Clinic series was 16%, and that of Thompson's was 25%. Patients with contralateral stenosis, who underwent carotid endarterectomy of the opposite side, had a stroke rate of 4% in this series. By contrast, for those patients with contralateral lesions who were not subject to elective operation, the stroke rate was 16% according to Thompson's series. The recurrent stenosis rate was 2.4% in the Cleveland Clinic series.

Neurological deficit is the most feared complication of carotid endarterectomy. Intraoperative efforts to minimize the occurrence have utilized a variety of techniques. General anesthesia is used by a majority of centers, because it depresses cerebral metabolism [24], and most surgeons prefer this anesthetic technique. Hypothermia enjoyed a period of popularity but has been discarded, as the alleged benefit was balanced by serious cardiac arrhythmias. Hypercarbia increases total cerebral blood flow, but hypocarbia has been used by others to increase regional blood flow in the ischemic cerebral cortex [25]. However, neither of these techniques has proven to be superior [26]. Many believe that by using general anesthesia and monitoring blood pressure, an indwelling shunt is not the most important factor in preventing stroke during carotid endarterectomy, but this factor is technical perfection [25-27]. The carotid artery is manipulated minimally prior to clamping. Every extraneous atheromatous fragment, which could be the nidus for thrombus, is removed during the endarterectomy. The proximal intima is divided sharply to provide a clean proximal end point. The distal feathery end of the atheroma must be teased away delicately from the remaining intima, and if there is any question of nonadherent distal intima, then this distal intima must be sutured to the wall of the artery. Finally, the arteriotomy is closed without creating a stenosis. Since technical perfection is achieved more easily without a shunt, its routine use is not favored. Kremen et al [28] had the follow-up survey clinically and by OPG-GEE. Twelve percent had a positive OPG examination. Three arteries (1.7%) demonstrated symptomatic recurrent stenosis. An additional 8.1% of the operative arteries had asymptomatic recurrent stenosis. A total recurrence rate of 9.8% was found. Because of this considerable silent recurrence rate, they recommended annual screening by OPG (Figure 4).

YEARS POSTOP	1	2	3	4	5	6	7	8	9	10	11	12
POSITIVE	2	0	4	1	1	4	2	1	1	0	0	1
NEGATIVE	58	19	17	15	19	6	5	3	6	3	2	3

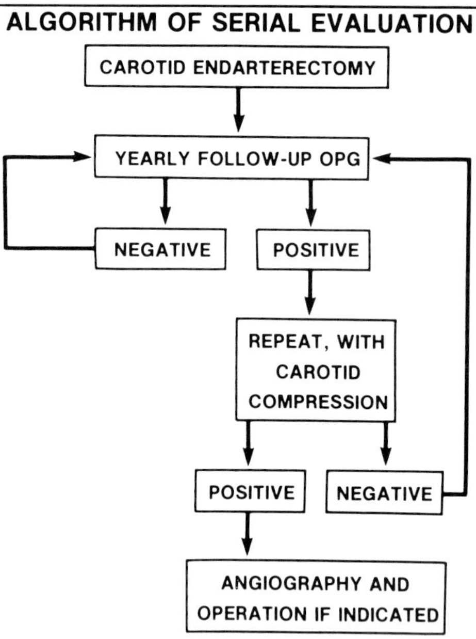

Figure 4. Summary of 173 arteries surveyed by ocular pneumoplethysmography. From Kremen et al [28].

According to Lindberg [29], if an acute carotid occlusion is operated on within one or two hours, it will be possible, in many cases, to restore cerebral blood flow before the brain has suffered irreversible damage. It has been found experimentally that occlusion of the middle cerebral artery will reduce the cerebral blood flow to 20-40%, but it can still be tolerated for two to three hours without irreversible damage [30,31]. The brain activity can be restored even after several hours of occlusion, despite cessation of neuronal activity [32,33]. In a review of emergency carotid endarterectomy for fluctuating neurological deficit by Menzer et al [34], the twelve patients with complete or near complete recovery of neurological function represented more than a three-fold improvement ($P > 0.01$). When compared with the natural history of a fluctuating neurological deficit, the data suggest that immediate operative intervention will result in better salvage. Another gratifying result was reported by Goldstone and Moore [35] in a neurologically unstable patient following emergency carotid artery surgery. On the basis of the experience with their twelve patients, Menzer et al [34] recommended an aggressive diagnostic and therapeutic approach for a patient with acute unstable cerebral vascular disease. When the operative and nonoperative groups were compared for neurological improvement vs. no change or deterioration, 70.6% (12 of 17) improved in the operative group, and 11.5% (3 of 26) improved in the nonoperative group ($P < 0.01$), whereas 6% (1 of 17) were worse or dead in the operative group, and 54.6% (14 of 26) were worse or dead in the nonoperative group ($P < 0.01$), Figure 5.

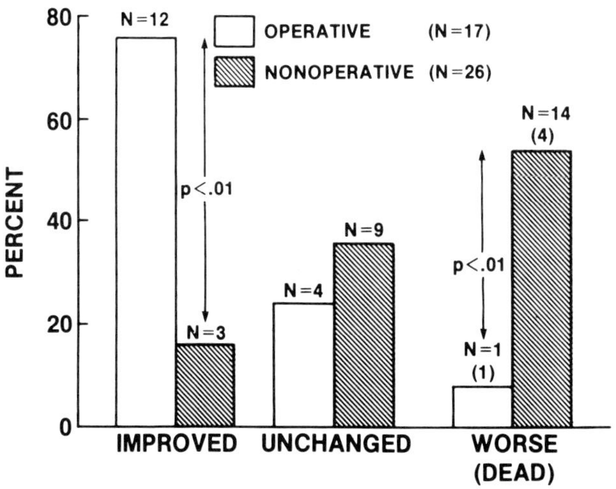

Figure 5. Stroke in evolution. From Mentzer et al [34].

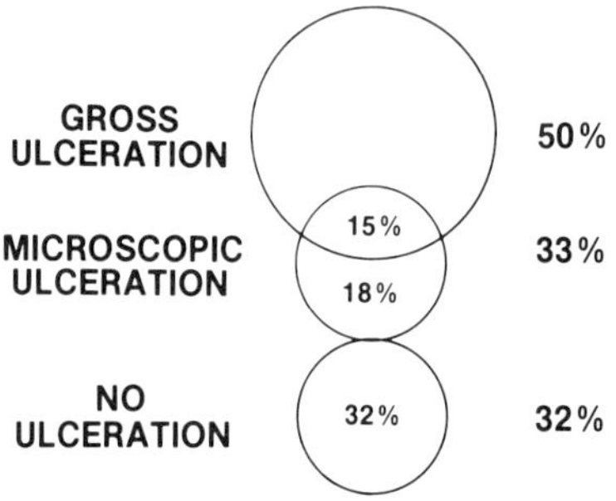

Figure 6. Results of pathologic analysis. From Bartynski et al [36]. Reprinted by permission of Amer J Surg.

Bartynski et al [36] investigated pathology of the ulcerating plaque in transient cerebral ischemia. The major portion of their study was related to pathological evaluation of the tissue removed at the operation. Three basic degrees of lesions were noted:

1. Gross ulceration which could be seen without magnification.
2. Microscopic ulcers which represented regions of intimal tears and breakdown with degeneration of subintimal structure.
3. No ulceration, either macroscopic or microscopic.

Microscopic ulcerations were seen in 50% of the specimens (Figure 6). These were often large and had characteristic grumous material in the excavation. Occasionally these ulcers were covered with a lining of endothelial cells which prevented subendothelial-blood contact. In 33% of the specimens, microscopic intimal ulceration was seen. Fifteen percent of these specimens also had gross ulcerations. They believe these intimal tears and subintimal necrosis represent important potential sites for arterial embolization.

According to the study made by Kroener et al [37], asymptomatic carotid bifurcation ulcerative plaque had a seven year stroke rate of 1%. On the basis of their study, prophylactic carotid endarterectomy was not felt to be justified for asymptomatic carotid bifurcation ulceration. However, the importance of asymptomatic carotid ulcer and the indication for prophylactic surgery have remained the subject of much debate. Groups of patients with asymptomatic bruits followed up by Thompson and Patman [38], Thompson et al [39], and Cooperman et al [40], and a group of patients followed up by Kartchner and McRae [41], in which hemodynamically significant stenosis was documented by noninvasive techniques, suggest an incidence of stroke in the range of 15-20% over a mean follow-up period of 2-5 years. These studies are often cited by advocates of prophylactic carotid surgery. On the other hand, data on the groups

Table 2B. Symptoms in Patients with Contralateral Stenosis Related to Percent Stenosis

	Percent stenosis				
	1-29	30-49	50-70	71-99	Total
Total patients	7	32	22	6	67
Number with TIA as new symptom	0	7	3	1	11
Number with CVA	1	0	2	0	3

From Podore et al [45].

of patients followed up by Humphries et al [42] and by Johnson et al [43], with stenosis greater than 50% determined angiographically on the contralateral to a surgically treated lesion suggest stroke rate on the order of 1% without antecedent symptoms, and argue against prophylactic surgery in these patients. Moore et al [44] studied seventy-two nonstenotic, ulcerated carotid lesions in 62 patients. Of twenty-nine patients with large, obvious ulcers or complex, cavernous ulcers, ten (34%) suffered strokes appropriate to the lesion within seventy-eight months of follow-up. None of these patients had appropriate antecedent ceberal symptoms. This 34% stroke rate by direct calculation gave a cumulative stroke rate of 87% at seventy-eight months when analyzed by life table method. As a result of this analysis, those authors advocated prophylactic endarterectomy for large or complex asymptomatic ulcers.

Podore et al [45] did a study on asymptomatic contralateral carotid artery stenosis. Sixty-seven patients with contralateral stenosis were observed (Table 2B). Twenty-eight of their lesions (42%) were at least 50% stenosed.

Table 3. Asymptomatic Carotid Bruit: Operative Mortality Following Carotid Endarterectomy (Total Experience = 20 Years)

Clinical category	No. of Patients	No. of operations	No. of deaths	Patient mortality	Procedure mortality
Frank stroke	296	358	20	6.8%	5.6%
Transient ischemia	575	737	7	1.2%	0.9%
Chronic ischemia	19	24	0	0	0
Asymptomatic bruit	132	167	0	0	0
Totals	1022	1286	27	2.6%	2.1%

From Thompson et al [46].

Table 4. Basic Patient Data

	Operated	Nonoperated
Number of patients	132	138
Age: range	42–82 years	39–86 years
Age: mean	64.7 years	65.7 years
Males	76 (57.6%)	74 (53.6%)
Females	56 (42.4%)	64 (46.4%)

From Thompson et al [46].

During the follow-up period, 14 patients (21%) subsequently developed symptoms referable to the contralateral carotid. Eleven of these patients (16.5%) developed classic TIAs, and all these patients underwent carotid endarterectomy. The average time span between the first and second procedure was twenty-three months, ranging from ten to forty-eight months. The other three patients (4.5%) suffered CVAs at six, ten and twenty-eight months respectively. Two of them died. The following guideline was established: Patients with contralateral artery stenosis should be advised to undergo stated carotid endarterectomies, if the surgeon's incidence of stroke and mortality is less than 3%.

Long-term follow-up on asymptomatic carotid bruits by Thompson et al [46] revealed some important data. Table 3 indicates entire experience of carotid endarterectomy and operative mortality of the total twenty-year experience. In two groups of patients with asymptomatic carotid bruits, one group had the operation, and the other group was followed without having the operation (Tables 4,5). Long-term follow-up data on the neurological status of the operated and nonoperated patients are shown on Tables 6–11.

Riles et al [48] studied comparison analyses of unilateral and bilateral carotid endarterectomies with five-year follow-up results (Figure 7). Postoperative neurological events were classified into three categories according to Owens [49].

Table 5. Data on Patients Having Endarterectomy

Number of patients	132
Number of operations	167
Operative mortality	0
Operation-related defects	
Transient	2 (1.2%)
Permanent, mild	2 (1.2%)

From Thompson et al [46].

Table 6. Long-Term Follow-Up Data on Operated and Nonoperated Patients with Asymptomatic Carotid Bruits

Patients	Asymptomatic	TIAs	Stroke		Months follow-up
			Nonfatal	Fatal	
Operated 132	120 90.9%	6 4.5%	3 2.3%	3 2.3%	6 to 184 Mean:55.1
Non-operated 138	77 55.8%	37 26.8%	21 15.2%	3 2.2%	to 180 Mean: 45.5 (ASX)
Significance	$p < 0.01$	$p < 0.01$			

From Thompson et al [46].

Table 7. Length of Follow-Up on Nonoperated Patients with Asymptomatic Carotid Bruits

Months followed	Long-term survivors	Long-term deaths	Total patients
0–12	19	12	31
13–24	14	5	19
25–36	9	6	15
37–48	11	6	17
49–60	9	6	15
61–72	5	3	8
73–84	6	1	7
85–96	7	2	9
97–108	1	1	2
109–120	2	1	3
121–132	0	2	2
133–144	1	4	5
145–156	2	1	3
180–200	2	0	2
	88	50	138

From Thompson et al [46].

Table 8. Causes of Long-Term Deaths

Causes of death	Operated	Non-operated
Cardiac	31	24
Cerebral	3	8[a]
Malignancy	4	1
Following other surgery	2	2
Generalized atherosclerosis	1	1
Uremia	1	1
Ruptured aortic aneurysm	1	0
Mesenteric infarction	0	3
Gastrointestinal hemorrhage	0	2
Burn	0	1
Emphysema	0	1
Auto accident	0	1
During arteriography	0	1
Cirrhosis	0	1
Undetermined	0	3
	43	50

From Thompson et al [46].
[a]Includes patients going from asymptomatic to TIAs, and nonfatal strokes dying later of cerebral causes.

1. Major stroke was designated if, in the postoperative course, a neurological deficit developed which interfered with the patient's vocation, ability to socialize or ability to care for himself.
2. Lesser deficit, not functionally disabling, but apparent from questioning or on neurological examination, and which failed to clear completely prior to discharge, were considered minor strokes.
3. Neurological deficits which came and went during the postoperative hospitalization were described as transient ischemic neurological deficits. These were recognized either immediately on recovery from anesthesia or occurred after a postoperative period of normalcy. These events include asymptomatic postoperative cerebral infarct detectable only by computed tomographic and radioisotope scans.

They reported major strokes in 1.9% and minor strokes in 2% for a total of 3.9%. Their data with literature comparison are shown on Table 12A, along with my own data. Operative mortality following endarterectomy in a large series is shown in Table 12B. As a rare complication, vocal cord paralysis following carotid endarterectomy has been described by Welch et al [50].

Table 9. Interval from Detection of Bruit to Onset of Ischemic Episode in Nonoperated Patients

Months interval	Patients with TIAs	Patients with strokes
0-12	10	15
13-24	9	2
25-36	5	3
37-48	3	2
49-60	3	0
61-72	1	1
73-84	4	0
85-96	1	0
97-108	1	0
109-120	0	0
121-132	0	1
Total patients	37	24
Range	1 to 99 months	1 week to 124 months
Mean interval	32.1 months	20.3 months

From Thompson et al [46].

In my series, there were three incidents of vocal paralysis noted. Two of them were temporary, and one patient remained paralytic. This patient had carotid endarterectomy and graft replacement for restenosis following vein patch graft. The surgical treatment of atherosclerotic occlusion of the innominate and subclavian arteries was reviewed and presented recently by Deriu et al [51]. Their surgical experience is summarized on Table 13. Contrary to their experience, my approach is by a lesser degree of surgery through applying axillary-axillary artery bypass. There was a postoperative follow-up after axillary-axillary bypass in my series of fifteen patients which showed satisfactory long-term patency rate. There was one patient who had reoperation at the eighth year postoperatively due to further arteriosclerotic occlusive disease at the donor site of axillary artery. Morbidity and mortality of this operation, in my experience, are extremely low with no postoperative mortality or major morbidity.

Cervical vertebral angioplasty for brain stem ischemia was reviewed recently by Imparato et al [52]. Symptoms, in order of frequency in their patients, are shown in Table 14, and the examples of commonly encountered combinations of lesions in Figure 8. In my experience, singular vertebral artery

Table 10. Length of Follow-Up on Patients Operated upon for Asymptomatic Carotid Bruits

Months followed	Long-term survivors	Long-term deaths	Total
6–12	11	9	20
13–24	16	2	18
25–36	12	5	17
37–48	9	4	13
49–60	7	3	10
61–72	9	5	14
73–84	8	3	11
85–96	2	5	7
97–108	1	4	5
109–120	4	1	5
121–132	1	2	3
133–144	5	0	5
145–156	1	0	1
157–168	2	0	2
181–192	1	0	1
Total	89	43	132

From Thompson et al [46].

Table 11. Types of Strokes Occurring in 24 Patients in the Nonoperated Group

Profound frank stroke, coma	6
Hemiplegia	7
Hemiparesis, severe	6
Hemiparesis, mild	2
Permanent blindness, partial	3

From Thompson et al [46].

Table 12A. Mortality and Incidence of Permanent Major and Minor Neurologic Complications after Carotid Endarterectomy

Source, year	Study interval	Patients/ Operations	Mortality/ Procedure number (%)	Neurologic deficits/ Procedure number (%)	Combined mortality and stroke incidence/ Procedure number (%)
West et al, 1979	1967–1975	147/186	1 (0.5)	7 (3.8)	8 (4.0)
Gundlach and Swenson, 1979	1969–1976	100/119	1 (0.8)	1 (0.8)	2 (1.6)
Carmichael, 1980	1968–1978	424/467	1 (0.2)	7 (1.5)	8 (1.7)
Hertzer and Beven, 1980	1976–1978	349/366	1 (0.3)	3 (0.8)	4 (1.1)
White et al, 1981	1973–1979	211/252	5 (2.0)	5 (2.0)	10 (4.0)
Owens	1973–1980	184/195	0 (0.0)	7 (3.6)	7 (3.6)
Chang	1976–1983	174/213	1 (0.5)	3 (1.4)	4 (1.9)

Table 12B. Operative Mortality Following Carotid Endarterectomy (Total Experience = 20 Years)

Clinical category	Patients	Operations	Deaths	Mortality	
				Patient	Procedure
Frank stroke	296	358	20	6.8%	5.6%
Transient ischemia	575	737	7	1.2%	0.9%
Chronic ischemia	19	24	0	0%	0%
Asymptomatic bruit	132	167	0	0%	0%
Totals	1022	1286	27	2.6%	2.1%

From Thompson et al [46].

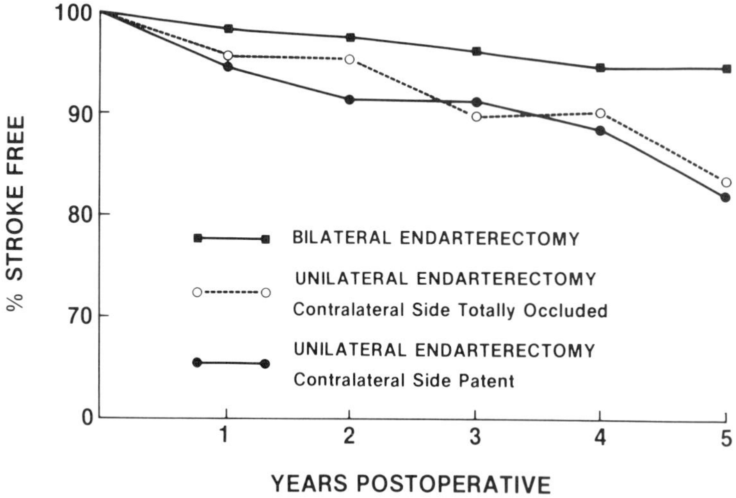

Figure 7. Comparison of late stroke incidence. From Riles et al [48].

Table 13. Surgical Treatment of Innominate and Subclavian Artery Atherosclerotic Occlusion

Operation	Patients no. (%)	Subclavian no. (%)	Innominate no. (%)
Carotid sub-clavian bypass	[a]22 (64.7%)	22 (81.4%)	0 (0%)
Aorto-carotid bypass	6 (17.6%)	0 (0%)	6 (85.7%)
Subclavian Endarterectomy	2 (5.8%)	2 (7.4%)	0 (0%)
Innominate Endarterectomy	1 (2.9%)	0 (0%)	1 (3.7%)
Exploration	1 (2.9%)	1 (3.7%)	0 (0%)
Others	2 (5.8%)	2 (7.4%)	0 (0%)

From Deriu et al [51].
[a]Five patients had a combined ipsilateral endarterectomy.

Table 14. Symptoms, in Order of Frequency, of 58 Patients with Vertebral Arterial Lesions with or without Associated Lesions Requiring Operations

Dizziness	26
Snycope	16
Transient extremity weakness	15
Headache	13
Aphasia	12
Unilateral amaurosis fugax	11
Hemiparesis	9
Confusion	4
Unilateral sustained visual loss	4
Bilateral sustained visual loss	3
Bilateral amaurosis fugax	3
Bilateral transient extremity weakness	2
Facial weakness	1
Ataxic gait	1

From Imparato et al [52].

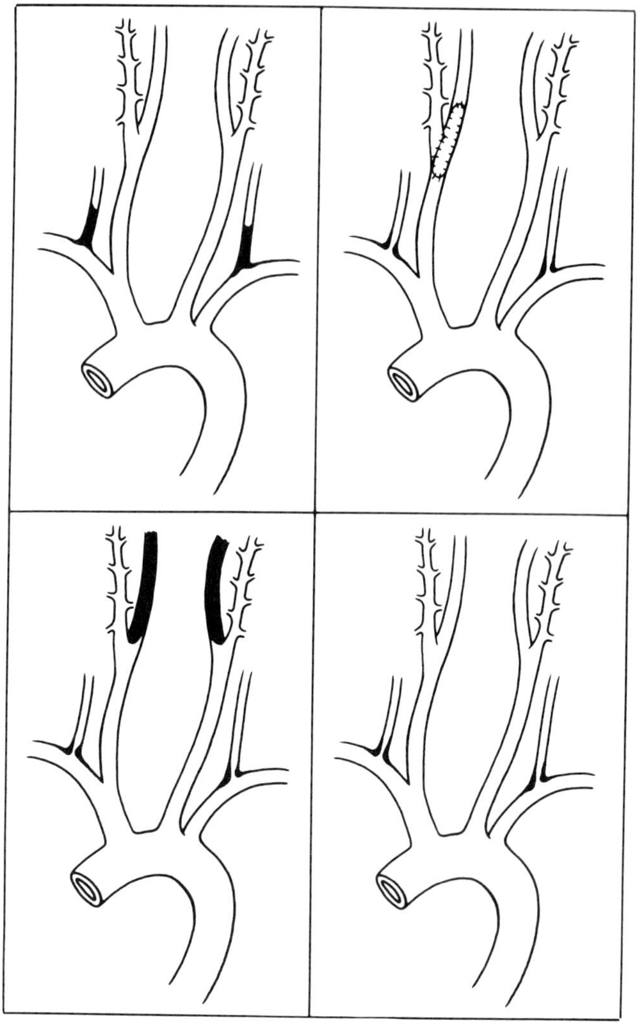

Figure 8. Lesion combinations most commonly encountered leading to unilateral vertebral angioplasty. From Imparato et al. [52].

revascularization is extremely limited. In two cases, endarterectomy and angioplasty with vein patch showed satisfactory long-term patency.

MATERIAL AND CLINICAL EVALUATION

This presentation is based on my personal experience with 276 cases of extracranial revascularization. Carotid endarterectomy was performed in 234 cases. In recent cases, for the past four years, there has been an increasing trend in the use of autogenous vein patch graft, which was done in 92 cases. The majority of the autogenous veins was from the saphenous vein. There were cases which utilized arm veins or external jugular veins. In the four-year follow-up, there was no evidence of aneurysmal formation from those arm veins or external jugular vein patch grafts. The indication for the vein patch was to avoid eventual luminal compromise following endarterectomy, and in clinical experience based on my series, there seemed to be better tolerance with the group of patients

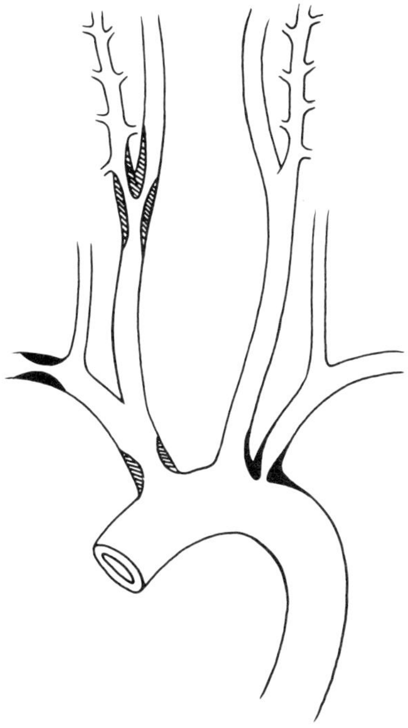

Figure 9. Multiple stenoses involving the proximal innominate artery, proximal subclavian arteries, and severe stenosis of the right carotid artery system.

who had patch graft in postoperative hypotension, in terms of carotid artery thrombosis. This may merely indicate luminal enlargement at the site of the distal internal carotid artery, which probably gives larger diameter of the artery. In the group which had endarterectomy without vein patch, there was major stroke in 1.4% and minor stroke in 0%. Hospital mortality was 1.4%. In seven years there was 0.7% restenosis in patients who had carotid endarterectomy and required reoperation. With better equipment for scientific and objective ways of following those patients postoperatively, more cases would be expected to be diagnosed as asymptomatic or symptomatic restenosis. With noninvasive vascular studies and further utilization of less invasive studies such as DSA, further delineation of the natural history of carotid artery disease will be clarified in the future. In the group which underwent carotid endarterectomy with vein patch, there was no major stroke. However, minor stroke was noted in 1%. There was

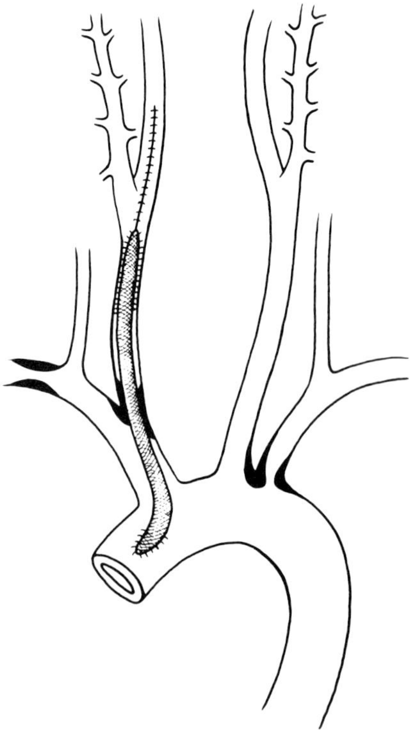

Figure 10. Patient in Figure 9 was treated with right carotid endarterectomy and ascending aorto–right common carotid artery bypass.

no operative or hospital mortality in these cases. In four-year follow-up, there was no known symptomatic restenosis which required surgical intervention. It is my policy and practice that all patients who are found to have carotid bruit are followed indefinitely. Those who have carotid endarterectomy are followed at regular intervals with necessary clinical evaluation and noninvasive vascular studies in our vascular laboratory. There was 1.2% incidence of isolated common carotid artery stenosis. In three cases, for the additional stenosis or occlusion of the common carotid artery in a patient with internal carotid artery stenosis with TIA, carotid endarterectomy was combined with aorto-common carotid artery bypass. The bilateral subclavian artery stenoses were considered to be asymptomatic other than hemodynamic deterioration (Figure 9). This problem was managed by doing carotid endarterectomy and ascending aortocarotid artery bypass (Figure 10). This patient had an asymptomatic postoperative period for over five years. In a similar situation of a patient without subclavian artery stenosis and who was undergoing a coronary artery bypass procedure, this was

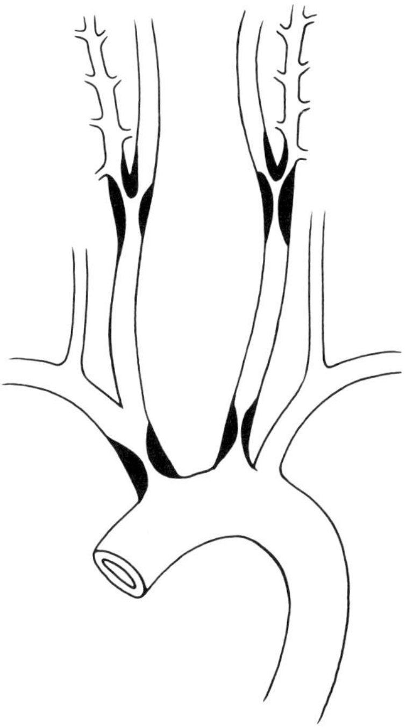

Figure 11. Multiple stenoses involving proximal innominate artery and proximal left common carotid artery at the origin in addition to severe bilateral bifurcation stenoses at the carotid artery system.

managed by concomitant carotid artery endarterectomy at the time of the coronary bypass and aorto-carotid artery bypass. In one patient who had bilateral internal carotid artery stenoses and common carotid artery stenosis with impending stroke, this severe problem was solved by bilateral carotid endarterectomies and ascending aorto-bilateral carotid artery bypass with reversed-Y Dacron graft. Patient was asymptomatic from the standpoint of TIA until the demise of patient in five years postoperatively (Figures 11, 12).

One patient had severe cerebral ischemic symptoms and was unable to stand or walk because of incapacitating dizzy spells. Aortic arch study showed complete occlusion of all major branches of the aortic arch at the origins except for left carotid artery system (Figures 13,14). Because of this extensive involvement with complete occlusion of the major branches at the origin, she was

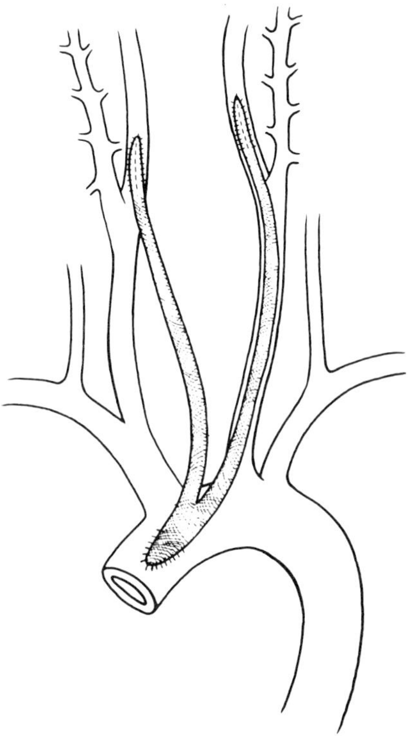

Figure 12. The patient with the problem shown in Figure 11 was managed with bilateral carotid endarterectomies and ascending aortobilateral carotid artery bypass with bifurcated Dacron Y graft.

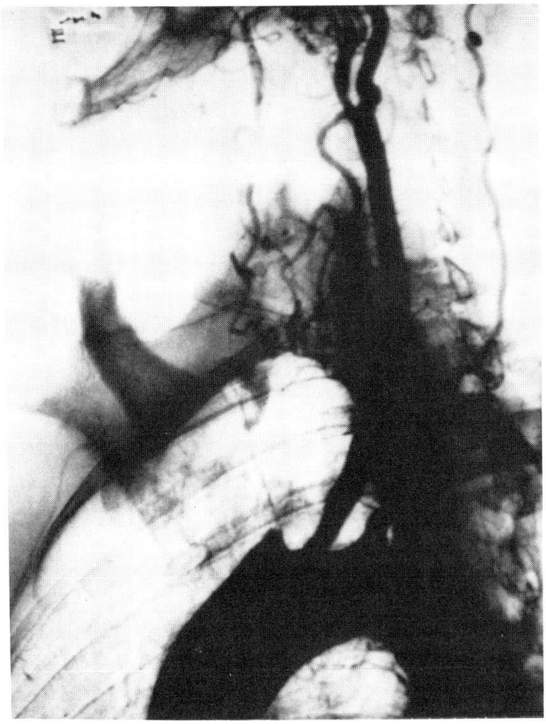

Figure 13. Aortic arch study showing complete occlusion of the innominate artery and left subclavian artery system. Only left common carotid artery system is coming off the aortic arch.

considered to be inoperable. This patient was reevaluated in our service. She was treated with reversed bilateral femorobilateral axillary artery bypasses (Figure 15), and became completely asymptomatic following this surgical procedure. In follow-up she remained asymptomatic until after two years postoperatively, when she developed arterial insufficiency of the right lower extremity with occlusion of the proximal superficial femoral artery. Because of competitive flow at the right femoroaxillary artery bypass and compromised lower extremity arterial circulation due to proximal superficial femoral artery stenosis, patient underwent right femoropopliteal artery bypass. Because of persistent septic gangrene of right foot, at third year after initial operation she underwent B-K amputation. At the present time she is asymptomatic from the standpoint of cerebral ischemic symptoms, and she is in a rehabilitation program for the prosthesis.

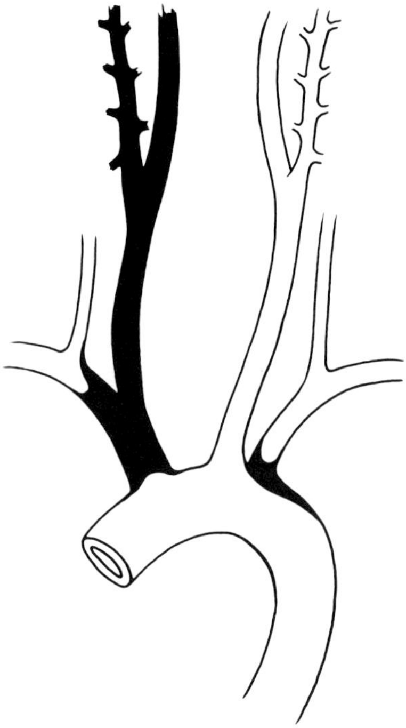

Figure 14. Schematic drawing of angiographic picture shown in Figure 13.

AXILLARY-AXILLARY BYPASS FOR SUBCLAVIAN ARTERY STENOSIS WITH SUBCLAVIAN STEAL SYNDROME AND ASSOCIATED ARTERIAL INSUFFICIENCY OF THE INVOLVED UPPER EXTREMITY

Long-term follow-up is encouraging in follow-up from one to eight years. There was one patient who had left subclavian artery stenosis with subclavian steal syndrome and profound ischemic change of the left upper extremity, and he underwent right axillo-left axillary bypass (Figures 16,17). He was doing well until about eight years after the initial operation. This time he came to the emergency room with severe arterial insufficiency of both upper extremities. The vascular work-up, including angiography, showed further progression of arteriosclerotic change at the donor side subclavian artery resulting in bilateral subclavian artery stenoses with equalization of the arterial pressure on both sides. In view of patent graft with bilateral subclavian artery stenoses, patient was managed with descending aorta left subclavian artery bypass. This, in turn, reversed the flow from the left side to the right side through the previously-made right axillo-left axillary bypass graft. Patient did well postoperatively

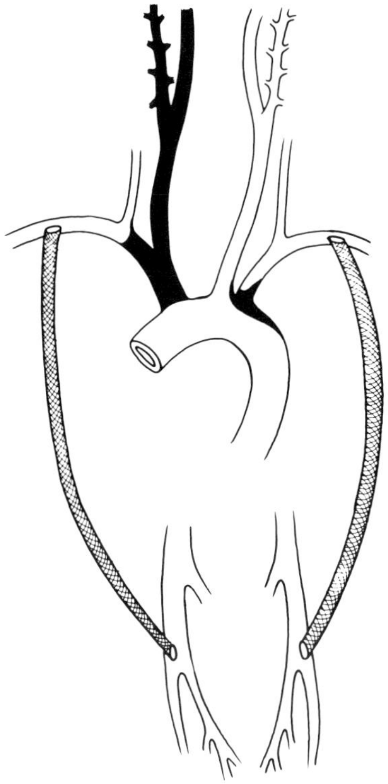

Figure 15. The condition described in Figures 13 and 14 was treated with reverse bypass to the subclavian artery system from the femoral artery system.

(Figure 18). However patient succumbed from exsanguination from the tear at the aortic anastomosis in the first twenty-four hours after surgery. Since this experience, the aortic anastomosis and major arterial bypass anastomosis have been reinforced with additional sutures and pledgets.

In a rare occasion, patient with subclavian steal syndrome had profound ischemic change of the involved side upper extremity. In this situation, the angiographic studies should extend beyond axillary artery down to the brachial system. One patient had this type of problem with multiple occlusions at the origin of the subclavian and brachial arteries. This was managed with left axillo-right axillary artery bypass and additional bypass with autogenous saphenous vein graft from the proximal brachial artery to the distal brachial artery beyond the second occlusion (Figure 19). In selected cases, the combined problem with TIA from carotid artery stenosis and additional impact from subclavian artery

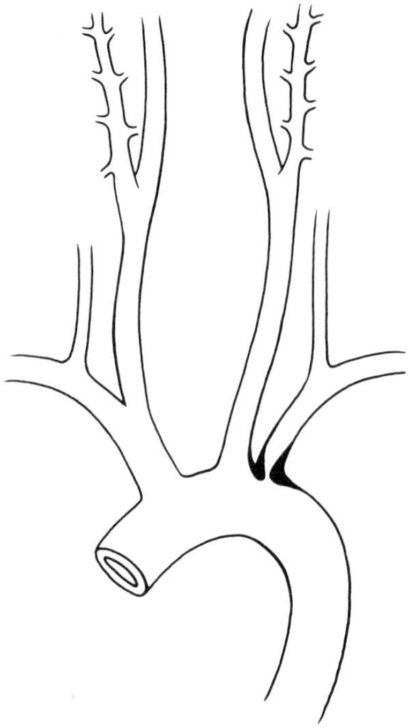

Figure 16. Severe stenosis of the left subclavian artery system at the origin with steal syndrome.

steal syndrome with arterial insufficiency of the involved side upper extremity, management may be confused. These eleven specially selected cases following noninvasive vascular studies and angiography were treated with concomitant endarterectomy and axillary-axillary artery bypass. On the other hand, as we have recently come to understand the underlying problems better, this type of concomitant surgical procedure is less frequent. Because of undue surgical risk in combining the carotid artery endarterectomy with peripheral vascular bypass procedure, this is a rare combination in our practice. We have encountered only one patient in that category.

One of the most important techniques for evaluating carotid artery and subclavian artery stenosis is multiple views of the arteries. Preoperative and pre-angiographic evaluation with noninvasive technique gives definite additional information for surgical judgment. Many times AP and lateral views show classical stenosis as illustrated in Figures 20, 21. On many occasions one view will give limited information as illustrated in Figure 22 which shows left

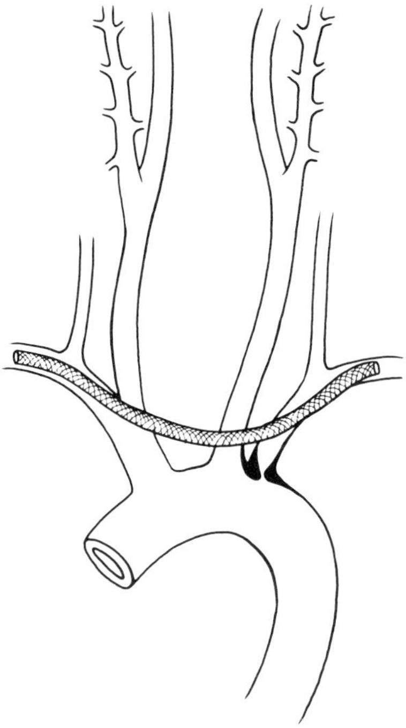

Figure 17. Condition with proximal subclavian artery stenosis with steal syndrome described in Figure 16 was treated with right axillo-left axillary artery bypass.

subclavian artery stenosis, as shown with arrows, and questionable stenosis of undetermined degree at the right carotid artery system, as shown with the triangular indicator. However, on the lateral view (Figure 23), the carotid artery stenosis is extremely critical with high-grade stenosis as shown with triangular indicators on the same patient's angiographic studies.

In my series, carotid artery aneurysm was of rare incidence. There were three cases operated on. Two patients had conventional endarterectomy and excision of aneurysmal wall on the anterior two-thirds; then this was repaired with angioplastic technique utilizing vein patch (Figure 24). A patient with carotid artery aneurysm involving the internal carotid artery with severe tortuosity was managed by doing resection and end to end anastomosis (Figure 25). In two patients, carotid body tumor was invading the carotid artery requiring resection of entire tumor and carotid artery.

The angiographic study of carotid body tumor is important for two reasons: The diagnostic feature of the tumor staining (Figure 26), and also this

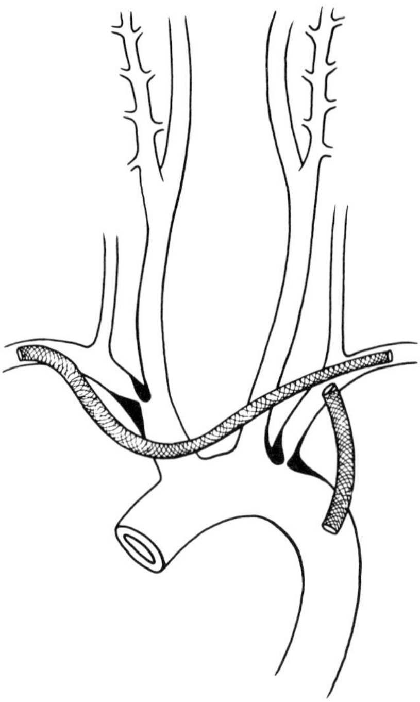

Figure 18. Due to progression of arteriosclerotic disease, the donor side subclavian artery developed severe stenosis. This was managed by additional bypass from descending aorta to the recipient subclavian artery. By doing this procedure, blood flow was reversed from the recipient subclavian artery to the donor side subclavian artery through the preexisting right axillo-left axillary artery bypass graft.

angiography, give further information of the underlying anatomical situation of the carotid artery system. Figure 27A shows an angiographic picture of patient who underwent left carotid endarterectomy and right axillary-left axillary bypass for subclavian steal syndrome. This patient came back five years after the initial operation with TIA. At that time his left carotid artery system was completely occluded from the origin with complete occlusion of the right internal carotid artery with retrograde filling with additional stenosis at the external carotid artery on the right side. Patient underwent right carotid endarterectomy, and one can see dominant vertebral artery with additional collateral circulation from the subclavian system on the left side. Right vertebral artery is small. During the operation on the right carotid artery, intraoperative shunting was carried out from the common carotid artery into the external carotid artery to give additional protection to the cerebral flow during the endarterectomy

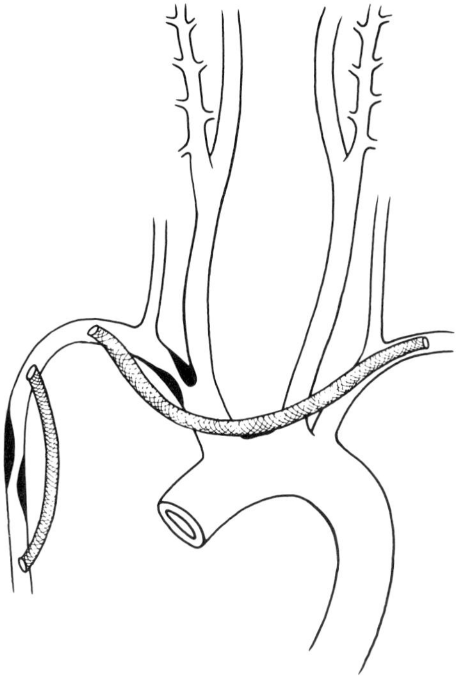

Figure 19. Patient with multiple stenoses involving the proximal subclavian artery and isp ipsilateral brachial artery occlusion. This was managed by left axillo-right axillary artery bypass with graft and then right axillary artery-distal brachial artery bypass with autogenous greater saphenous vein graft.

procedure. The patient kept smoking but was asymptomatic. Three years later he came back with occasional episodes of TIAs. Repeated DSA study showed complete occlusion of bilateral carotid artery system with still functioning axillary artery-axillary artery bypass graft (Figure 27B). Patient is still alive and well otherwise, with antiplatelet treatment and no evidence of infarction.

A patient who previously underwent thoracic aorto-left subclavian artery bypass, descending aortobilateral femoral artery bypass and distal revascularization developed arterial insufficiency of the right hand [47]. The angiographic study showed open bilateral internal carotid arteries (Figure 28). However, this time the right subclavian artery stenosis had progressed further with steal syndrome and arterial insufficiency of the right upper extremity. Subsequently patient underwent left axillo-right axillary artery bypass. In the following two years patient underwent bilateral carotid endarterectomies on separate

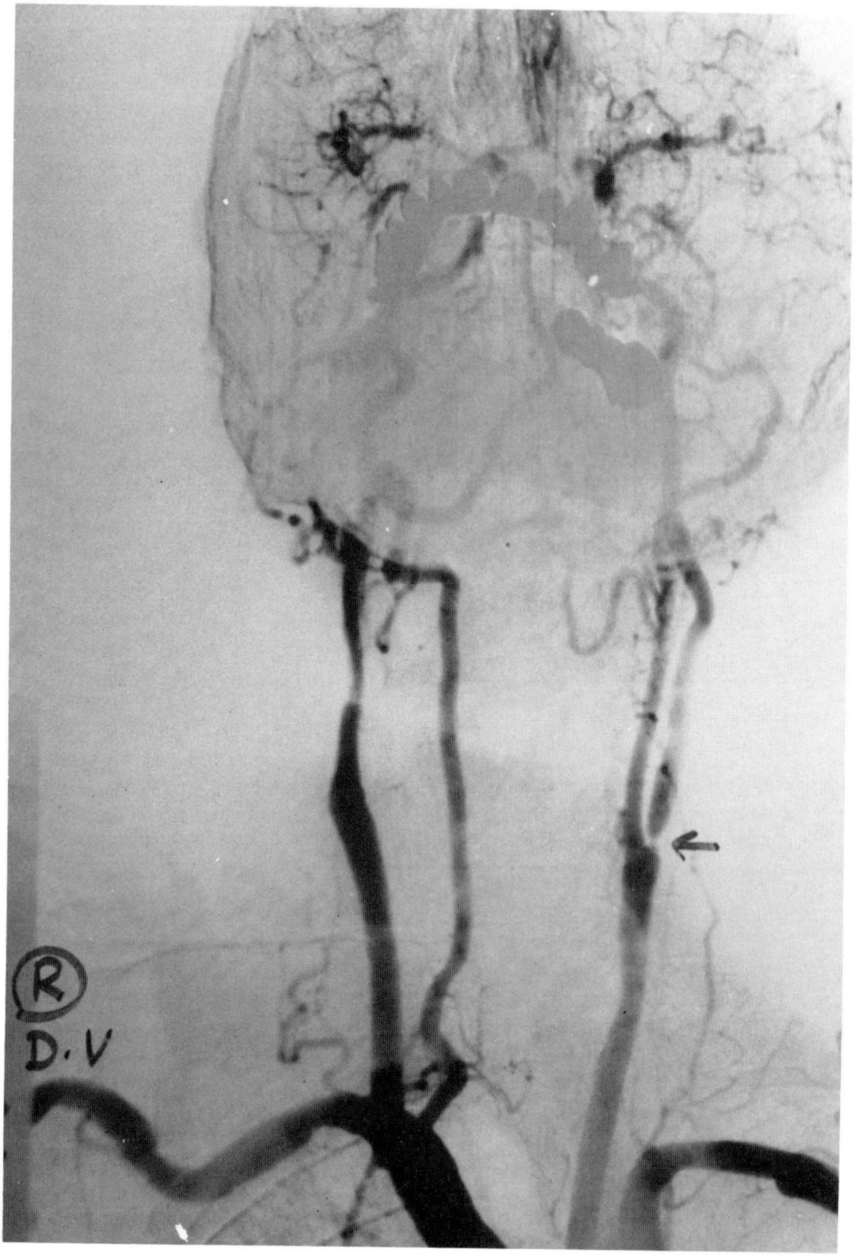

Figure 20. Conventional aortic arch study, P–A view, showing high degree of stenosis at the origin of left internal carotid artery (arrow).

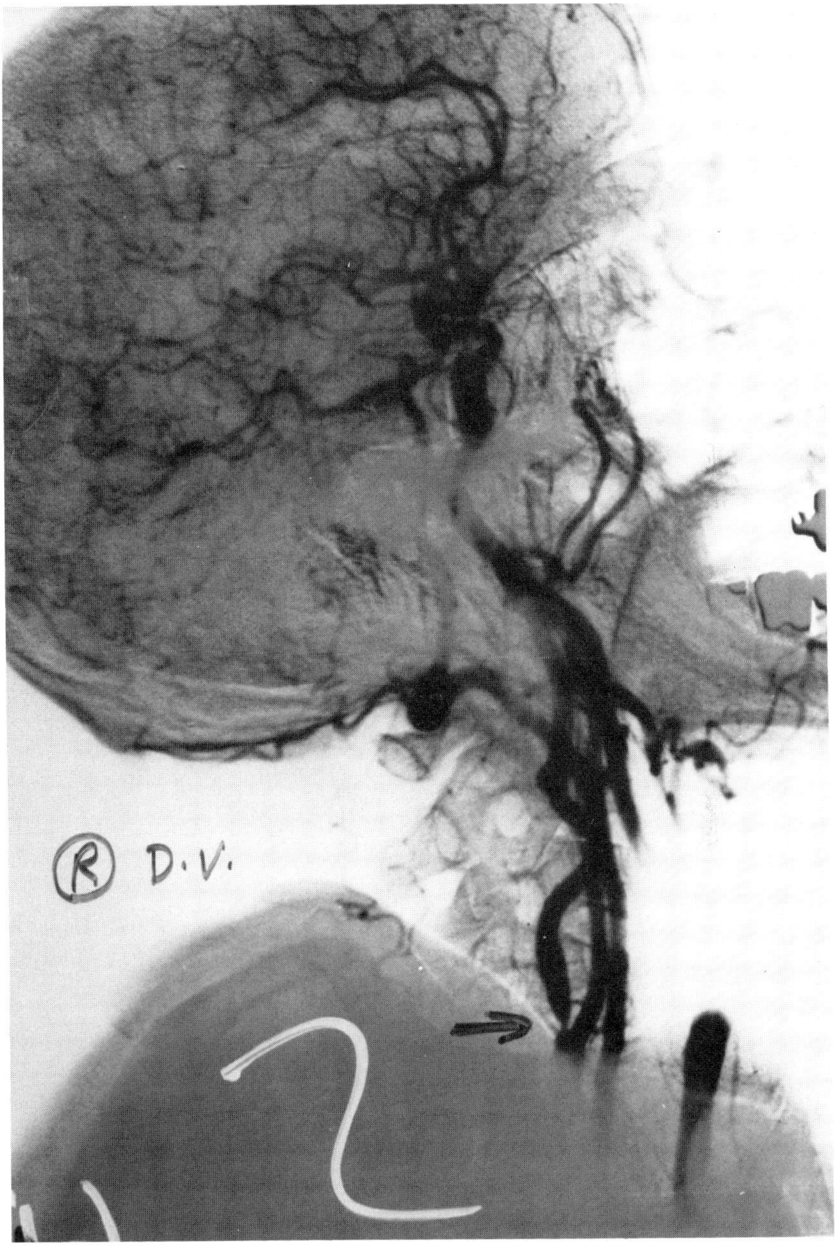

Figure 21. Lateral view of aortic arch study showing severe stenosis (arrow) on the same patient as in Figure 20.

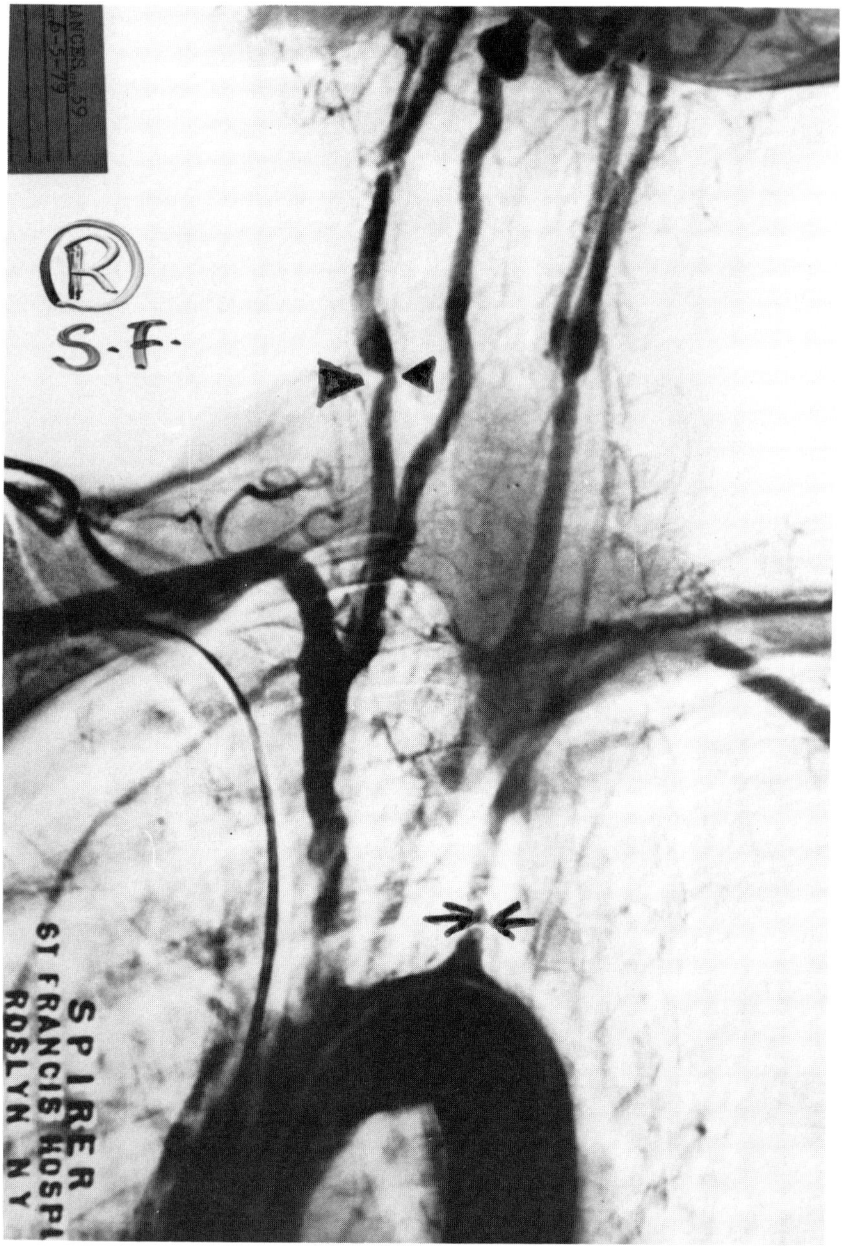

Figure 22. Aortic arch study showing severe stenosis at the left proximal subclavian artery (arrows), and right carotid artery stenosis (triangular arrows).

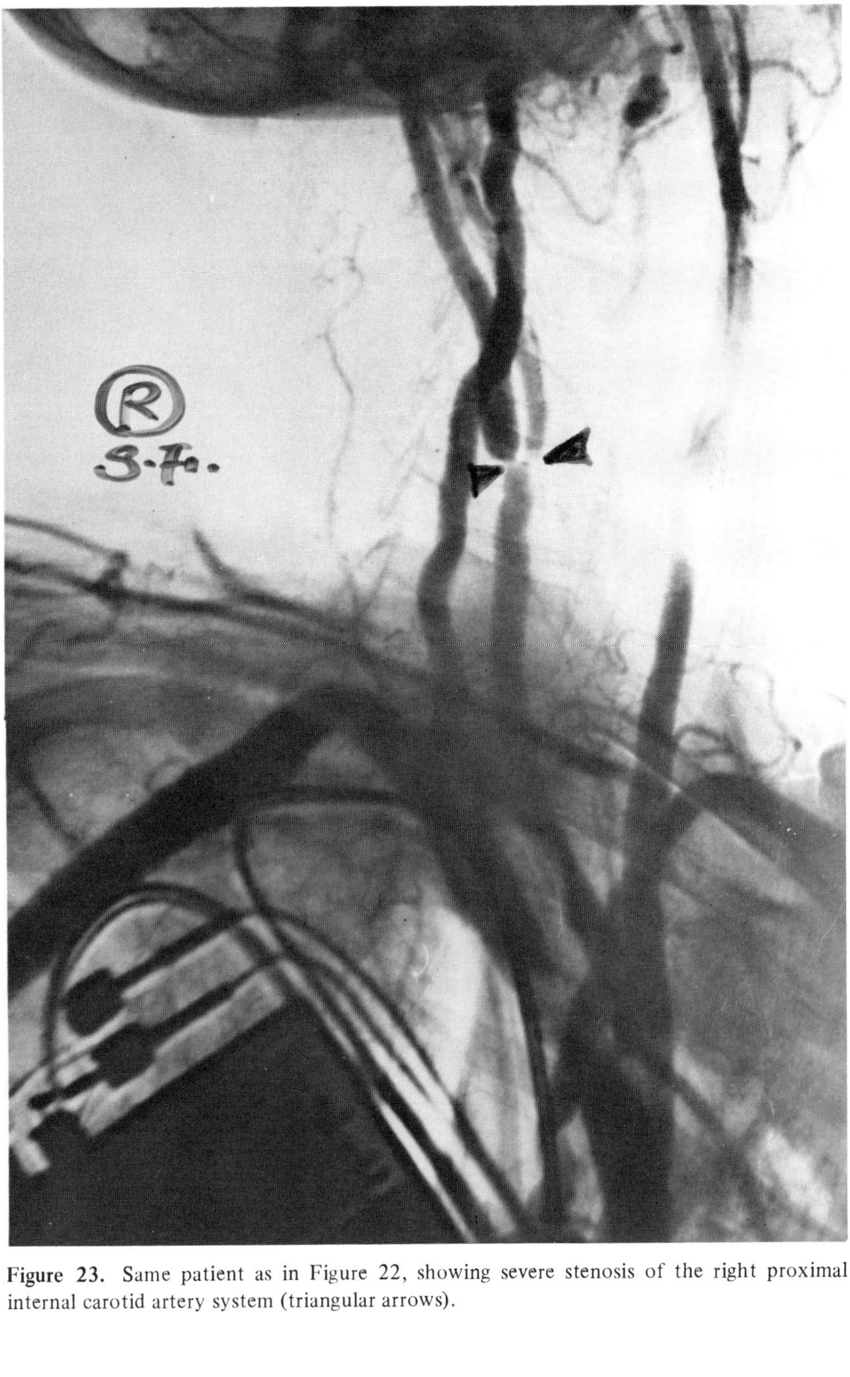

Figure 23. Same patient as in Figure 22, showing severe stenosis of the right proximal internal carotid artery system (triangular arrows).

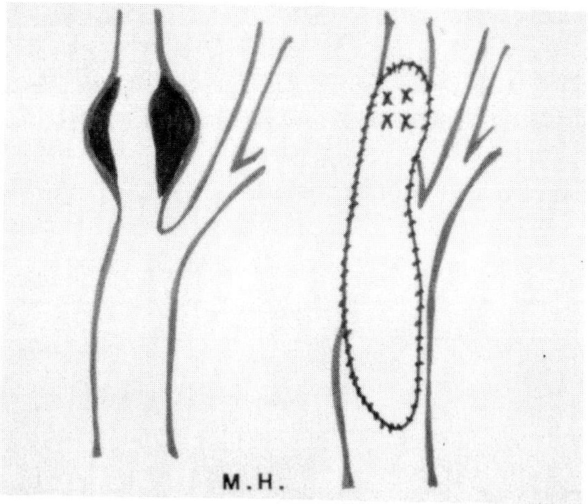

Figure 24. Severe stenosis of the internal carotid artery system being treated with endarterectomy and angioplasty using autogenous vein patch. The tacking stitches of the distal intima at the internal carotid artery should be proximal to the distal angle of the arteriotomy. Therefore the vein patch can prevent possible luminal compromise.

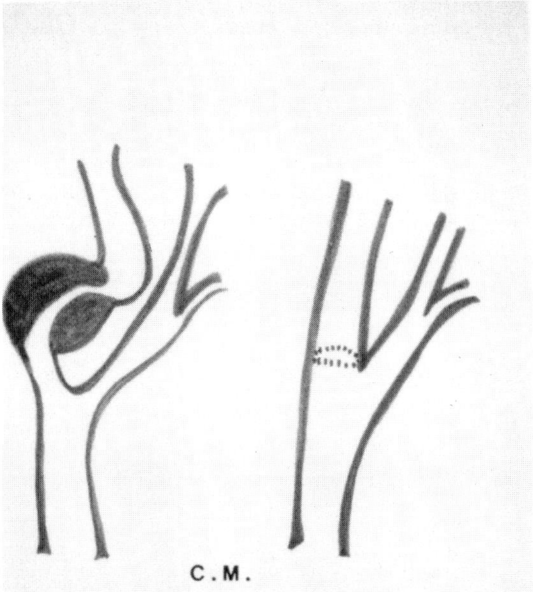

Figure 25. If the tortuosity of the internal carotid arteries is severe, then this portion can be resected with or without additional endarterectomy of the remaining artery, and then end-to-end anastomosis.

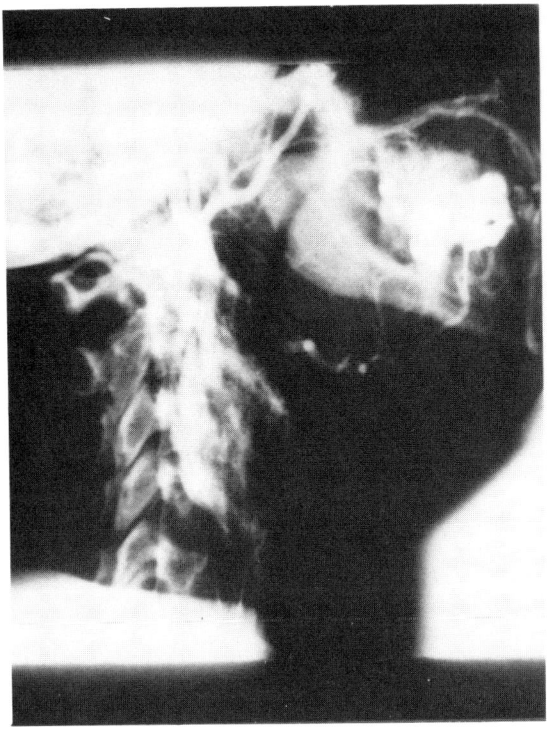

Figure 26. The aortic arch study showing massive tumor staining at the neck in a case of large carotid body tumor.

occasions. This patient shows classical example of progression of arteriosclerotic disease involving multiple systems.

In April, 1983, a patient was brought back to New York after she had massive myocardial infarction and cardiogenic shock. Patient needed permanent pacemaker. During the period of cardiogenic shock, patient thrombosed right femoral-popliteal artery bypass graft with severe ischemic change of right lower limb. Because of fresh myocardial infarction, the necessary revascularization for the right lower extremity ischemia was not possible, and at a later date patient has major amputation due to progression of septic gangrene of the right leg. Currently, the patient has permanent pacemaker and prosthesis of right leg, with all other grafts functioning.

In terms of technical aspect, carotid artery endarterectomy with patch may demand further operative time. However, the early clinical comparison

a

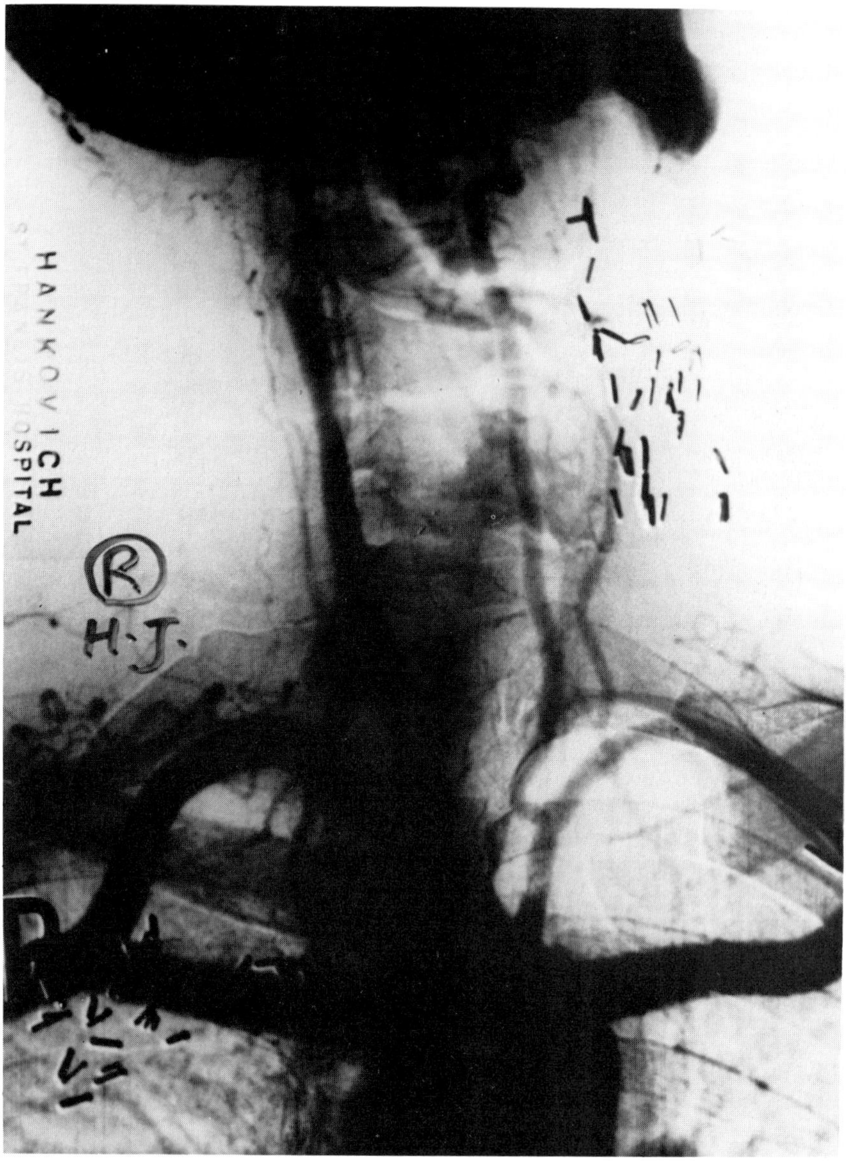

Figure 27A. Patient, who had axillary-axillary artery bypass for subclavian artery stenosis and steal syndrome and left carotid endarterectomy, came back five years postoperatively with complete occlusion of entire left carotid artery system and stenosis of the right carotid artery. The angiography shows patent axillary artery-axillary artery bypass graft and absence of left carotid artery system.

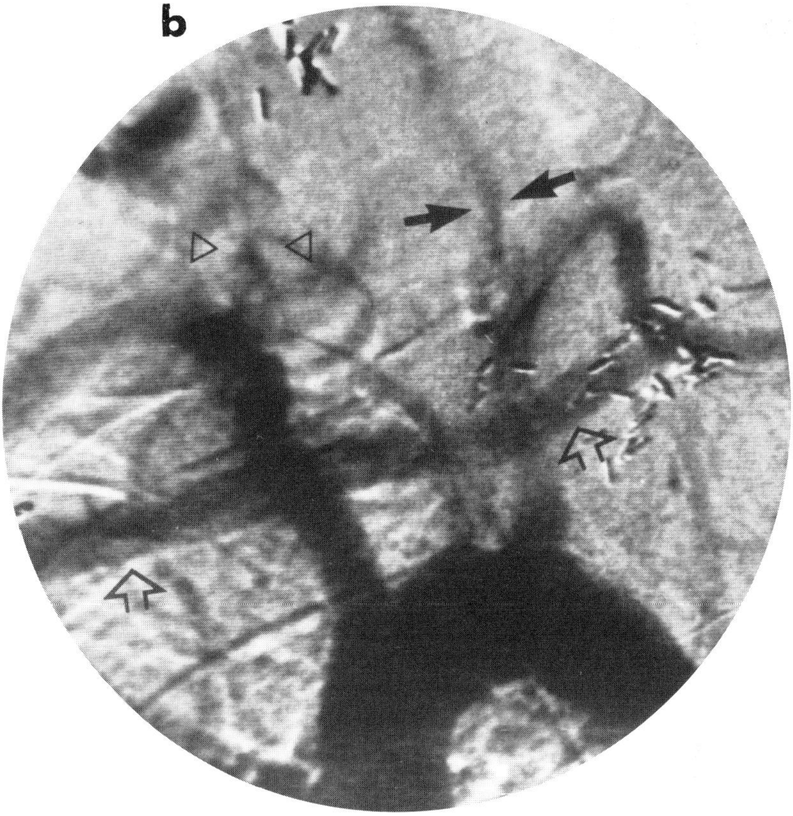

Figure 27B. The patient in Figure 27A returned three years after right carotid endarterectomy. At this time the DSA study shows patent axillary–axillary artery bypass graft (open arrows), and absence of entire bilateral carotid artery system (triangular arrows on the right side and arrows on the left side).

of my own series with two groups of patients, one with vein patch and one without vein patch, showed some clinical impression that the group of patients with patch graft had better results. This evaluation will require further investigation with a longer follow-up to give statistical merit. This is not the intention of this presentation (Tables 15,16).

In a patient (Figure 29) who developed recurrent stenosis after carotid endarterectomy and vein patch, it was found to be technically impossible to redo the endarterectomy alone because of severe adhesion and ulceration at the

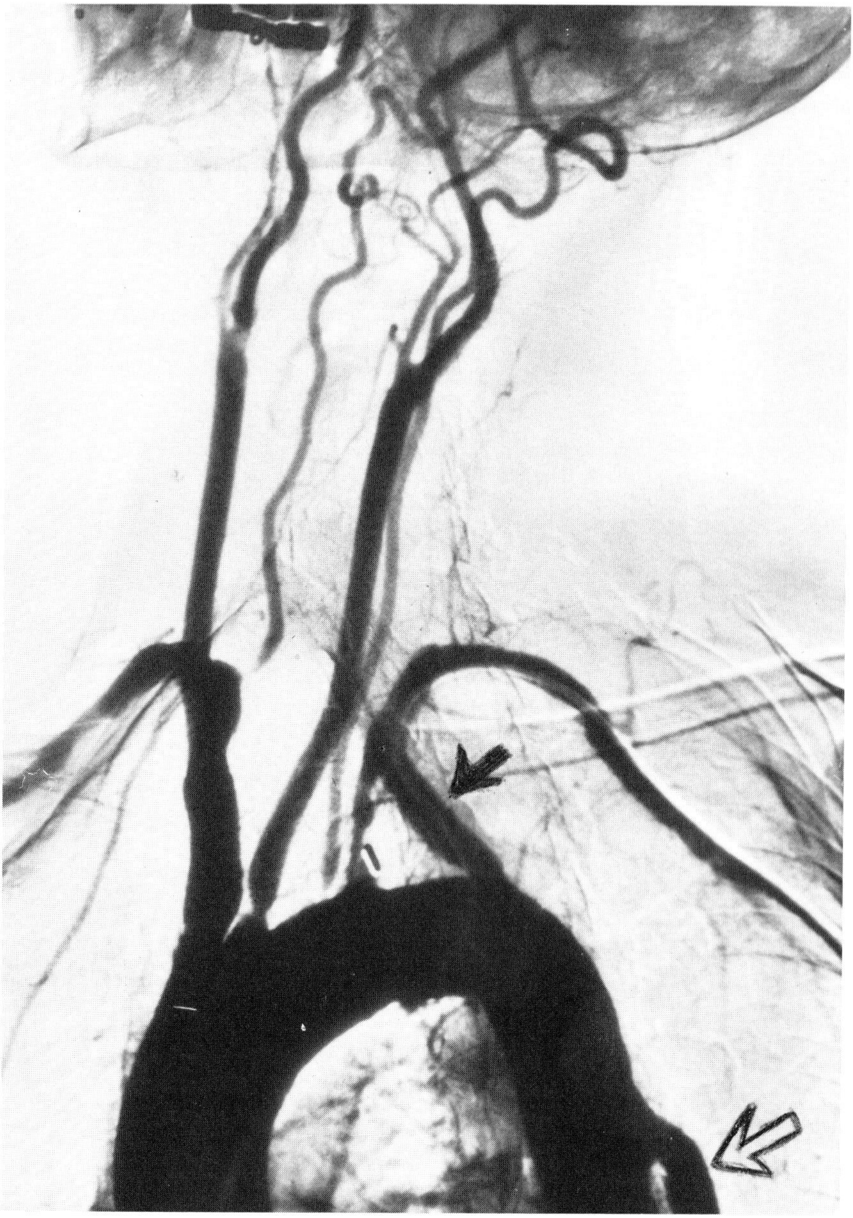

Figure 28. Aortic arch study showing patent descending aorto-left subclavian artery bypass graft (arrow), and patent descending aortobilateral femoral artery bypass graft (open arrow).

Table 15. Carotid Endarterectomy Without Patch

Major stroke	1.4%
Minor stroke	0%
Restenosis	0.7%
Mortality	1.4%

Table 16. Carotid Endarterectomy with Patch

Major stroke	0%
Minor stroke	1.4%
Restenosis	0%
Mortality	0%

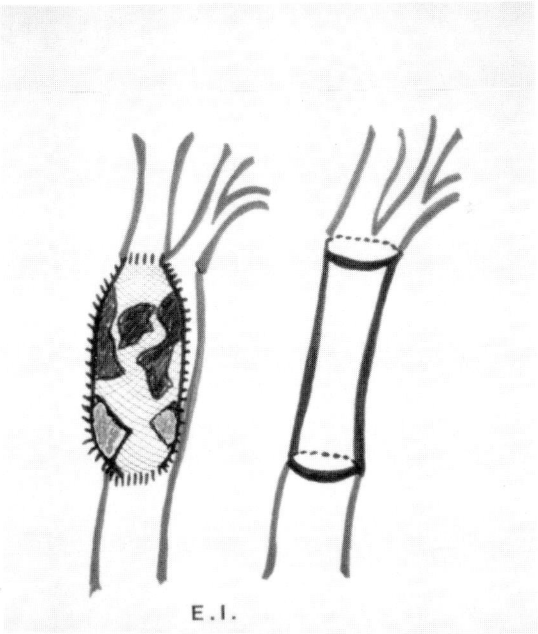

Figure 29. Patient with restenosis of the carotid artery three years after endarterectomy and vein patch graft. This was managed with resection of the involved segment of the carotid artery and old patch graft, and graft replacement.

vein patch. This was resected, and graft replacement was carried out with satisfactory outcome.

SURGICAL TECHNIQUE FOR CAROTID ENDARTERECTOMY AND VEIN PATCH ANGIOPLASTY

Carotid artery surgery requires employment of every detail of surgical principles and meticulous surgical skill. Technique of cerebral protection and other principles have been stated in the introduction and discussion of this paper. The following steps are routine in my surgical technique: All operations were performed under general endotracheal tube anesthesia in normotensive and normocarbic conditions. During the operation patient was monitored with EKG and arterial pressure through intraarterial catheter. In all cases routine intraoperative shunting was used. No attempt was made to measure stump pressure for the purpose of selective shunting in this series. EEG monitoring was not done on a routine basis. After satisfactory general endotracheal tube anesthesia under proper monitoring, entire neck, chest and appropriate lower or upper extremity are prepped with Betadine wash. A semivertical incision is made along the anterior border of the ipsilateral sternocleidomastoid muscle. The incision is deepened by sharp and blunt dissection, retracting the muscle laterally to expose the carotid sheath. The branch of the internal jugular vein, the facial vein, is ligated and divided, and the internal jugular vein is retracted laterally along with muscle. Careful dissection then begins to expose and free the common carotid artery. Care is taken to avoid injury to the underlying, structure, mainly the vagal nerve. As the dissection approaches distally at the bifurcation, 1% Xylocaine solution is infiltrated into the carotid body in order to prevent possible fluctuation of BP and pulse rate. Only after this, is further careful dissection carried out to expose the external carotid arteries. Sometimes the first branch, and rarely the second branch, of the external carotid artery is divided after ligation to aid further dissection and to rotate the artery for the benefit of internal carotid artery exposure. At this point the hypoglossal nerve is identified and preserved intact. In the case of high carotid artery bifurcation, the hypoglossal nerve can be freed further by ligating small arterial and venous branches around the nerve with small hemoclips. Ligation of these small venous and arterial branches around the hypoglossal nerve will give further room to free the internal carotid artery. Extreme care should be given to manage the arterial system gently to avoid undue stress on the atheromatous plaque with possibly unstable ulcerating plaque, which has already compromised the arterial lumen. This would minimize possible dissection or embolization. Rubber vessel loop is placed around the external carotid artery. The dissection of the internal carotid artery should be higher than the distal extent of the atheromatous plaque on palpation. This is extremely important for complete endarterectomy and revascularization. The distal internal carotid artery can be freed gently up to the base of the skull. It has been my experience that it is rarely necessary to resect the mandible or to divide the digastric or stylohyoid muscles. At this point a segment of the greater saphenous vein is obtained by a vertical incision on the distal or proximal part of the lower extremity, depending on the venous condition. If patient has a history of intermittent claudication or other signs of arterial insufficiency, it is not our policy to remove the saphenous vein. For other indications, such as impending problem with eventual coronary revascularization, saphenous vein is again preserved. In this situation arm vein is used (antecubital, cephalic, or basilic vein). If the arm vein is not available, then the neck veins (external jugular vein or branch of internal jugular vein, such as facial vein) are used. It is not my policy to use a prosthesis for angioplastic patch purpose, for a variety of reasons. A most important concern is possible restenosis and source of embolization faster than with autogenous vein patch graft. When vein is obtained, patient is heparinized systematically.

Following heparinization, arteriotomy is made extending from the common carotid artery proximal to the atheroma. This arteriotomy is then extended distally to the internal carotid artery distal to the atheromatous plaque, until the normal arterial wall is noted within the rim of maximum safety of surgical repair. It is also important to have enough of the distal internal carotid artery to make sutures for angioplasty later on. Every necessary dissection should be done before the arteriotomy is made. A shunt is then introduced into the common carotid artery. Care is taken to remove all possible atheromatous debris or air in the shunt by flushing the pulsatile flow through the shunt. Then the distal end of the shunt is introduced into the distal internal carotid artery. Prior to the insertion of the shunt cuff, care is taken to irrigate the arterial lumen of the internal carotid artery with heparinized normal saline solution (2000 units and 500 cc. of normal saline solution). The appropriate shunt clamp or rubber tourniquet is applied around the shunt and artery proximally and distally. At this time the shunt is checked carefully to make certain that there is no air bubble or cholesterol debris in the shunt. This is carried out by using two Kelly clamps, one proximally and one distally on the shunt, and by opening one at a time until the shunt is checked out clearly. Circulation is restored through the shunt. Endarterectomy is carried out under direct vision and not in a hasty manner. The procedure is initiated by finding appropriate dissection line. Sharp resection is carried out at the normal part of the carotid artery proximally. Then dissection is carried out distally around the orifice of the external carotid artery. Further dissection is carried out carefully to the internal carotid artery to the point where the atheroma feathers out to a thin tail. If the distal internal carotid artery does not feather out, then sharp transection of the intima is made at the point where the least involvement is seen. The proximal end of

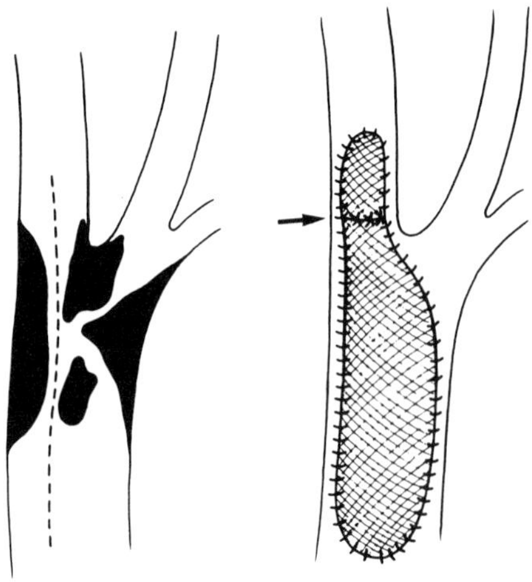

Figure 30. Patient with carotid artery stenosis and multiple ulcerations treated with endarterectomy and angioplasty with autogenous greater saphenous vein patch graft. The arrow indicates the tagging suture of the distal intima, proximal to the distal anastomosis of the angioplasty vein patch, to prevent luminal compromise.

the distal intima of the internal carotid artery is then tacked down with 6–0 Prolene sutures in interrupted or continuous fashion. It is important that this end point is proximal to the distal angle of the arteriotomy on the internal carotid artery, as shown on Figure 30 with arrow. In this way vein patch will be able to prevent possible compromise of the internal carotid artery lumen over the area of tacking suture. The endarterectomy is now completed by doing the final step of direct and indirect endarterectomy of the orifice and proximal portion of the external carotid artery. The arterial lumen is irrigated with a copious amount of heparinized normal saline solution. A small peanut sponge on a stick is useful to peel off loose atheromatous debris from the arterial wall. Care is taken to irrigate under and around the shunt at the point of insertion to the common and internal carotid arteries. Vein patch, in reversed manner, is then applied to the arteriotomy. The angioplastic sutures should be started at the distal corner on the internal carotid artery under direct vision with 5-0 or 6-0 Prolene in interrupted and continuous fashion. Once the distal corner is completed, the sutures are made continuously toward the proximal artery on the lower part of the arteriotomy. At the mid-portion of the suturing another suture can be started, or the same suture can be continued around the proximal corner. At the final steps of the suturing the shunt is clamped and removed, first from the common carotid artery. Then the shunt is completely removed from the distal internal carotid artery. During the final few stitches, proximal pulsatile flush is done, re-clamp applied to proximal artery, then external carotid clamp is released temporarily, and the internal carotid artery clamp is released temporarily. The arterial lumen is then irrigated. Finally the internal carotid artery clamp is released again. In this way the air or possible free debris in the arterial lumen will again be flushed out. As the suturing progresses, the artery will be distended by back flow from the internal carotid artery, until the last possible air has escaped. The suturing is completed, and then the internal carotid artery is close clamped with atraumatic, double bubble Fogarty clamp. Circulation is restored to the external carotid artery and then to the internal carotid artery in a sequential manner. The suture line is inspected, and arterial pulses are checked on the common, internal and external carotid arteries. With these careful surgical steps, it is extremely rare to find a situation requiring intraoperative angiography. The heparin is neutralized in a ratio of 3000 units to 40 mg of Protamin. Careful hemostasis is carried out with electric coagulation and Weck clips. The neck incision is closed in layers using 2-0 Vicryl or Dexan sutures for the inner layers and 4-0 sutures for the skin in a subcuticular manner. In a similar fashion incisions for vein patch are also closed. Sterile dressings are applied with 4×8 combine, and folded sterile towel is applied around the neck without much compression. It is not routine to use a drain in this operation except for an unusual situation such as excessive oozing, or when operation is for restenosis. All patients take antiplatelet agents (Persantine and ASA) up to day of hospital admission, which is normally one or two days prior to surgery. This medication is resumed the day after surgery, when patient is allowed to take PO medication or diet. Dressing is removed in twenty-four hours. Patient is given pre and postoperative antibiotics routinely. The neck incision heals without problem. Infection at the neck incision is extremely rare. Patient is monitored postoperatively in the recovery room and in the intensive care unit. Hypertension is treated with intravenous nitroprusside drip. Care is taken to prevent hypotension by careful management of intake and output, and necessary agent. If patient has bilateral carotid artery stenoses, this is followed with the following principles:

1. Routinely the symptomatic side is operated on first, if the degree of stenosis is high on both sides. Then the asymptomatic side is watched

Table 17. Patients Operated for Acute Occlusion of One Carotid Artery

Case	Age (sex)	Symptom	Contralateral carotid artery	Procedure causing occlusion	Stump pressure during operation	Time from operation until symptom	Time from symptom until reoperation	Results
1	71 (F)	TIA + Paresis	Severe stenosis	Angiography	unknown		1.0	Remission
2	57 (M)	TIA	Stenosis	TEA	Unknown	20	2.0	Remission
3	60 (M)	TIA	Occluded	TEA	Unknown	1	1.5	Unchanged
4	66 (M)	TIA	Operated	TEA	> 75 mm Hg	1	1.0	Died
5	66 (M)	TIA	Normal	Resection of aneurysm	22 mm Hg	6	1.0	Remission
6	58 (F)	TIA	Stenosis	TEA	55 mm Hg	2	1.0	Unchanged

From Lindberg [29].

or operated on, on a semi-elective basis, depending on the patient's problem or condition.

2. If patient has a higher degree of severity of stenosis at the contralateral side with higher hemodynamic deterioration, the asymptomatic side is operated on first to give the best possible benefit for hemodynamic protection during the operation, and the symptomatic side is done at the same admission, in a week's time.

Patient is normally discharged in three to seven days after surgery, if patient had unilateral carotid endarterectomy. Postoperatively, I follow all patients in the vascular clinic with clinical evaluation and noninvasive vascular studies at regular intervals in conjunction with follow-up by a team consisting of internist or cardiologist and neurologist. Sometimes a patient with uncontrollable TIAs or amaurosis fugax is found to have a high degree of stenosis with or without severe ulceration, and such a patient is given intravenous anticoagulation therapy, and surgery is done on an urgent basis. It is known that acute carotid artery occlusion can be treated surgically if it can be corrected within one to two hours after the first sign of deterioration, according to Lindberg [16]. His experience is shown on Table 17.

AXILLARY ARTERY-AXILLARY ARTERY BYPASS

This is the most commonly used extra-anatomic bypass procedure for subclavian artery stenosis and steal syndrome with or without arterial insufficiency of the involved upper extremity. All the operations are done under general endotracheal general anesthesia with upper extremities placed at the side of the trunk to relax the pectoral muscles. The entire neck and chest are prepped and draped in sterile fashion using Betadine painting. A transverse incision is made on the anterior chest wall on each side approximately two-fingers' breadth below the clavicle. The pectoralis major muscle is split along the direction of the muscle fibers. The neurovascular bundle is divided in between ligatures if necessary. The pectoralis minor muscle is retracted laterally. The axillary vein is freed and retracted inferiorally. Care is taken to preserve the brachial plexus intact. The axillary artery is freed from the proximal and then the distal portion. The axillary artery is freed first on the donor side and then to the receiving artery. Tunnel is made in semi-U shape over the sternum subcutaneously. Patient is given systemic heparin intravenously. End-to-side anastomosis is made between the side of the axillary artery on the donor side and end of 10 mm PTFE graft. The earlier cases in this series were done with Dacron graft. However the last half of the series was done using PTFE. Following completion of the proximal anastomosis at the donor site, the graft is then brought through the tunnel over the sternum into the receiving axillary artery in U shape. Care should be taken to insure that the graft lies in a natural manner without tension to the artery. Such tension may give sudden interruption of the anastomosis at early postoperative period and also may compromise the axillary venous drainage, In the last twenty-six cases, one patient had sudden onset of acutely expanding hematoma due to interruption of the suture line in one month postoperatively. This required emergency surgical repair.

Care is taken to evacuate all possible air or clot in the graft before the second anastomosis is completed. Then circulation is restored first to the distal then to the proximal axillary artery in a sequential manner. Heparin is then neutralized with Protamin. Incision is closed in layers using absorbable sutures. Skin is closed in subcuticular manner, and dressing is applied in the usual manner. The dressing is removed in twenty-four hours postoperatively. Patient is given Persantine and ASA postoperatively. Patient is normally discharged from the hospital from four days to a week after the surgery, and then is followed as an out-patient with necessary noninvasive follow-up studies. This type of extra-anatomic bypass is an operation of choice in a given situation. Rarely, when this is not possible, proximal anastomosis is done at the aorta and on an extremely rare occasion, from the common carotid artery.

SUMMARY

From this material, and that of other authors in this section, the indications and basic principles of surgical treatment for cerebral vascular disease are much clearer at this time. However, in my experience and opinion, surgery for asymptomatic carotid bruit is controversial. For practical purpose, at this time, asymptomatic bruit is evaluated with noninvasive vascular studies. If noninvasive vascular studies reveal significant hemodynamic deterioration, and that particular patient is to undergo a major surgical procedure, I consider surgical repair of that carotid artery stenosis necessary prior to major surgical intervention. As of this time, it has not been routine practice to perform angiographic studies for asymptomatic carotid artery bruit, especially if there is no evidence of hemodynamic deterioration. Currently that group of patients is followed on a regular basis with repeated noninvasive vascular studies as necessary. With the current sophistication of noninvasive vascular studies and the availability of DSA, further definition and the natural history of asymptomatic carotid bruit will be clarified in the future of our practice.

For symptomatic cerebral vascular disease, we suggest the following clinical course:

> If the clinical picture shows a stable pattern, this group of patients should undergo elective work-up. If elective work-up, including vascular

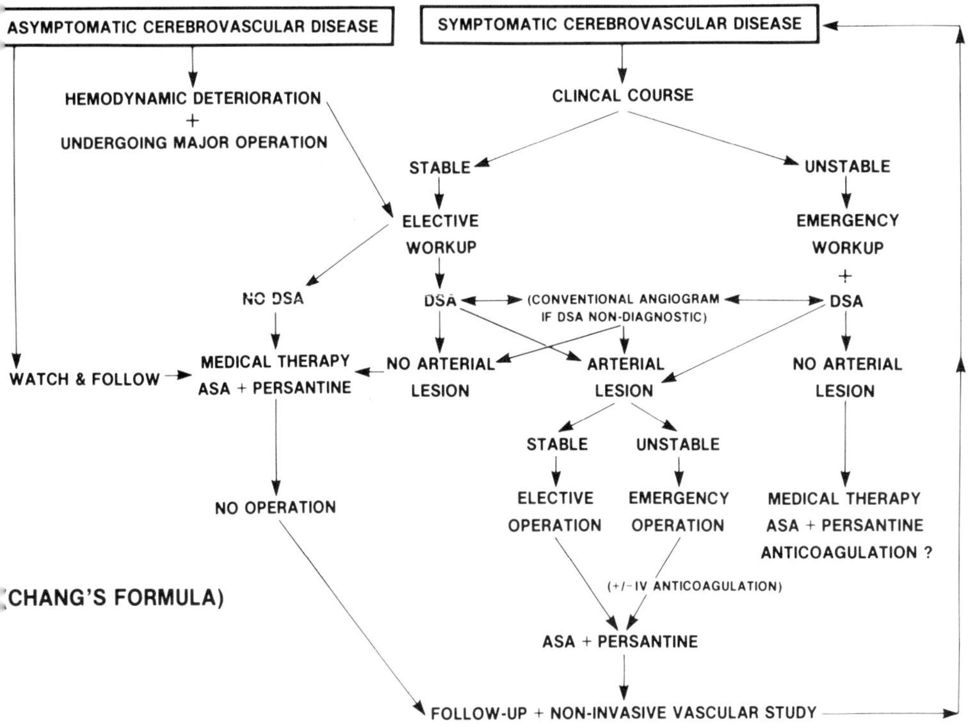

Figure 31. Author's current policy of practice for cerebrovascular disease.

studies, shows no evidence of hemodynamic deterioration, and patients have no history of amaurosis fugax, this group is watched further with subsequent evaluation. However, if the elective work-up showed underlying carotid artery stenosis and/or clinical evidence of TIA, we proceed with DSA. If this study does not correspond to the clinical picture or the findings of noninvasive vascular studies, then patient is subjected to conventional aortic arch study. If this angiographic study shows no definite arterial lesion, then patient is followed further. If the arterial lesion is confirmed with angiographic study, then proper surgical treatment should be planned. If patient's clinical condition is stable, the patient should be scheduled for elective surgery. However, if clinical condition is not stable, and patient has a high degree of stenosis with possible impending thrombosis or stroke, such a patient should be scheduled for emergency

Table 18. Indications for Operation

Indication	Patients	Percent
Focal transient cerebral ischemia	117	35
Asymptomatic carotid stenosis	83	25
Previous completed stroke	50	15
Vertebrobasilar syndrome	49	15
Two or more factors	36	10
Total	335	100
Preceding another peripheral vascular procedure	51	15
Preceding myocardial revascularization	49	15
Combined with myocardial revascularization	5	1
Total	105	31

From Hertzer and Lees [11].

operation. This type of patient may require preoperative intravenous anticoagulation therapy, if CT scan shows no evidence of acute infarction.

When patient has suspected symptomatic cerebral vascular disease and is clinically unstable, patient should go through emergency work-up and DSA. Again, application of conventional aortic arch study should be considered, if DSA study is nondiagnostic or does not correspond to the clinical suspicion of noninvasive vascular study results. If this emergency work-up fails to show responsible arterial lesions, then this kind of patient should be watched with medical therapy. Until proven otherwise, it is our policy to treat such patients with ASA and Persantine. In selected cases, anticoagulation therapy may have to be considered, depending on the patient's clinical condition.

All patients are followed indefinitely on a regular basis with necessary noninvasive vascular studies. This is summarized in Figure 31, modified from the outline made by Goldstone and Moore [35].

It is my opinion that if the main surgeon and medical center staff have technical excellence performing carotid artery surgery, with minimum morbidity and mortality, further expansion of surgical indication may be possible (Table 18).

REFERENCES

1. Stanton PE Jr, Rosenthal D, McClusky DA, Lamis PA. Hemodynamic assessment and surgical correction of the kinked internal carotid artery. Southern Medical J 74:11:1348–1352, 1981.
2. Broadbent WH. Absence of pulsation in both radial arteries, vessels being full of blood. London Tr Clin Soc 8:165–170, 1875.
3. Chiari H. Ueber das Verbalten das Teilungswinkels des carotis Communis bei der Endarteritis chronica deformans. Verh Dtsch Ges Pathol 9:326–330, 1906.
4. Strully JJ, Herwitt ES, Blankenberg HW. Thrombo-endarterectomy for the thrombosis of the internal carotid artery in the neck. J Neurosurg 10: 474–478, 1953.
5. Eastcott HHG, Pickering GW, Rob CG. Reconstruction of internal carotid artery in a patient with intermittent attacks of hemiplegia. Lancet 1954 (2):994–998.
6. Cooley DA, Al-Naaman YD, Carton CA. Surgical treatment of atherosclerotic occlusion of common carotid artery. J Neurosurg 13:500–505, 1956.
7. DeBakey ME, Crawford ES, Cooley DA, Morris GC Jr, Garrett HE, Fields WS. Cerebral arterial insufficiency: one to 11-year results following arterial reconstructive operation. Ann Surg 161:821–845, 1965.
8. Ennix CL Jr, Lawrie GM, Morris GC Jr, et al. Improved results of carotid endarterectomy in patients with symptomatic coronary disease; an analysis of 1546 consecutive carotid operations. Stroke 10:122–125, 1979.
9. Riles TS, Kopelman I, Imparato AM. Myocardial infarction following carotid endarterectomy; a review of 683 operations. Surg 85:249–252, 1979.
10. Keats AS. Anesthesia for carotid endarterectomy. Cleveland Clinic Quarterly 48:1:68–71, 1981.
11. Hertzer N, Lees CD. Fatal myocardial infarction following carotid endarterectomy. Ann Surg 194(2):212–218, 1981.
12. DeWeese JA, Rob CG, Satran R, et al. Results of carotid endarterectomies for transient ischemic attacks—Five years later. Ann Surg 178:258, 1973.
13. Thompson JE, Austin DJ, Patman RD. Carotid endarterectomy for cerebrovascular insufficiency: long-term results in 592 patients follow-up for thirteen years. Ann Surg 172:663–679, 1970.
14. Sundt, TM, Sharbrough FW, Piepgras DG, Kearns TP, Messick JM, O'Fallon WM. Correlation of cerebral blood flow and electroencephalographic changes during carotid endarterectomy. Mayo Clin Proc 56:533–543, 1981.
15. Barnett HJM. A randomized trial of aspirin and sylfinpyrazone in threatened stroke. New Engl J Med 299:53–59, 1978.
16. Fields WS, Lemak NA, Frankowski RF, Hardy RJ. Controlled trial of aspirin in cerebral ischemia. Stroke 8:301–306, 1977.
17. Reuther R, Dorndorf W. Aspirin in patients with cerebral ischemia and normal angiograms in nonsurgical lesions: results of a double blind trial. In J Breddin, W Dorndorf, D Loew, R Marx (eds.), Acetyl-salicylic Acid in

Cerebral Ischemia and Coronary Heart Disease, pp. 97–106, Stuttgart, New York, F. K. Schattauer Verlag, 1978.
18. Moncada S, Vane JR. Arachidonic acid metabolites and the interactions between platelets and blood vessel walls. New Engl J Med 300:1142–1147, 1979.
19. Ross R, Glomset JA. The pathogenesis of atherosclerosis. N Engl J Med 295:369–377; 420–425, 1976.
20. Grundy BL, Sanderson AC, Webster MW, Richey ET, Procopio P, Karanjia PN. Hemiparesis following carotid endarterectomy: comparison of monitoring methods. Anesthes 55:462–466, 1981.
21. Lees CD, Hertz NR. Postoperative stroke and late neurologic complications after carotid endarterectomy. Arch Surg 116:1561–1568, 1981.
22. Thompson JE, Austin DJ, Patman RD. Carotid endarterectomy for cerebrovascular insufficiency: Long-term results in 592 patients followed up to 18 years. Ann Surg 172:663–678, 1970.
23. Ott DC, Cooley DA, Chapa L, et al. Carotid endarterectomy without temporary intraluminal shunt: study of 309 consecutive operations. Ann Surg 191:708–713, 1980.
24. Wells BA, Keats AS, Cooley DA. Increased tolerance to cerebral ischemia produced by general anesthesia during temporary carotid occlusion. Surg 54:216, 1963.
25. Baker WH, Dorner DB, Barnes RW. Carotid endarterectomy: Is an indwelling shunt necessary? Surg 82:3, 321–326, 1977.
26. Baker WH, Rodman JA, Barnes RW, et al. An evaluation of hypocarbia and hypercarbia during carotid endarterectomy. Stroke 7:451, 1976.
27. Ehrenfeld WK, Hamilton FN, Larson CP, et al. Effect of CO_2 and systemic hypertension on downstream cerebral arterial pressure during carotid endarterectomy. Surg 67:87, 1970.
28. Kremen JE, Gee W, Kaupp HA, McDonald KM. Restenosis or occlusion after carotid endarterectomy. Arch Surg 114:608–610, 1979.
29. Lindberg B. Acute carotid occlusion. Indication for surgery? J Cardiovas Surg 21:315–320, 1980.
30. Sundt TM, Jr, Waltz AG. Cerebral ischemia and reactive hyperemia. Studies of cortical blood flow and microcirculation before, during, and after temporary occlusion of middle cerebral artery of squirrel monkeys. Circ Res 28: 426–433, 1971.
31. Sundt TM, Jr, Sharbrough FW, Anderson RE, Michenfeld JD. Cerebral blood flow measurements and electroencephalograms during carotid endarterectomy. J Neurosurg 41:310–320, 1974.
32. Hayakawa T, Waltz AG. Immediate effects of cerebral ischemia: evolution and resolution of neurological deficits after experimental occlusion of one middle cerebral artery in conscious cats. Stroke 6:321–327, 1975.
33. Heiss WD, Hayakawa T, Waltz AG. Cortical neuronal function during ischemia. Effects of occlusion on one middle cerebral artery on single-unit activity in cats. Arch Neurol 33:813–820, 1976.
34. Mentzer R, Jr, Finkelmeier BA, Crosby IK, Wellons HA. Emergency carotid

endarterectomy for fluctuating neurologic deficits. Surg 89(1):60–66, 1981.
35. Goldstone J, Moore W S. Emergency carotid artery surgery in neurologically unstable patients. Arch Surg 111:1284–1291, 1976.
36. Bartynski WS, Darbouze P, Nemir P, Jr. Significance of ulcerated plaque in transient cerebral ischemia. Amer J Surg 141:353–357, 1981.
37. Kroener JM, Dorn PL, Shoor PM, Wickbom IG, Bernstein EF. Prognosis of asymptomatic ulcerating carotid lesions. Arch Surg 115:1387–1392, 1980.
38. Thompson JE, Patman RD. Endarterectomy for asymptomatic carotid bruits. Surg Digest 7:9–14, 1972.
39. Thompson JE, Patman RD, Talkington CM. Asymptomatic carotid bruit: long-term outcome of patients having endarterectomy compared with unoperated controls. Ann Surg 188:308–316, 1978.
40. Cooperman M, Martin EW, Jr, Evans WE. Significance of asymptomatic carotid bruits. Arch Surg 113:1339–1340, 1978.
41. Kartchner MM, McRae LP. Noninvasive evaluation and management of the asymptomatic carotid bruit. Surg 82:840–847, 1977.
42. Humphries AW, Young JR, Santilli PH, et al. Unoperated asymptomatic significant internal carotid artery stenosis: A review of 182 instances. Surg 80:695–698, 1976.
43. Johnson N, Burnham SJ, Flanigan DP, et al. Carotid endarterectomy: A follow-up study of the contralateral nonoperated carotid artery. Ann Surg 188:748–752, 1978.
44. Moore WS, Boren C, Malone J, et al. Natural history of nonstenotic asymptomatic ulcerative lesions of the carotid artery. Arch Surg 113:1352, 1978.
45. Podore PC, DeWeese JA, May AG, Rob CG. Asymptomatic contralateral carotid artery stenosis: A five-year follow-up study following carotid endarterectomy. Surg 88:748–752, 1980.
46. Thompson JE, Patman DR, Talkington CM. Asymptomatic carotid bruit: Long-term outcome of patients having endarterectomy compared with unoperated controls. Ann Surg 188(3):308–316, 1978.
47. Chang JB. Surgical treatment of aorto-iliac artery disease. Angiology 32(2): 73–105, 1981.
48. Riles TS, Imparato AM, Mintzer R, Baumann FG. Comparison of results of bilateral and unilateral carotid endarterectomy five years after surgery. Surg 91(3):258–262, 1982.
49. Owens ML, Wilson SE. Prevention of neurologic complications of carotid endarterectomy. Arch Surg 117:551–555, 1982.
50. Welch E, Geary JE. Vocal cord paralysis following carotid endarterectomy. J Cardiovas Surg 20:393–394, 1979.
51. Deriu GP, Ballotta E. The surgical treatment of atherosclerotic occlusion of the innominate and subclavian arteries. J Cardiovas Surg 22:532–538, 1981.
52. Imparato AM, Riles TS, Kim GE. Cervical vertebral angioplasty for brain stem ischemia. Surg 90(5):842–852, 1981.

3

Aortic Aneurysm

6
Abdominal Aortic Aneurysm Management

Anthony M. Imparato

The surgical management of abdominal aortic aneurysms has evolved rapidly over a period of thirty years since Dubost et al. reported the successful resection of such an aneurysm in 1952. In rapid succession appeared confirmation of the feasibility of the operative procedure, the availability of artificial blood vessel substitutes and most recently the description of the technique of nonresective treatment for extremely poor-risk patients in whom vascular continuity is provided by axillofemoral bypass grafting.

In rapid succession the indications for surgical intervention have evolved, and the beneficial effects of elective surgical procedures upon the survival of afflicted patients was confirmed.

PATHOLOGY

Abdominal aortic aneurysms are almost universally associated with arteriosclerotic disease. Although commonly referred to as atherosclerotic, the distribution of aneurysmal dilatation is characteristic involving the immediate infrarenal aorta extending to the bifurcation into common iliac arteries and frequently involving both common iliac arteries, the process, however, ending abruptly at the bifurcation of the common iliac arteries. Rarely is the immediate bifurcation transgressed by the aneurysmal process, although there is on occasion an associated hypogastric artery aneurysm starting usually half to one centimeter beyond the origin of that vessel. The aneurysm is most commonly fusiform with degeneration of the wall extending beyond the intima into the media, there being as well laminated thrombus within the aneurysmal sac, seemingly an attempt on the part of the body to maintain an appropriate-sized lumen. Variations of the pathologic process include the so-called inflammatory aneurysm where the wall is thick, white and of almost cartilagenous consistency with intimate adherence of the duodenal wall (3rd and 4th portions) to the belly of the aneurysm. Additional variations include involvement of one or both of the renal arteries which may originate directly from the aneurysm wall. Less frequently the suprarenal abdominal aorta is involved in the fusiform dilatation with the renal and mesenteric vessels originating from aneurysm. On rare occasion there is diffuse aneurysmal dilatation of the entire abdominal aorta and iliac arteries, and even more rarely with associated involvement of the thoracic aorta.

Calcification of the intima and media of the common iliac, external iliac and hypogastric arteries is quite common creating problems in vascular control. Universally there is atheromatous degeneration involving the intimal layers of the iliac vessels and aorta posing the hazard of distal embolization.

Ruptures of the infrarenal abdominal aorta when they occur are usually found at the left posterolateral wall, while erosions through the entire thickness of the aneurysm wall down to the spinous ligaments may remain contained for long periods of time.

Although most abdominal aortic aneurysms encountered in this day of early diagnosis of the condition are found in the asymptomatic stage, any acute or chronic condition of the abdomen or lumbar spine may be simulated by an abdominal aortic aneurysm. Approximately one-third of aneurysms are detected by the patients who become aware of abdominal pulsations. The remainder are either discovered by physical examination or by investigations for other abdominal conditions by the use of roentgenograms obtained for investigation of the urinary tract, of the gastrointestinal tract or of the arterial system.

When rupture occurs the clinical picture becomes striking with pain either of the abdomen or back or both being a prominent feature frequently associated with shock, electrocardiographic changes and an expanding pulsating abdominal mass.

Variations of free rupture occur with fistula formation into the gastrointestinal tract, when there may be painless and either intermittent or at once exsanguinating gastrointestinal bleeding. Another type of rupture with fistula formation occurs when the aneurysm ruptures into the inferior vena cava producing a clinical picture frequently of acute congestive heart failure with an associated arteriovenous fistula bruit, if one will listen to the abdomen with a stethoscope. A third variant of rupture is that which occurs posteriorly with exposure of the lumbar vertebral ligaments sometimes producing back pain and sometimes not.

The nature of the pain may be characteristic with a sensation of tearing in the back, mid-abdomen or pelvis with radiation into the flank or groins. On the other hand there may be a picture simulating intestinal or renal colic.

DIAGNOSIS

Diagnosis of abdominal aortic aneurysm depends upon constant awareness of the fact that individuals over the age of 50 with abdominal or back pain of whatever charateristic may harbor an abdominal aortic aneurysm. Approximately 80% to 90% of aneurysms can be diagnosed or at least strongly suspected on physical examination and confirmed with either a lateral roentgenogram of the abdomen, a sonogram or a CAT scan of the abdomen. The latter two procedures usually give an accurate estimate of the size and location of the aneurysm with the CAT scan being more accurate, the sonogram tending to underestimate its size although giving an accurate representation of the remaining lumen within the thrombus.

There exists considerable controversy regarding the role of routine angiographic study in the evaluation and management of abdominal aortic aneurysm. The angiogram fails to reveal the true size of the aneurysm but does outline the renal and mesenteric vessels, the outflow vessels in the pelvis and extremities and leads to an apparently increased number of surgical procedures associated with the aneurysms including renal arterial reconstructions, mesenteric and perhaps the lower extremity reconstructions which, however, are not clearly associated with either increased survival following the operative procedure or decreased morbidity directly associated with the operation. Although there are reports of the lack of complications associated with angiographic studies of the aortic aneurysms, catheter studies have been associated with both embolization and death. The advent of the digital subtraction study employing intravenous administration of contrast material (DIVA) has eliminated the mechanical complications of inserting catheters into the aneurysm and have permitted a liberalization of the indications for angiographic studies employed by those who indicate selective angiography. The absence of pulses in the groin or anywhere in the lower extremity, uncontrolled hypertension, rapidly failing renal function, any syndrome suspected of representing visceral ischemia, and chest x-rays indicating the possibility of there being an associated upper abdominal or thoracic aortic aneurysm constitute indications for angiographic study.

There is one important contribution provided by the routine angiographic study, and that is the detection of the large marginal colonic artery connecting the inferior mesenteric and superior mesenteric arteries, indicating obstructive disease of the superior mesenteric artery, with a large portion of the colonic circulation being by way of the inferior mesenteric artery, which is ordinarily sacrificed during the aneurysm operation. The problem of colonic ischemia, however, can be managed by careful palpation of the superior mesenteric artery to determine its patency, by estimating the vigor of inferior mesenteric retrograde flow when that vessel is patent within the aneurysm, measuring its retrograde pressure, and by carefully preserving the hypogastric arteries during the operative procedure.

INDICATIONS FOR OPERATION

The abdominal aortic aneurysms that are smaller than 5 centimeters in diameter rarely rupture. The peak of rupture appears to be in the 6- to 7-centimeter transverse diameter range. In the absence of severe cardiac pulmonary or uncontrolled renal failure, elective surgical intervention is indicated for aneurysms that are 5 centimeters in transverse diameter or larger.

For those patients who have minimal findings to suggest associated atherosclerotic disease, evaluation of coronary circulation and of cerebral circulation become of paramount importance. Those patients who die following elective abdominal aortic aneurysm operations usually do so from acute myocardial infarction. Perioperative strokes, although occurring with lesser degrees of frequency than formerly, still occur from time to time. Two basic approaches have been utilized to cope with the problem. Routine coronary and cerebral angiographic studies are performed by some, while others attempt to estimate the operative risk by noninvasive studies, including estimates of left ventricular function by gated pool determinations and of cerebral circulation by employing oculoplethysmography or Doppler imaging of the carotid arteries.

The Cleveland Clinic data, in which routine coronary angiographic studies are performed and coronary revascularization procedures are done for specific indications, suggest that both perioperative and latent myocardial infarcts might be decreased in number. The effect of a radical approach to carotid artery disease is not well documented.

TECHNIQUE OF EXCISION OF ABDOMINAL AORTIC ANEURYSMS

The procedure for excision of abdominal aortic aneurysms varies somewhat from clinic to clinic but appears to involve the basic principle evolved by Dr. Creech, of leaving the posterior wall of the aneurysm in situ and replacing the aneurysm with a plastic prosthesis.

Care is taken to avoid a number of surgical problems, which include damage to adherent venous structures, prevention of distal embolization of atherosclerotic or thrombotic debris, preventing hypotension and shock upon restoration of circulation, avoiding ischemic injury of the colon and protecting the kidneys from developing renal insufficiency.

The rupturing abdominal aortic aneurysm introduces unique problems including obtaining control of the abdominal aorta above the site of rupture, restoring the circulating volume and restoring often severely impaired renal function.

Special technical problems include obtaining additional proximal exposure of the supra-aortic infrarenal segment by division of the left renal vein, transplantation of the inferior mesenteric artery in the presence of superior mesenteric arterial occlusion, upon the need to sacrifice a hypogastric artery or upon the detection of a large marginal artery on a preoperative angiographic study. Technical problems may occur in association with common iliac artery aneurysms. These can almost always be managed by careful technique at the iliac bifurcation. Rarely does a need arise to implant the distal limb of the prosthesis in the femoral arteries.

POSTOPERATIVE COMPLICATIONS THAT ARE UNIQUE TO THE ANEURYSM

Complications include the development of ischemic colon syndromes, the development of graft infection and, very rarely, late embolization to the lower extremities. Lower extremity ischemia may supervene as a result of intraoperative embolization or from either late postoperative embolization or in situ thrombosis in the femoral tibial arteries at sites of severe occlusive atherosclerotic disease.

The late complications, occurring usually years later, include the development of false aneurysms with either frank rupture retroperitoneally or with rupture into the duodenum producing aortoduodenal fistulae with gastrointestinal hemorrhage. Associated infections of prostheses are probably the most serious of all late complications, rarely resulting in retrieval of the patient.

As survival of aneurysm patients becomes prolonged, one begins to see the development of aneurysmal disease in other parts of the body. The popliteal site probably represents the most common associated site, while involvement of the suprarenal segment is another less common but important site of progression of aneurysmal disease.

RESULTS

The increased survival of patients who undergo elective abdominal aortic aneurysm intervention is clear-cut. Their increased susceptibility to cardiac and cerebrovascular insufficiency problems also appears to be well-documented and indicates a need for close follow-up for many years following elective aneurysm operation.

Immediate survival figures are excellent with most series reporting 5% or less mortality for elective procedures. The survival for ruptured abdominal aortic aneurysms is extremely variable, ranging from 60 to 80% down to approximately 25%. The high mortality from ruptured aneurysms appears to justify an aggressive attitude towards nonruptured aneurysms.
135:332-336, 1952.

BIBLIOGRAPHY

Connelley TL, McKinnon W, Smith RB, Perdue GL. Abdominal aortic surgery and horseshoe kidney. Arch Surg 115:1459, 1980.

Cooley DA, DeBakey ME. Surgical treatment of aneurysms of the abdominal aorta by resection and restoration of continuity with homograft. Surg Gynecol Obstet 97:257, 1953.

Crawford ES, Schuessler JS. Thoracoabdominal and abdominal aortic aneurysms involving celiac, superior mesenteric, and renal arteries. World J Surg 4: 643-652, 1980.

Creech O. Endoaneurysmorrhaphy and treatment of aortic aneurysm. Ann Surg 164:935-946, 1966.

Dubost C, Allary M, Oeconomos N. Resection of an aneurysm of the abdominal aorta. Arch Surg 64:405, 1952.

Gerbode F. Ruptured aortic aneurysm. A surgical emergency. Surg Gynecol Obstet 98:579, 1954.

Imparato AM, Berman IR, Bracco A, Kim GE, Beaudet R. Avoidance of shock and peripheral embolism during surgery of the abdominal aorta. Surg 73(1):68-73, 1973.

Kwann JH, Connolly JE, Molen RV, et al. The value of arteriography before abdominal aneurysmectomy. Amer J. Surg 134:108-114, 1977.

Julian OC, Grove WC, Dye WS, Olwin J, Sadove M. Direct surgery of arteriosclerosis resection of abdominal aorta with homologous aortic graft replacement. Ann Surg 138:387-399, 1953.

Leather RP, Shah D, Goldman M, Rosenberg M, Karmody AM. Non-resective treatment of abdominal aortic aneurysms, use of acute thrombosis and axillo-femoral bypass. Arch Surg 114:1402-1406, 1979.

Rámirez AA, Riles TS, Imparato AM, Megibow AJ. CAT scans of inflammatory aneurysms: new technique for preoperative diagnosis. Surg 91(4):390-393, 1982.

Raskin MM, Cunningham JB. Comparison of computed tomography and ultrasound for abdominal aortic aneurysms: A preliminary study. J Comput Tomogr 2:21–23, 1978.
Robicsek R, Daugherty HK, Mullen DC, Tam W, Scott WP. The value of angiography in the diagnosis of unruptured aneurysms of the abdominal aorta. Ann Thorac Surg 11:538, 1971.
Smith RF, Szilagyi DE. Ruptured abdominal aortic aneurysms: Problems of diagnosis and management. Ann Surg 154(suppl):175–181, 1961.
Szilagyi DE, Smith RF, Elliott JP. Temporary transection of the left renal vein: A technical aid in aortic surgery. Surg 65:32, 1969.
Thompson JE, Hollier LH, Patman RD, Persson AV. Surgical treatment of abdominal aortic aneurysms: factors influencing mortality and morbidity—A 20-year experience. Ann Surg 181:654-661, 1975.
Voorhees AB, Jaretski A, Blakemore AH. Use of tubes constructed from Vinyon "N" cloth in bridging arterial defects: A preliminary report. Ann Surg 135:332-336, 1952.

7
Management of Thoracoabdominal Aortic Aneurysms

George J. Reul, Jr., and Denton A. Cooley

The surgical management of thoracoabdominal aneurysms is one of the most challenging problems in vascular surgery [1-6]. The potential for complications is great, since most thoracoabdominal aneurysms involve the blood supply to vital organs of the abdomen, thorax, and nervous system. As most aneurysms are manifestations of generalized aortic and vascular disease, reconstruction may be difficult because of the poor quality of anastomotic sites. The pathology and clinical presentation are complex. The etiology and type of aneurysm determine the method of treatment. Currently, diagnostic techniques have been perfected so that an accurate diagnosis can be made and treatment can be tailored to the diagnosis [7]. The surgery is usually extensive, but if simple principles are employed, the morbidity and mortality can be decreased markedly. This chapter discusses the techniques we employ to adhere to these simple principles.

DEFINITION

There is some confusion regarding the definition of a thoracoabdominal aneurysm. A thoracoabdominal aneurysm includes any aneurysm that is anatomically present in the thorax and abdomen. It usually bridges the diaphragm and should be distinguished from high, abdominal aortic aneurysms, where the aneurysm involves the suprarenal abdominal aorta and does not cross the diaphragm. Since most suprarenal abdominal aortic aneurysms are approached through a thoracic incision, these are usually included as thoracoabdominal aneurysms. In some instances, only the abdominal or thoracic portion of the aneurysm is resected, leaving a portion behind to preserve circulation to vital structures such as the spinal cord. Double aneurysms, in which a thoracic aneurysm and an infrarenal abdominal aneurysm are present with the suprarenal portion not involved, should be excluded. Probably the most confusing type of aneurysm is the "mega" aneurysm, which involves the ascending aorta, arch, descending thoracic aorta, and abdominal aorta. These aneurysms usually are Type I dissecting aneurysms, which involve the entire aorta and arise from a tear in the ascending aorta with distal dissection. The "mega" aneurysm may also result from medial necrosis or weakness with massive dilatation of the entire aorta.

TYPES OF THORACOABDOMINAL ANEURYSMS

Most thoracoabdominal aneurysms are manifestations of atherosclerosis (Table 1). The true atherosclerotic aneurysm is nondissecting and usually involves the distal thoracic aorta at about the midportion and extends into the suprarenal aorta; it may or may not involve the infrarenal abdominal aorta to the iliac arteries. These aneurysms are large, filled with debris and clots, and may be very thick- or thin-walled. They are usually of a more chronic nature. Expansion and rupture into the retroperitoneum, chest, or abdomen are frequent. As with other aneurysms, they most commonly are associated with hypertension and atherosclerosis in other areas.

Table 1. Types of Thoracoabdominal Aneurysms

1. Atherosclerotic
2. Dissecting
   - Type I — Originating in the ascending aorta and extending into the iliac arteries
   - Type III — Originating at the left subclavian artery and extending into the infrarenal aorta or iliac arteries
3. "Mega" aneurysm
4. Mycotic
   - Salmonella
   - Syphilis
5. Mucocutaneous syndrome
6. Coarctation aneurysm

The second most common aneurysm is the dissecting type, which is usually of atherosclerotic origin or associated with cystic medial necrosis. A large percentage of dissecting aneurysms of the descending aorta, which originate at the left subclavian artery (Type III), extend below the diaphragm into the abdominal aorta and may have an exit point anywhere along the course of the abdominal aorta including the iliac arteries. The Type I thoracic aneurysm, in which the entrance tear originates in the ascending aorta and extends through the entire aorta, may present as a "mega" aneurysm. Marfan's syndrome may be associated with dissecting aneurysms or large dilated aorta, although these are generally atherosclerotic in origin.

Other types of thoracoabdominal aneurysms may be caused by infections such as salmonellosis, either acute or chronic, or syphilis. Mycotic aneurysms from embolization are very rare. Aneurysms from mucocutaneous syndrome may occur in the younger age group and are quite rare, as are aneurysms from coarctations of the abdominal aorta.

ANESTHETIC MANAGEMENT

Because most patients with thoracoabdominal aneurysms also have coronary artery disease or other atherosclerotic lesions, because of the vital organs involved, and because of the rapid and severe hemodynamic changes which occur during repair, good anesthetic management is essential. This implies adequate monitoring and access to the venous system for rapid infusion of fluids. The most important aspect in anesthetic management is the regulation of blood volume and pressure during the various periods of the operation. Mannitol is usually given prior to cross-clamping of the aorta. Marked hypertension, which usually occurs at the time of cross-clamping depending upon the level of the clamp, must be avoided, since damage to the cerebral and myocardial systems might occur. Trimethaphan or nitrates can be used to avoid the hypertension. Just prior to release of the aortic cross-clamp, it is important to administer adequate volume replacement, or severe hypotension may result, requiring reclamping the aorta several times. These long episodes of hypotension may result in spinal cord paralysis, renal failure, or myocardial infarction. On the other hand, release of the clamp at the time of hypertension may cause excessive bleeding of the anastomoses.

SURGICAL TREATMENT

The approach to treatment of thoracoabdominal aneurysms depends upon the etiology and the exact anatomy involved. The primary goal of the surgeon

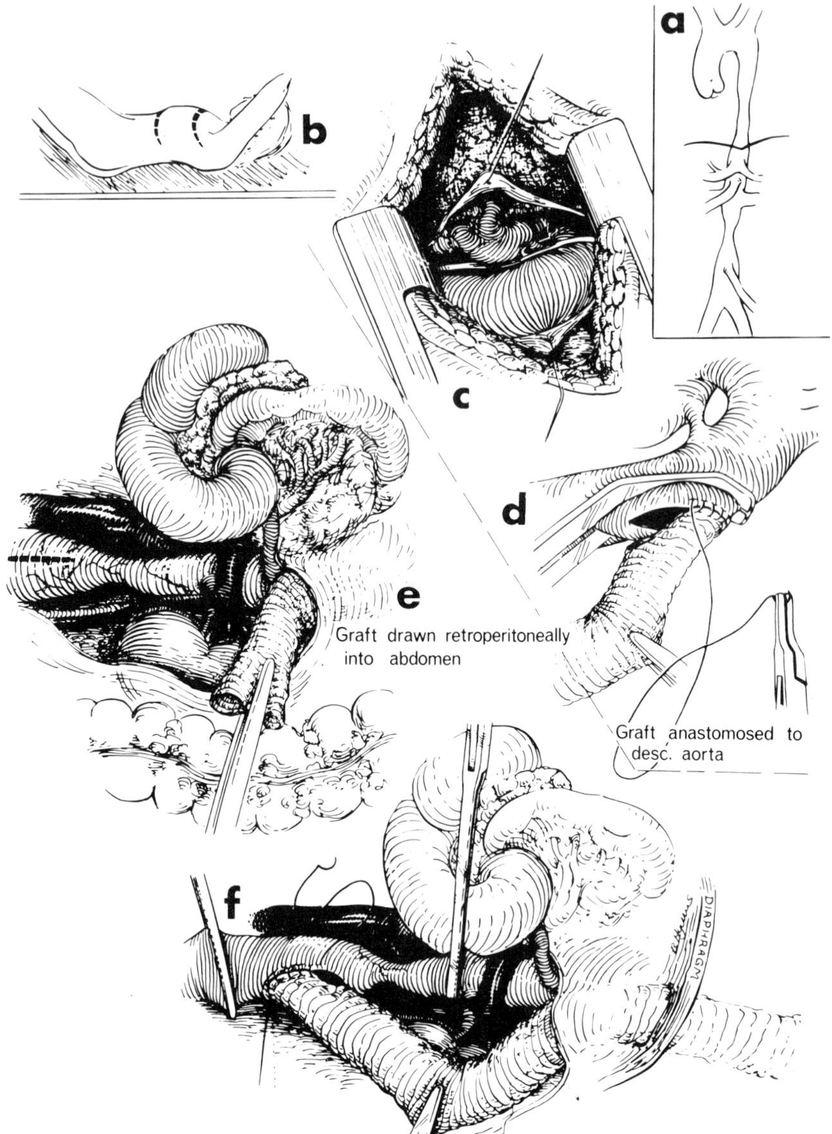

Figure 1. The approach to a thoracoabdominal coarctation is shown. The same approach is utilized for thoracoabdominal aneurysms. **(a)** The areas of coarcted segment of infrarenal and supraceliac portions of the thoracic aorta are shown. **(b)** A transthoracic incision, which is standard for a thoracoabdominal approach, is made through the seventh

is to eliminate the most vascular portion of the aneurysm which may rupture. Thus, in the presence of a "mega" aorta or with multiple aneurysmal areas, a staged repair is done. The most important area is repaired first. In most cases, this is the ascending aorta where the risk of rupture is greater.

If an isolated thoracoabdominal aneurysm is present, a standard surgical approach can be utilized. Most thoracoabdominal aneurysms arise at the mid-thoracic aorta and extend either above the suprarenal or the infrarenal abdominal aorta. In these cases, a thoracoabdominal incision is made (Figure 1). The patient is placed in the supine position with the left thoracoabdominal area elevated. A midline abdominal incision is made first. The lower extent of the incision depends upon whether or not the iliac arteries are involved. The upper portion is extended into the left thorax by transecting the costal margin and extending the incision usually into the seventh interspace. If more proximal control is desired, a higher incision can be made. The incision is carried down through the diaphragm up to the abdominal aorta avoiding the phrenic nerve. The viscera are then elevated to the right side by incising along the peritoneal reflection. The spleen, stomach, tail of the pancreas, and left colon are elevated through the retroperitoneal space to the right of the patient. The left kidney can be elevated with the rest of the viscera, although it is preferable to leave the left kidney in the renal fossa to avoid bleeding. If this is done, the left renal vein may be transected to gain accurate control of the aneurysm, although in most instances it can be left intact and the graft tunneled beneath the renal vein. Once the viscera have been elevated, the true extent of the aneurysm can be seen. The entire abdominal aorta can be exposed. Proximal exposure is done by retracting the lung anteriorly. The thoracic aorta is encircled by a tape in a portion of relatively normal aorta. The distal aorta is also encircled.

At this point, it is essential to assess the exact extent of the aneurysm so that provisions for repair can be made. The important areas of concern are the spinal cord, the kidneys, the distal circulation of the lower extremities, and the visceral circulation (liver and intestines). Damage to the spinal cord can occur because of loss of blood supply to the spinal cord or ischemia of the spinal cord by aortic occlusion during repair. It is essential to retain some blood supply to

---

intercostal space extending through the costal margin and into the midline. If proximal control is necessary, an incision is made through the fourth intercostal space. (c) The incision through the fourth intercostal space is demonstrated, showing the proximal portion of the thoracic aorta and the lung retracted anteriorly. (d) A bypass graft is placed to the thoracic aorta at the level of the ligamentum arteriosus. (e) The abdominal portion of the incision is shown with the spleen, duodenum, and tail of the pancreas reflected anteriorly. The left kidney is retained in the left renal fossa. The left renal vein is seen. The graft is drawn retroperitoneally to the area of infrarenal abdominal aorta, where it will be anastomosed to the area of the dotted line. (f) The anastomosis is completed to the infrarenal aorta.

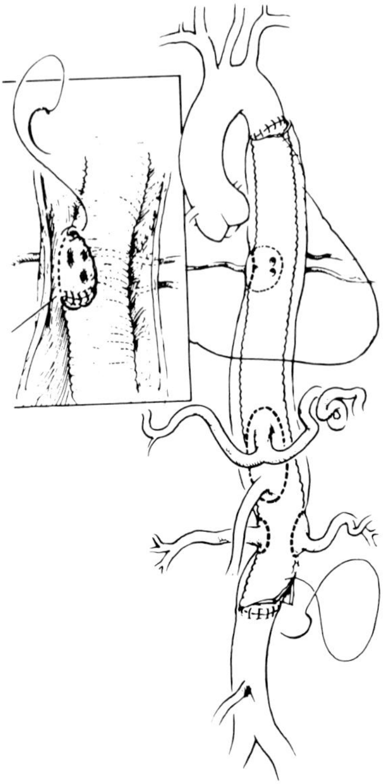

Figure 2. A large thoracic aneurysm involving the descending thoracic aorta and extending to the infrarenal abdominal aorta is shown. Since the aneurysm crosses the area of large spinal arteries, special repair of the spinal arteries is necessary and is shown in the inset. After occlusion of the aorta proximally and distally, the inner portion of the aneurysm is examined for large clusters of spinal arteries. If present, they are reanastomosed to the aortic graft by removing a portion of the graft and anastomosing the spinal arteries on the inside of the aortic aneurysm. The spinal arteries, therefore, have been retained. The remainder of the repair is completed by placing the celiac axis and superior mesenteric artery as a separate implant onto the aortic graft. The renal arteries are implanted separately. The clamp may be removed at the end of each anastomosis to provide flow to the structures bypassed. The distal anastomosis is completed in the infrarenal abdominal aorta, and normal aortic continuity is reestablished. The principles of suturing the graft inside the aneurysm and placing units or individual vessels to the graft from inside the aneurysm are demonstrated.

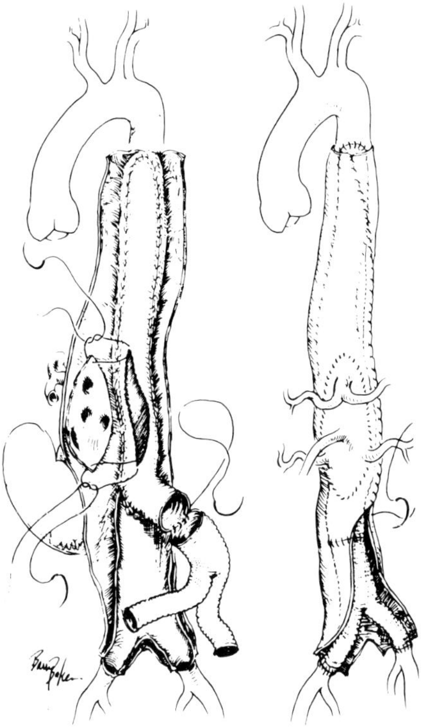

Figure 3. Another technique for preserving the spinal arteries is illustrated. A large thoracoabdominal aneurysm is shown extending from the midthoracic aorta to the iliac arteries. A large number of spinal arteries can be seen along the course of this aneurysm; therefore, the graft is placed as a large tongue or patch over the posterior wall of the thoracic aorta, and a running continuous suture is used to include the entire posterior wall of the thoracic aorta. The celiac axis, superior mesenteric, left and right renal arteries are reimplanted as one unit to the inside of the graft with a running suture. The distal portion of the graft is sutured over the upper abdominal aorta. A bifurcation graft is sutured to this graft and then to the iliac arteries to reestablish distal aortic continuity. On the right is shown the completed anastomosis with the entire posterior wall of the thoracic and abdominal aorta retained to the level of the iliac grafts. This technique demonstrates the principle of preserving the spinal arteries and of using a single anastomosis for all the visceral vessels. This is not our usual technique and is applied to selected aneurysms only.

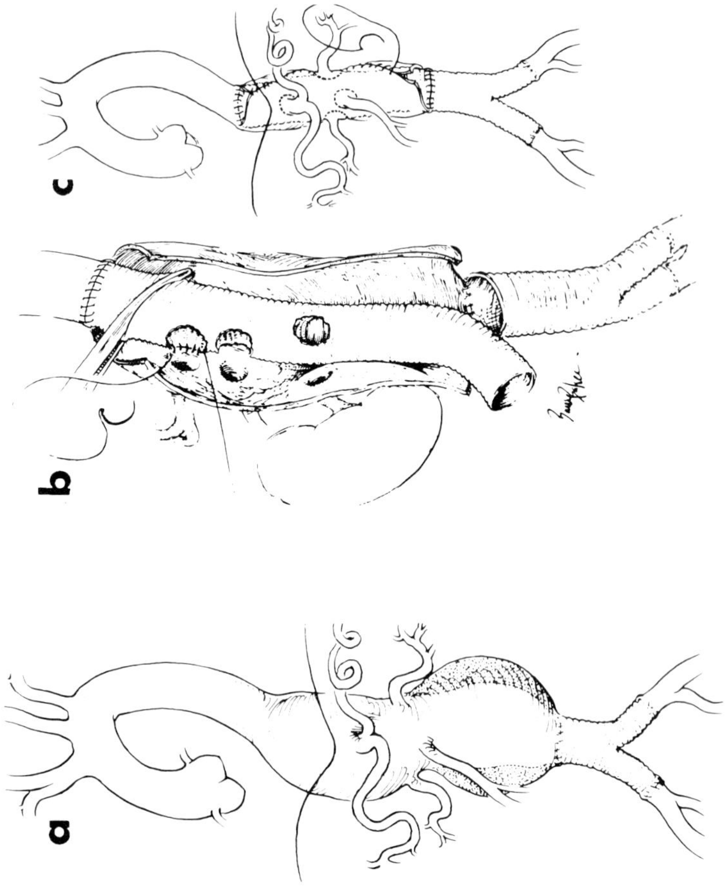
c
b
a

Figure 4. **(a)** Diagram of a thoracoabdominal aneurysm is shown. A previous aortoiliac bypass had been done from the infrarenal abdominal aorta. The anastomosis was placed too far distally, and a pseudoaneurysm developed at the proximal portion beneath the renal arteries. In addition, there was a large thoracoabdominal aneurysm present. **(b)** Approach to the aneurysm was through a thoracoabdominal incision, and the proximal anastomosis was accomplished just above the diaphragm to the proximal portion of the aneurysm. Separate buttons of graft have been removed, and the celiac axis, superior mesenteric, and right renal arteries are shown being reimplanted separately to the graft from inside the thoracic aneurysm. Separate implantation was necessary in this particular case because of the large area between the buttons and the poor tissue between these areas. Single running sutures are used for each anastomosis, and the clamp may be moved down the aortic graft following each anastomosis to provide instant flow to the completed areas. **(c)** The finished anastomoses are shown from the outside. The old aneurysm is wrapped around the aorta, and the graft is attached to the previously placed iliac graft to reestablish normal aortic continuity. Each artery has been reimplanted separately inside the aneurysm. This technique demonstrates the principle of separate implantation which allows for good hemostasis, since a double layer of aorta is used on the anastomosis.

the spinal cord, and in most instances the largest spinal arteries are located from levels T-10 through L-2. These arteries can be either reimplanted separately or retained by placing the proximal aortic graft over the arteries as a tongue up into the area of relatively normal aorta (Figures 2 and 3). In some instances if the diseased aorta extends beyond this area, the aorta must be resected and these arteries reimplanted as one separate unit onto the graft. In most instances, they can be retained.

After the proximal thoracic aorta is cross-clamped, the aneurysm is opened, and the location and importance of the spinal arteries are assessed by backbleeding of the intercostal and lumbar arteries into the aneurysm. The proximal anastomosis is completed including and avoiding closure of the spinal arteries, or the spinal arteries may be reimplanted. A running 3-0 or 2-0 polypropylene suture is usually utilized for the proximal anastomosis. A woven Dacron graft preclotted with albumin and autoclaved is used. Heparin is always given in a 1 mg/kg dose prior to cross-clamping of the aorta.

The celiac artery, superior mesenteric artery, right renal artery, and the left renal artery are identified next in the aneurysmal sac as orifices, with or without backbleeding. The debris and clot of the aneurysm are removed. The celiac axis, superior mesenteric artery, and right renal artery usually can be reimplanted as one unit onto the graft. A corresponding plug of graft is removed, and the elliptical portion of the aorta with the celiac axis, superior mesenteric artery and right renal artery is sutured to the graft with one continuous polypropylene suture inside the aneurysm. The left renal artery is reimplanted next, usually separately or as the same unit. The clamp may be released after each anastomosis, placing it distal to each new anastomosis and restoring circulation to the vital areas more rapidly; however, in most cases excessive backbleeding is avoided by one aortic clamping episode for the visceral vessels. Care must be taken not to allow air and debris to enter these arteries and to insure that adequate backflow is present with satisfactory orifice size and no arteriosclerotic obstruction. In some instances, orificial endarterectomy is necessary if the vessels are occluded by atherosclerosis. Separate reimplantation of each artery should be avoided because of the nature of the vessels and the time involved in this type of anastomosis (Figure 4). The distal graft is then attached to the aorta below the renal arteries or to the iliac arteries with a bifurcation graft, depending upon the anatomy present.

Using this technique, proper protection of the spinal cord and renal and visceral arteries is accomplished. If the patient is metabolically stable, approximately 30 minutes of proximal aortic occlusion are usually safe for preservation of the kidneys, viscera, and spinal cord (Table 2).

The remaining portion of the aneurysm is then sewn over the graft. The viscera are replaced in the abdominal cavity, and the abdomen is closed. Heparin is reversed with protamine. Care must be taken to avoid excessive bleeding and

Table 2. Cross-Clamp Time Related to Paraplegia in Aneurysms of the Descending Thoracic Aorta

Clamp time (minutes)	Number[a]	Paraplegia (%)
< 30	104	2.9
> 30	84	13.0
< 45	169	6.5
> 45	19	16.0
< 60	184	7.0
> 60	4	25.0

[a]Total number of patients = 188

hypertension which would necessitate massive blood transfusion and could cause hypothermia and, often, very severe complications. A cell saving device may be utilized for autotransfusion in selected cases [8].

Other alternative methods which are available for treatment of thoraco-abdominal aneurysms are utilized only in special cases. These include bypass grafts with individual bypasses to the arteries and bypass grafts for retrograde perfusion. The standard direct approach, however, is quite simple and results in the fewest complications.

COMPLICATIONS

One of the most serious complications associated with repair of thoraco-abdominal aneurysms is paraplegia from spinal cord ischemia. This occurs in approximately 6 percent of the patients who have large thoracoabdominal aneurysms extending from the midthoracic aorta distally. It can be avoided in most patients by retaining or reimplanting the spinal arteries and avoiding cross-clamp times over 30 minutes. In our experience, it is not avoided by the use of shunts or pumps to provide distal flow during aortic occlusion [9,10]. Measurement of spinal cord ischemia by evoked potential as done by Cunningham and Spencer appears promising if the techniques can be simplified and applied to all patients [11]. The fact remains that some aneurysms are so large with involvement of the spinal arteries that paraplegia cannot be avoided.

Another serious complication which may occur is acute renal failure; however, this is usually temporary and can be treated medically as long as there is no evidence of mechanical renal artery obstruction from the operation. Adequate renal perfusion can be ascertained by a postoperative renal scan. If there is oliguria or anuria and the potassium rises to unsafe levels or fluid management becomes difficult, early hemodialysis is indicated.

Pulmonary complications are fairly common since retraction of the lung is necessary, and most of these patients have decreased respiratory function due to obstructive emphysema. Phrenic nerve paralysis and the post-thoracotomy chest also limit respiratory function somewhat.

Postoperative bleeding is another avoidable complication. Accurate anastomoses are obtained by suturing the graft inside the aneurysm utilizing a double layer of aorta at the anastomotic sites. Avoidance of hypertension and adequate heparin reversal are essential. Retroperitoneal bleeding can be minimized by proper dissection in planes with avoidance of trauma to the spleen. Proper blood component therapy and avoidance of hypothermia also prevent excessive bleeding.

Intestinal and liver infarction are extremely rare, but may occur from embolization of debris into the arteries or unrecognized occlusion of the distal arteries. If it occurs from prolonged ischemia, usually renal failure and paraplegia also occur. If suspected, early exploration should be done to assure patency of the anastomoses. Postoperative ileus and/or diarrhea may be associated with ischemic colitis secondary to sigmoid ischemia or embolic debris in the mesenteric arteries.

RESULTS

Results of thoracoabdominal aneurysm repair correlate directly with the size of the aneurysm, the location of the aneurysm, and the generalized condition of the patient. We have made no special mention of ruptured thoracoabdominal

Table 3. Principles of Surgical Treatment of Thoracoabdominal Aneurysm

1. Proper anesthetic management
2. Thoracoabdominal incision through 7th intercostal space
3. Retroperitoneal reflection to the right
4. Woven Dacron tube graft (preclotted and autoclaved)
5. Systemic heparinization (1 mg/kg)
6. Proximal and distal aortic occlusion
7. Preservation of large spinal arteries
8. Establishment of aortic continuity
9. Assurance of adequate visceral and renal flow
10. Direct anastomosis to aortic graft surturing inside the aneurysm
11. Hemostasis

aneurysms, since the surgical management is the same as that for chronic or acute aneurysms; however, the mortality is higher because of obvious complicating factors. From 1955 through 1982, we operated upon 143 patients for thoracoabdominal aneurysms. Most patients were in the older age group (55-65 years) and had other complicating factors. With the use of present day anesthetic management and simplified techniques (Table 3), the mortality for abdominal aneurysm resection has decreased from 33 percent during the first 10 years (1955-1965) to 10 percent in 107 patients operated upon in the past 10 years (1971-1981). The most common cause of death has been myocardial infarction.

Patients should be observed for aneurysms which may occur in other areas, since approximately 12 to 20 percent will have new aneurysms during the follow-up period. Other complications of arteriosclerosis such as coronary artery disease and cerebrovascular insufficiency are very common.

CONCLUSION

A thoracoabdominal aneurysm is a severe threat to life. If left untreated, 90 percent of patients with a diagnosis of thoracoabdominal aneurysm will die. The direct approach to repair of the aneurysm, as well as special care in anesthetic management and in handling the visceral and spinal arteries, are essential for good results. Utilizing a simple approach for removal of the aneursymal sac most likely to rupture and restoration of normal circulation to the arteries arising from the aneurysm are the goals of surgical treatment.

REFERENCES

1. Crawford ES, Snyder DM, Cho GC, Roehm JOF. Progress in treatment of thoracoabdominal and abdominal aortic aneurysms involving celiac, superior mesenteric and renal arteries. Ann Surg 188:404, 1978.
2. Crawford ES, Snyder DM. Treatment of aneurysms of the aortic arch: A progress report. J Thorac Cardiovasc Surg 85:237, 1983.
3. Pierce WS, Vincent WR, Fitzgerald E, Miller FJ. Coarctation of the abdominal aorta with multiple aneurysms. Ann Thorac Surg 20:687, 1975.
4. Selle JG, Robicsek F, Daugherty HK, Cook JW. Thoracoabdominal aortic aneurysms. A review and current status. Ann Surg 179:763, 1974.
5. Stoney RJ, Wylie EJ. Surgical management of arterial lesions of the thoracoabdominal aorta. Amer J Surg 126:157, 1973.
6. Webster MW. Thoracoabdominal aortic aneurysms. In CD Campbell, (ed.), Aortic Aneurysms: Surgical Therapy, pp. 115–138. Mount Kisco, NY, Futura Publishing Co., 1981.

7. Wheeler WE, Beachley MC, Ranniger K. Angiography and ultrasonography. A comparative study of abdominal aortic aneurysms. Amer J Roentgenol 126:95, 1976.
8. Winton TL, Charrette EJP, Salerno TA. The cell saver during cardiac surgery: Does it save? Ann Thorac Surg 33(4):379, 1982.
9. Culliford AT, Ayvaliotis B, Shemin R, Colvin SB, Ison OW, Spencer FC. Aneurysms of the descending aorta: Surgical experience in 48 patients. J Thorac Cardiovasc Surg 85:98, 1983.
10. Donahoo JS, Brawley RK, Gott VL. The herparin-coated vascular shunt for thoracic, aortic and great vessel procedures. A ten-year experience. Ann Thorac Surg 23:507, 1977.
11. Cunningham JN Jr, Lashinger JC, Merkin HA, Nathan IM, Colvin S, Ransohoff J, Spencer FC. Measurement of spinal cord ischemia during operations upon the thoracic aorta: Initial clinical experience. Ann Surg 196:285, 1982.

4

Aortoiliac Artery Occlusive Disease

8
Surgical Management of Aortoiliac Occlusive Disease

D. Emerick Szilagyi

This chapter summarizes the concepts and practices that I follow in treating patients with aortoiliac occlusive disease. No attempt is made to be comprehensive and include approaches different from those I utilize. Emphasis will be placed on those details that are important in everyday clinical practice rather than to present the unusual.

For all practical purposes, the term aortoiliac occlusive disease is equivalent to aortoiliac atherosclerosis. Atherosclerotic involvement of the aortoiliac arterial tree has distinctive characteristics. The disease process is most advanced in the iliac arteries and may indeed originate in them. In 90 percent of the cases the disease is multifocal, that is the aorta and both iliac arteries are involved to varying degrees. Multifocal disease always is progressive at variable rates. The ultimate result of the progression is complete obliteration of the aortic bifurcation. In contrast, isolated iliac atheromas are usually stable.

CLINICAL DIAGNOSIS

The diagnosis of aortoiliac occlusive disease can always be made on purely clinical grounds, that is, on the basis of the findings of history and physical examination. Sophisticated instrumentation is very rarely necessary. There are, however, certain historical pitfalls, particularly as regards symptoms and signs of degenerative arthritis (particularly of the hip), intervertebral disc disease, spinal cord disease, and other types of degenerative neuromuscular diseases. Situations in which nonvascular conditions must be ruled out arise with progressively greater frequency, since almost any complaint that involves difficulty in using the lower extremities and is associated with some discomfort or pain on exercise will be first considered to be due to vascular diseases by many internists. Careful analysis of the symptomatology and physical findings usually yields the correct diagnosis in these diseases.

ANGIOGRAPHY

When diagnostic doubt exists, angiographic visualization of the arterial tree is usually mandatory to settle the diagnostic problem, regardless of the firmness of the clinical diagnosis. The referring physician usually will not be satisfied with a negative opinion unless supported by the objective evidence of roentgen studies. But even in cases in which the diagnosis is clinically entirely clear, angiographic visualization is essential for the appropriate planning of the surgical procedure. It has been advocated that, in complete absence of both femoral pulses, aortography is not necessary, but I do not accept this tenet. Even in these cases, the exact anatomical distribution and extent of the occlusive disease can be established only with the help of good roentgen images. In all other cases, obviously, angiographic exploration of the arterial tree from the level of the renal arteries, at least to the midcalf, is an indispensable part of operative planning.

Our primary angiographic technique for peripheral arterial studies is translumbar aortography. Two principal variants of technique are employed, depending on the level of aortic puncture. In the technique of high puncture the tip of the translumbar needle is aimed at the level of the upper border of the first lumbar vertebra, and in the low puncture technique the tip of the needle is directed to the midportion of the third lumbar vertebra. The high puncture technique is used only in cases in which the femoral pulses are absent, or questionably palpable, or when visualization of the visceral arteries is particularly important. In other cases, the low puncture technique is employed, always care being taken to opacify the renal arteries. Transfemoral percutaneous arteriography is resorted to when details of anatomical characteristics of an atherosclerotic imvolvement are desired below the level of the common femoral artery, and, in particular, in the infragenicular distributions of the popliteal artery. In some cases of poor-risk patients with good femoral pulses, the angiographic examination is limited to the percutaneous femoral arteriogram.

In all angiographic efforts, it is of the utmost importance to obtain exposures of good quality. For this purpose one must have a system of multiple exposures, the number of roentgenograms being large enough to cover a time span of about 20 seconds. Our cassette changer accommodates eight 36 x 17 inch cassettes that can be exposed at intervals of from 1.5 to 2.5 seconds.

The relative merits of the translumbar as compared with the transfemoral catheter technique, as well as the procedural details of the method are amply discussed is an earlier publication of mine [1].

USE OF INDIRECT DIAGNOSTIC METHODS

The role of indirect or noninvasive methods of diagnosis has been stressed by some in recent years. I have a very adequate flow laboratory available for consultation, but seldom use it for diagnostic assistance in aortoiliac occlusive disease. The most common clinical situations in which indirect methods may be useful are as follows: Incongruity between degrees of anatomic changes and symptomatology (the tests used would be treadmill exercise and segmental arterial pressures); difficulty in evaluating physical signs (ultrasound pulse detection); coincidental nonvascular disease and early aortoiliac occlusive process (waveform analysis, segmental arterial pressures).

In a large majority of instances, I find aortography necessary for a firm therapeutic decision, regardless of the results of the indirect tests.

OPERATIVE INDICATIONS

As with all surgical disease, the decision to perform a therapeutic procedure for aortoiliac atherosclerosis is dependent on the assessment of the factors of severity of symptoms, type and degree of anatomical change and the availability of technical procedure suitable for the risk factors. All these considerations are highly favorable for the surgical management of aortoiliac occlusive disease. Procedures are available for the correction of all the variants of pathological anatomy for a wide range of degrees of risk. As a result, during the past decade the operative indications for aortoiliac occlusive disease have broadened at both ends of the spectrum. On the side of early involvement in good-risk patients, surgical treatment is often recommended for intermittent claudication of only moderate severity even though true disablement is not present. This position is justified not only by the very low operative mortality and morbidity and the persistence of good results but also by the circumstances that, as already mentioned, multiple occlusive lesions are almost always progressive. At the other end of the spectrum, very few cases of advanced disease are unsuitable, because of impaired operative risk, for some modified corrective procedure.

SURGICAL TECHNIQUE

There are two classic modalities available for the correction of aorto-iliac occlusive disease: thromboendarterectomy and grafting. Endarterectomy is the older and unquestionably the more physiological procedure. For technical reasons, I have used this corrective technique only in those cases in which the occlusive process had not extended, to any significant degree, beyond the point of the bifurcation of the common iliac artery, and which, therefore, may be regarded as early or moderately advanced examples of atherosclerosis.

In this procedure, the aortoiliac segment is approached through a long mid-line incision and appropriate control of the inflow and outflow is obtained. The removal of the intimal complex is performed under direct vision, through longitudinal arteriotomies. The right common iliac artery and the aorta are opened through a continuous incision. Particular care is taken in the dissection of the distal extremity of the occluding lesion at or near the iliac bifurcation. A clean line of break-off must be achieved at the level of the external iliac artery. In order to reduce the total occlusion time, the arteriotomy in the aorta and the right common iliac artery is closed before carrying out the endarterectomy of the left common iliac artery.

In regard to grafting procedures, the most common technical variant is the aortobifemoral bypass utilizing, in my practice, Helanca Dacron prosthesis. This is the standard operation for about 95 percent of the patients, comprising all cases of acceptable risk and unsuited for endarterectomy. Axillofemoral bypass procedures and femoral–femoral cross-over bypass grafts will be described presently.

It should be noted that unilateral operations in the aortoiliac area in good-risk patients are now rarely performed in my practice, since it has been learned that the less affected side almost always progresses to a significant symptomatic stage or complete obliteration within a matter of months or very few years after the first side has been repaired.

A variant of the bypass technique is used when the aortic occlusive process is far advanced or when associated aneurysmal change has to be dealt with. In these instances the diseased aorta is transected and the proximal anastomosis is carried out in an end-to-end fashion to the aorta or the iliac artery respectively. This procedure is often designated as an exclusion bypass.

Two technical features in the performance of aortofemoral bypass grafting must be emphasized. It is of the utmost importance to explore the common femoral artery whenever angiographic evidence of disease in that area is present. In case of an intimal occlusive process, careful endarterectomy must be carried out in order to provide an ample and free outflow into the deep femoral system. The second technical detail of great importance is that the proximal or aortic anastomosis must always be placed in an area of the aorta that is as nearly normal as one can find. This usually necessitates the placement of the proximal anastomosis very close to the level of the renal arteries.

End-to-side aortic reconstruction has been criticized on the assumption that this type of anastomosis reduces blood flow and tends to induce aneurysmal changes at the anastomotic side. It has been shown that the flow reduction is on the order of five percent, which is of no significance in a biologic system [2]. In my experience, in over a thousand such operative cases, serial postoperative aortograms showed an incidence of aneurysmal changes at the anastomosis of about .2%.

A special case of aortoiliac occlusive disease is that in which the thrombotic process has extended to the level of the renal arteries. In these cases, special precautions must be observed to be able to provide a satisfactory proximal site for an end-to-end anastomosis. During the thromboendarterectomy of the aortic stump, the aorta must be clamped above the renal arteries and the renal arteries must be protected by separate small clamps. At times the left renal vein may have to be transected.

A more recent grafting procedure is the bilateral axillofemoral bypass graft. This technique is used in poor-risk patients with advanced disease and in cases in which a previous aortic operation, or sometimes multiple previous operations, have failed. The procedure can be simplified by constructing only one axillary anastomosis and by making the shaft of the graft Y-shaped to supply both common femoral arteries. The immediate and early (up to two years) success rate of this procedure is highly satisfactory (in our hands, 85-90 percent). We have no firm figures for late patency rates, but they run about 10 percent below those for aortobifemoral bypasses.

In cases in which serious disease is present in one iliac area, but both the aorta itself and the opposite iliac trunk are still patent and there is a good contralateral femoral pulse, a cross-over femoro-femoral graft may be justified. In our limited experience with 16 such grafts the late (after 3 years) patency rate has been around 40 percent.

The type of prosthesis I use was developed in my laboratory. It has a taffeta weave of specially treated, elasticized Dacron fibers, and is smooth-walled (uncrimped). It has the advantages of lightweight construction, thus minimizes bulk and high porosity.

SPECIAL PROBLEMS OF CASE SELECTION

In the selection of cases for surgical treatment, certain special problems occur that deserve consideration. One of the most frequent problems of this type is the simultaneous occurrence of aortoiliac and femoropopliteal occlusive disease. A typical example is that in which there is extensive aortoiliac disease with complete obliteration of the one iliac axis and advanced stenotic changes in the other iliac trunk; at the same time bilateral superficial femoral arterial occlusion is present. Experience has shown that the correction of the aortoiliac component takes precedence, and that in 85 to 90 percent of the cases the repair of the aortoiliac occlusive process alone is all that is necessary. In the rare instance in which the femoropopliteal component requires surgical attention, the repair is done at a later stage.

Another common problem in this category is the association of symptomatic femoropopliteal occlusive disease with the aortoiliac involvement, in which the justification for surgical correction is questionable. The clarification of the need for correction may be helped by one or more of the methods of indirect flow measurement. The very important question of whether the blood pressure in the external iliac trunk is sufficient to maintain patency in a femoropopliteal graft can be answered accurately by measurement through direct puncture of the common femoral artery. In case of doubt, surgical intervention may be delayed, and the progression of the aortoiliac involvement serially observed.

At times the surgeon's hand can be forced in such a situation. Although no significant advance may be noted in the aortoiliac lesion, the patient may develop incipient gangrene of the foot due to progression of the femoropopliteal involvement. A prophylactic aortoiliac bypass operation is carried out in preparation for a right femoropopliteal autogenous vein bypass.

A somewhat related problem is that of the patient who has relatively trivial symptoms of claudication, which to him are subjectively important, and disease of such early involvement as to make major direct surgical attack unjustified. In these cases I have cautiously begun to test the effectiveness of dilatation.

Although complete obliteration of the abdominal aorta almost always is best handled with transection of the aorta for an end-to-end anastomosis, when significant collateral circulation around the obstruction is present, an end-to-side bypass procedure without permanent interruption of the continuity of the aorta is preferable.

Before presenting the results we have obtained with aortofemoral bypass operations, some comments on the method of collecting our follow-up data appear to be in order. Obviously, the reliability of the data on results is dependent on the thoroughness and accuracy of the follow-up methods and on the care with which the data are tabulated. During the past 25 years we have stored our follow-up data in a vascular registry, which provides facilities for careful observation of every patient who has ever been under our care. The patients are seen in the clinic every year, or reports from their personal physicians are requested at yearly intervals. The postoperative patency of the operations is ascertained by aortography before discharge and, thereafter, at intervals as indicated.

We made a careful analysis of our follow-up data in 471 cases of aortofemoral and iliofemoral Dacron bypass operations performed for aortoiliac occlusive disease from 1955 to 1971. At the end of the first year of observation, the patency rate was 98.3 percent. This figure includes the immediate postoperative failures but does not include the operative deaths. Thereafter there was a rather steady but slow deterioration of the patency rates, which ranged from 1 to 11 percent and averaged 3.5 percent. At the end of the fifth-year interval, 93.1 percent of the cases showed patent grafts, and at the end of the tenth-year interval, 71 percent of the cases were still open. The rate of patency at the end of 14 years was nearly 50 percent. There was a sudden drop between the 14th and 15th years to a zero rate of patency, but this is unquestionably the result of the very small number of cases observed during this interval, and therefore cannot be regarded as statistically significant. By the end of the 13th postoperative year, the total late cumulative mortality was 28.5 percent.

The follow-up results of aortoiliac endarterectomy, accumulated and tabulated in the same manner as described for the bypass procedure, disclosed a patency rate of 88.8 percent at the end of the first year of observation. Thereafter, the rate showed a deterioration closely comparable to that seen for the bypass operations, namely a deterioration of nearly 3 percent per year. Again, the 15-year patency rate is just below 50 percent. The late cumulative mortality rate was 36.8 percent.

It can be readily seen that the results with the two procedures are strikingly similar with a very slight advantage for the bypass grafts. It must be stressed, as was mentioned before, that the aortoiliac endarterectomies in our practice were performed in cases less advanced than those in which bypass grafting was carried out. It is safe to say, therefore, that if there is any bias in the comparison it is in favor of the endarterectomies. From the point of view of some details of statistical methodology, several critical points can be raised about the interpretation of these results. There is little doubt, however, that the two series are large enough and the observations extended over a long enough period of time to allow a meaningful comparison of the results of the two procedures. With all the necessary reservations in mind, one can thus conclude that both operations were eminently satisfactory and little choice can be made between them from the point of view of late results. Since bypass grafting represents an operation that is less traumatic, technically simpler, and more widely applicable than endarterectomy. I have come to prefer this procedure as a standard operative intervention.

REFERENCES

1. Szilagyi DE, Smith RF, Elliott JP, Hageman JH. Translumbar aortography: A study of its safety and usefulness. Arch Surg 112:399–408, 1977.
2. Szilagyi DE, Whitcomb JG, Schenker W, Waibel P. Laws of fluid flow and arterial grafting. Surg 47:55–73, 1960.

9
Management of Failed Aortofemoral Artery Bypass

George J. Reul, Jr., and Denton A. Cooley

Aortobilateral femoral artery bypass has withstood the test of time as the procedure of choice for the treatment of aortoiliac occlusive disease. There are minimal complications, and long-term patency rates are good, especially when compared to other vascular procedures. The attrition rate from coronary disease and cerebrovascular disease adds significantly to the postoperative and long-term mortality. Failure of one or both limbs of the aortofemoral bypass graft may occur in the immediate postoperative period or anytime in the follow-up period. Repeat surgical treatment requires special application of vascular surgical principles combined with individualizing the approach to each unique problem, particularly with consideration of the cause for failure, the clinical symptoms, the state of the jeopardized limb, and the generalized condition of the patient.

DIAGNOSIS IN THE EARLY POSTOPERATIVE PERIOD

The diagnosis of failure of one or both limbs of an aortobilateral femoral bypass graft may be difficult in the immediate postoperative period. In most cases, there is severe vasospasm with discoloration and livedo reticularis of the lower extremities. This is due to hypothermia induced by the surgery, the hemodynamic state, and the metabolic results of cross-clamp release of the abdominal aorta. If the patient is very obese, it may be difficult to palpate the femoral pulses as well as to obtain good Doppler signals. It may, also, be difficult to obtain pulses or good Doppler readings in the peripheral arteries of the foot and ankle because of severe vasospasms, distal small vessel disease, or femoropopliteal occlusive disease. If, however, these changes persist or become more severe three to six hours after surgery, the diagnosis becomes easier. In most cases of graft occlusion, instead of the blotchy cyanosis of the lower extremities, the lower extremity is pale, painful, and paralyzed, The diagnosis of acute graft failure is confirmed by the clinical signs and loss of arterial Doppler signals. An aortogram may be harmful because some of these patients are in borderline renal failure or are metabolically unstable, and the procedure may exacerbate these problems. Renal function can be evaluated by renal scan. Reexploration can be delayed somewhat, but it should be delayed no more than 8 to 12 hours if acute graft occlusion is suspected.

CAUSES OF ACUTE GRAFT OCCLUSION

The causes of acute graft occlusion are most commonly problems with outflow and/or inflow. These may be caused by judgment and technical errors, embolization, external entrapment, or metabolic factors. Problems with outflow of the graft are probably the most common problems. The distal femoral portion of the graft may be anastomosed to a small profunda branch which has very little outflow and is not adequate to maintain patency. If endarterectomy is done to this type of vessel, there may be an inadequate endarterectomy with an obstructive flap or dissection. If the superficial femoral artery was patent with a proximal plaque, the graft may have been placed too far proximally, so that the superficial femoral occluded. Debris or clot may have been present to decrease the outflow.

All of these problems of outflow can be avoided by assuring an adequate distal anastomosis. The anastomosis in most cases should be done to provide the maximum amount of outflow possible. If the superficial femoral artery is patent on arteriography and the profunda femorus artery is patent, then the graft should be placed overriding both the superficial femoral and profunda femorus arteries so that adequate flow may be present. In most cases of advanced arteriosclerosis, there is a plaque overriding the superficial femoral artery. If this is opened into the femoral artery so that the graft may act as a patch graft, then adequate distal outflow can be obtained. If there is very little backflow in the profunda femorus artery, a localized endarterectomy or a direct endarterectomy with onlay patch must be done. Proximal flow into the iliac segment is also essential if there was previous patency, in that, at least one of the two bypass limbs should provide retrograde flow into the iliac to perfuse the pelvic structures including the penis and sigmoidal arteries of the colon. If retrograde perfusion is not allowed to both iliac arteries and they were patent preoperatively, then ischemic colitis with possible sigmoid gangrene and perforation, impotency, or even necrosis of the gluteal muscles may occur.

Inflow problems may occur in patients with a very small proximal aorta, especially in elderly women with severe calcific plaques. Adequate inflow into the graft can be assured by flushing the graft and observing the amount of bloodflow present at the time of the first operation. If the anastomosis is carried out just below the renal arteries, in most cases, adequate short-term and long-term outflow can be assured. There usually is a soft, disease-free area at that site for proper anastomosis. If not, a proximal endarterectomy can be done. We prefer an end-to-end anastomosis of the proximal aorta because it provides for better outflow.

Mechanical factors may be involved with early failure. These include kinking of the graft, especially when an end-to-side anastomosis is done. If the graft is too tight, kinking of the distal vessels at the crotch of the graft or flattening of one limb may occur. Entrapment by the inguinal ligament may occur. If the graft is too loose, kinking of the graft occurs when the bowel is replaced. Embolization of debris from the proximal aorta may completely occlude the graft or cause distal embolization with "trash foot." This can be avoided by temporarily clamping the supraceliac aorta at the diaphragm and removing the debris prior to the proximal aortic anastomosis.

We prefer to use systemic heparin during aortofemoral procedures to avoid clotting problems (1 mg per kg). If the graft is not flushed properly, clot may occur inside the graft. With proper management of the operation, this should never occur. Some patients may have severe polycythemia with thrombocytosis and may have excessive clotting. This is extremely rare and may be assessed at the time of surgery by clotting of the graft. Excessive thrombosis may also result from a thrombotic reaction to the use of heparin. These patients may have clotting of their entire vascular system with the administration of heparin and are very difficult to manage.

Metabolic causes of early graft occlusion include severe hypotension from prolonged clamping and hypothermia. In addition, myocardial infarction or other causes of low cardiac output must be considered. Most of these causes of acute or early graft occlusion can be avoided.

CAUSES OF LATE GRAFT OCCLUSION

Late graft occlusion may be caused by progression of distal disease in the native arteries, intimal hyperplasia of the graft, especially at the site of the neointima and graft junction, and distal embolization from the graft or proximal aorta. In some cases, the neointima from the graft may embolize by trauma at the time of other surgical procedures or aortography or even by blunt abdominal trauma or violent activities involving severe vibrations to the grafts.

Material failure of the graft or suture material may result in pseudoaneurysm and thrombosis or dilatation of the graft. Graft aneurysm or thrombosis may result from improper graft structure. Pseudoaneurysm may occur at

Table 1. Failed Aorto-Femoral Bypass

Causes of Failure
Technical and judgmental errors
Progression of distal disease
Intimal hyperplasia of graft
Embolization
Material failure
Pseudoaneurysm
Proximal-distal
Infection
External entrapment
Trauma
Metabolic factors

the proximal and distal anastomosis. When it occurs distally in the femoral arteries, thrombosis may result because of the large amount of turbulence in the aneurysm and progression of the distal disease. Some aneurysms can be blamed upon suture failure if the wrong suture is selected or improperly handled during repair. The prosthetic graft to the artery anastomosis is dependent upon the integrity of the suture during the life of the patient. Other causes of pseudoaneurysm are pulling away of the graft material by constant stretching and/or by weak arterial walls. Pseudoaneurysm of the proximal aorta may result in rupture into the duodenum with aortoduodenal fistula or rupture into the retroperitoneum. In addition, it may result in thrombosis of the distal aorta.

External entrapment of the graft may occur by severe scar tissue and fibrosis or by a very tight inguinal ligament in a small inguinal canal. Infection is the cause of graft failure, which is not a concern of this present discussion.

Lastly, metabolic factors such as hypercoagulability, Collagen's disease, or diabetes mellitus with severe distal disease, hyperlipidemias, and other generalized conditions may result in either progression of the disease in the distal arteries or in the graft itself.

Similar problems with respect to outflow and inflow of the graft are causes of failure in the late stage as with the acute stage (Table 1). Once again, it must be emphasized that technical skill and judgment based on experience and common sense must be utilized for each individual vascular procedure to prevent late failure.

SURGICAL MANAGEMENT OF ACUTE GRAFT OCCLUSION

The surgical management depends upon whether or not failure of the aorto-femoral bypass is in the immediate postoperative period. It obviously depends upon the cause of the failure and the general condition of the patient. The indications for reoperation are usually the same as those for the first operation, once the risk is taken into consideration along with the anatomical situation. Most patients who have an acute thrombosis of one or both limbs of the aorto-femoral graft should have immediate repair. Patients who develop a failure in the late follow-up should have repair based upon the severity of the disease process, generalized condition, and anatomical situation. The type of operation is also tailored on these principles.

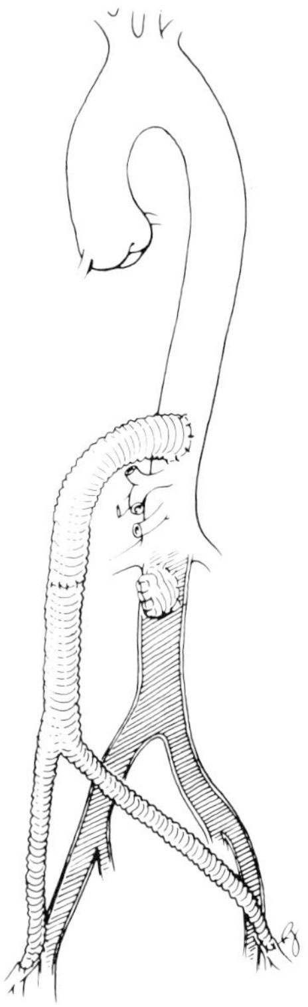

Figure 1. A graft has been placed from the supraceliac abdominal aorta at the level of the diaphragm and above the celiac artery. This is an area that is relatively free of plaque and easily accessible for inflow to the femoral arteries for reoperation. The graft may be placed in the anterior preperitoneal space or retroperitoneally. The supraceliac anastomosis avoids the area of the infrarenal aorta which may be fibrotic from previous operations or infected.

At the time of acute occlusion of an aortobilateral femoral graft, the patient is prepped as if a repeat aortofemoral bypass graft is to be done with the exception of those in whom the performance of a distal femoropopliteal bypass may be anticipated, at which time the entire lower extremity should be prepped. The groin of the affected side is explored first, with the hope that abdominal exploration will not be necessary. Fogarty catheters are inserted proximally to establish the amount and quality of the proximal flow and to establish whether or not there is an inflow problem. A large Fogarty catheter is necessary for this, and suction or clamps may be used to remove fibrin, depending upon the amount of time from the first operation to the second. Care must be taken not to embolize debris down the contralateral limb if only one limb is obstructed. If both limbs are obstructed, then both groins can be opened at the same time and a clamp placed on the contralateral limb to prevent embolization of more debris distal to the distal anastomosis. If it is apparent that an inflow problem is present, in that the proximal flow is very poor, then abdominal reexploration is usually necessary to establish the cause for the proximal failure. In most instances, the graft will have to be replaced at a higher level with performance of an endarterectomy or choice of a different site for the proximal graft. The aorta may be occluded at the supraceliac portion at the diaphragm to allow a more proximal anastomosis. If this is not possible, in rare instances, inflow may be provided by a supraceliac aortic graft (Figure 1), axillobilateral femoral graft, or ascending aorta-to-femoral graft (Table 2). If only one graft limb is involved and there is a proximal problem, then a femoral-femoral cross-over graft may be utilized from the contralateral limb to the affected limb (Figure 2). This cannot be done if there is no distal disease on the donor side. In any event, good proximal flow must be obtained.

Table 2. Failed Aorto-Femoral Bypass

Options for inflow	
Aorta	
Infrarenal	Abdominal
Supraceliac	Abdominal
Ascending	Thoracic
Old graft	
Proximal cuff	
Ipsilateral side	
Contralateral side (cross-femoral)	
Extra-anatomic	
Axillary artery ± cross-femoral	

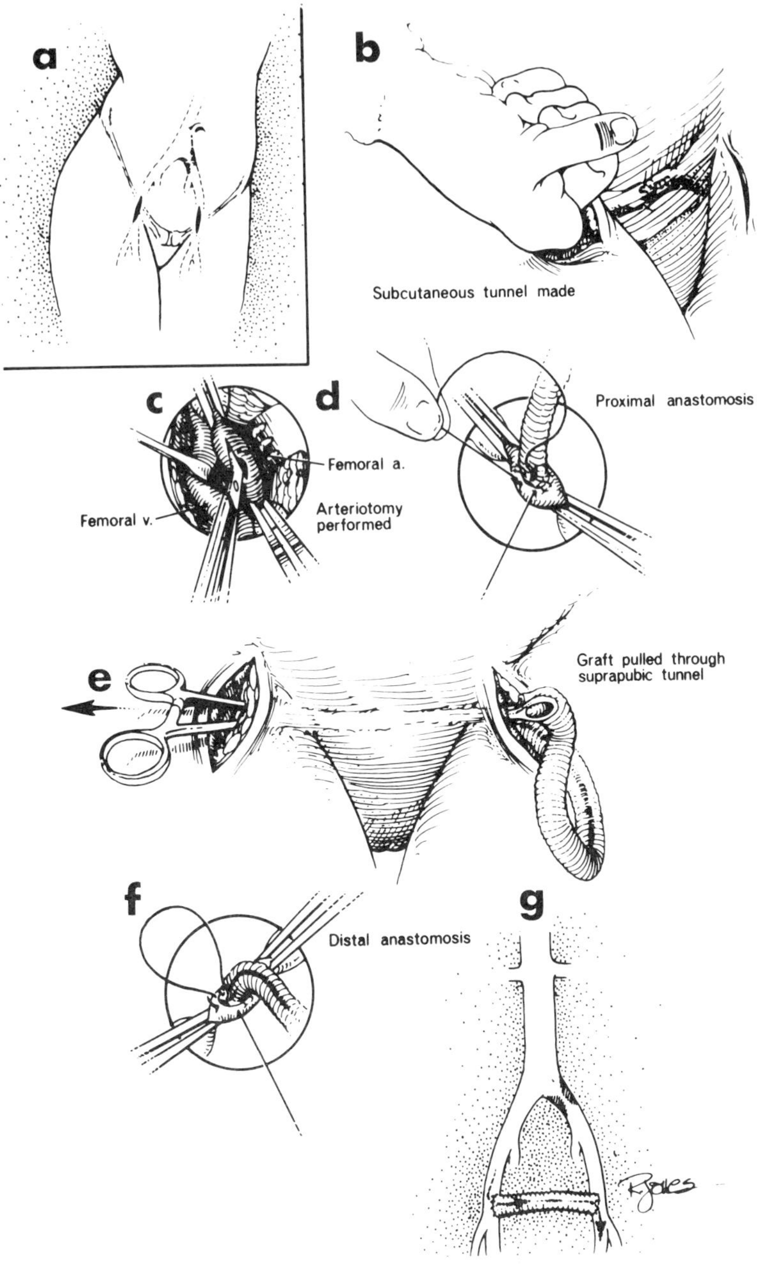

Figure 2. The technique of placement of femoral-femoral graft. This may be useful if one of the graft limbs is thrombosed and cannot be opened. A double velour Dacron graft can be placed from the contralateral limb to the femoral artery in the technique shown. Tunneling should be done behind the pubis to avoid trauma to the graft when pressure is exerted. The graft should be placed loosely so that not too much tension is present. This allows for body flexion.

Next, the outflow portion of the graft must be examined and thrombectomy done to all distal vessels. The graft should be opened to the area of the anastomosis, and the anastomosis inspected. In most instances, the cause of failure may be apparent by visual inspection. This can be corrected by a number of different techniques to reconstruct the femoral artery and outflow tracts (Figure 3). If there is a very small profunda femorus artery and the superficial femoral artery is completely occluded, then a femoropopliteal or femorotibial bypass may be indicated to obtain distal flow. All attempts should be exerted to preserve the profunda femorus artery.

SURGICAL MANAGEMENT OF LATE GRAFT OCCLUSION

As is the acute occlusion, the treatment of late occlusion should be directed toward achieving good outflow and inflow. After adequate arteriograms are done, the lesion can be accurately assessed. In most instances, one limb only is occluded, and there usually is poor distal runoff in that lower extremity. Even though there is no retrograde filling of the femoral artery or there are no collateral branches present on arteriogram, reconstruction can be successful depending on the situation. Exploration of the femoral area of the occluded limb is the direct approach. Once proximal control of the formerly placed graft is obtained, the distal vessels can be identified. In some instances, the scar is so dense that they cannot be adequately dissected. As long as proximal control is present, distal control can be established internally without dissection by Fogarty catheters or metal dilators placed in the distal vessels to occlude the back bleeding. Since some type of reconstruction most often is necessary, it is better to isolate the profunda and superficial femoral arteries along with the proximal iliac artery for some length so that adequate lengths of arteriotomy can be done. The graft is usually opened over the lesion; and if there is obstruction, the incision is extended into the arteries involved. Profundaplasty may be necessary. This can be accomplished either by endarterectomy with patch graft or direct patching beyond the last occlusive plaque. If the superficial femoral artery is completely occluded, the graft can be placed directly to a profundaplasty (Figure 3f). The profundaplasty can be extended down the entire length of the profunda femorus artery if necessary. We have utilized double velour Dacron patch grafts for this reconstruction, although a vein graft is an alternative. We prefer to save the saphenous veins for distal femoral bypass if necessary. If the superficial femoral artery is occluded, it can be opened by either a patch graft or a direct graft of Gore-tex or vein. The proximal common femoral or iliac artery should be preserved if possible. A direct onlay graft over the entire common femoral artery into the superficial femoral or profunda femoral artery is the best procedure (Figure 3b). However, any number of methods can be utilized to obtain flow to the superficial femoral, profunda femorus, and proximal common femoral or

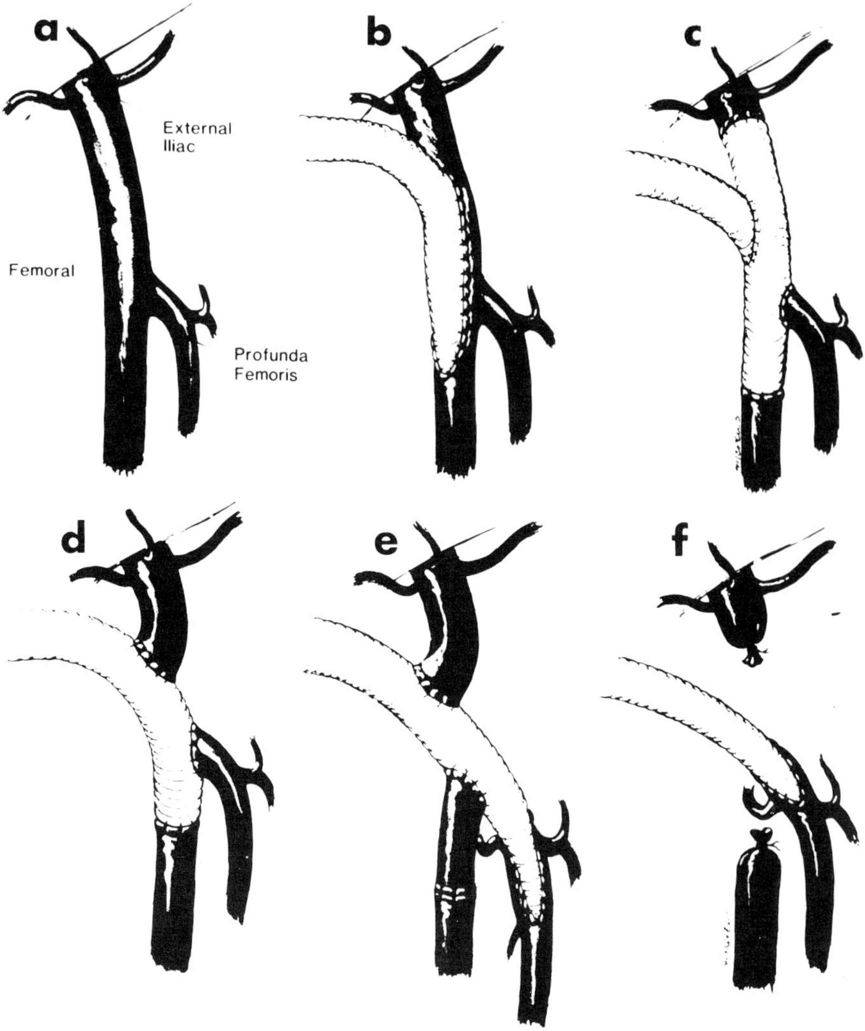

Figure 3. The types of femoral artery reconstruction. **(a)** The normal anatomy is illustrated. The external iliac artery ends at the inguinal ligament. There are multiple collaterals providing the pudendal branches in this area and attempts should be made to preserve them. Usually the plaque is quite thick at that area and may regress more proximally. The common femoral artery is shown. The profunda femorus and superficial femoral artery are its distal branches. **(b)** The ideal placement of an aorto-femoral graft is shown to be overriding the superficial femoral and profunda femorus termination of the common femoral artery. The graft acts as an onlay patch for any plaques at the orifice of the superficial femoral and good retrograde perfusion is assured. **(c)** Total occlusion of the common femoral artery is present. The orifice of the profunda and superficial femoral artery were, likewise, involved with atherosclerotic plaque. An interposition graft of 8-mm double velour

Patients	Grafts	Mean implant	Closures	Patency
105	210	43.9 mo.	4	98.1%

Clinical Results

FILAMENTOUS VELOUR FEMOROFEMORAL GRAFTS
March 3, 1971 through February 1, 1979

Patients	Grafts	Mean implant	Closures	Patency
65	67	32.5 mo.	7	89.6%

FILAMENTOUS VELOUR AXILLOFEMORAL GRAFTS
May 20, 1970 through February 1, 1979

Patients	Grafts	Mean implant	Closures	Patency
54	84	30.0 mo.	18	78.3%

Figure 4. Comparison of aorto-femoral bypass grafts, femoral–femoral bypass grafts, and axillo–femoral bypass grafts is shown as reported by Ray et al. The patency rate of the aorto–femoral grafts is superior. The patency rate of the axillo–femoral grafts is acceptable but poor when compared to the longer follow-up and the better results in the aorto-femoral group. The femoral–femoral grafts are, likewise, favorable. The closure rate is much higher than the aorto–femoral grafts.

---

was placed from the common femoral artery just at the origin of the external iliac to the superficial femoral artery after a nondiseased portion of the superficial femoral artery was obtained. An endarterectomy was then done to the profunda femorus artery, and a good portion of the profunda femorus artery attached to the interposition graft. Inflow was from the previously placed aortic graft. Arterial continuity has been established in the three major vessels in the groin. **(d)** In a similar situation to c, complete occlusion of the common femoral artery and its branches was found. The limb of the inflow graft, either from the femoral-femoral or aorto–femoral area, was placed end-to-end to the superficial femoral artery. The common femoral artery was reimplanted after endarterectomy to the proximal portion of the graft. The profunda femorus artery was also reconstructed and placed into the graft. A patch graft could have been used if necessary. **(e)** Another variation for this procedure, in which a long profundaplasty was necessary, is shown. The inflow portion of the graft was placed end-to-end to the superficial femoral artery with a long patch graft overriding the superficial femoral artery to open up all of its branches. The patch graft was placed to the area of artery that was free of disease. The remainder acted as a patch graft to enlarge the orifice. The superficial femoral artery was reimplanted. The common femoral artery was, likewise, reimplanted. **(f)** In cases where the superficial femoral artery is completely occluded throughout its course and the external iliac and common femoral artery are, likewise, occluded proximally, ligation of both of these arteries may be necessary. End-to-end anastomosis of the inflow portion of the graft, after profundaplasty, was done.

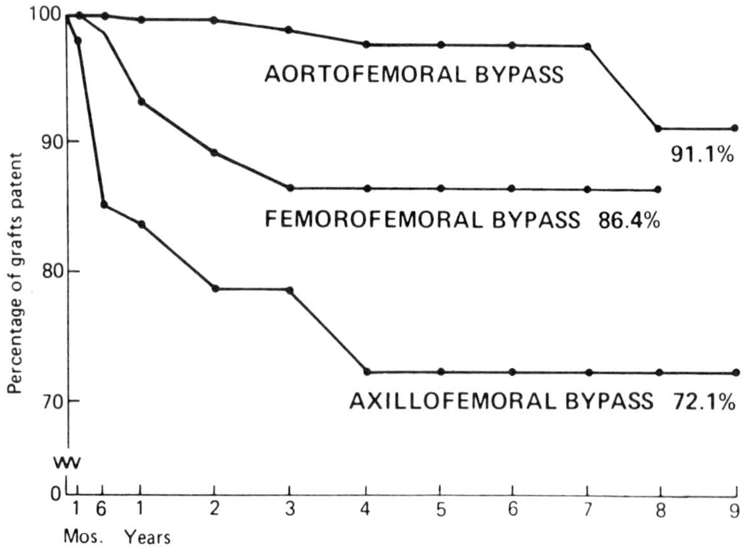

Figure 5. An actuarial table demonstrates the patency rates of aorto-femoral bypass grafts, femoral-femoral bypass grafts, and axillo-femoral bypasses from Ray et al. Note the sudden drop in patency rate at 7 years. We have not experienced this in our patients. The graft occlusion rate is 1 to 3 percent per year.

iliac artery (Figure 3). These can be reimplanted separately to the graft or as units whenever possible. If the superficial femoral artery is blocked and there appears to be inadequate profunda and common femoral runoff, the femoropopliteal bypass can be done utilizing the saphenous vein or a 6 mm Gore-tex graft. Aortopopliteal artery bypass should be avoided, since some revascularization at the groin level should be attempted to reestablish blood supply to the profunda femorus artery and/or the distal iliac artery for retrograde perfusion.

A proximal inflow portion of the graft can usually be reestablished by Fogarty catheter passage in the graft and removal of the old clot and debris. If there is no primary inflow problem, the graft will have adequate flow to maintain the distal bed. As much of the neointima should be removed as possible. Proximal inflow entrapment may occur at the inguinal ligament especially with fibrosis; therefore, the inguinal ligament should be incised to assure adequate inflow. In the rare occasion when adequate inflow cannot be established by thrombectomy procedure, a femoral-femoral cross-over graft may be utilized if the ipsilateral side has good forward flow and there is no significant distal obstruction on the donor side. We have avoided the use of axillofemoral bypass grafts and reversed them only rarely for treatment of infected cases, if there is no other possible treatment. The patency rate of the axillofemoral grafts is poor compared to the other methods and the complications much greater (Figures 4, 5).

If both aortofemoral limbs are occluded, we prefer to use the direct approach to the abdominal aorta. An abdominal incision is made, retroperitoneal structures reflected to the right, and the aorta identified. In most instances, the proximal aortic anastomosis can be retained and a small cuff of the old graft utilized for the bypass graft. If there is a proximal inflow problem, then a new anastomosis must be done proximal to the obstruction. In some instances, a supraceliac graft can be placed at the supraceliac aorta just below the diaphragm (Figure 1). This graft can be tunneled through either the anterior peritoneum or retroperitoneum to the femoral arteries. In some instances, tunneling is difficult because of multiple procedures, then femoral-femoral grafts or extra anatomic grafts can be utilized.

RESULTS

At the Texas Heart Institute from 1955 through 1982, 400 patients underwent 573 procedures for failed aortofemoral bypass grafts. During the more recent period from 1971 to 1983, 2,160 patients underwent aortofemoral or aortoiliac bypass grafts. An additional 1,757 patients underwent abdominal aneurysm resection, approximately one-third having aortoiliac or aortofemoral reconstruction. The actual percentage of failure of these grafts from 1971 through 1982 was only 5.7 percent. In the entire series, 26 percent of the reoperations were done in the acute period on the first day following surgery. Another 9 percent were reoperated from the first day to 30 days following surgery. Late graft failure occurred from 30 days to three years and six months in another 36 percent. Thus, approximately 71 percent of the patients had reoperation within the first 3½ years. The remainder of the reoperations was distributed relatively equally, averaging 1 percent or 3 percent per year over the next 20 years. There were another 173 multiple operations, 115 second reoperations, 38 third reoperations, 15 fourth reoperations, and 5 fifth reoperations. Multiple reoperative procedures were done at longer intervals from the previous procedures when compared to the first reoperation group.

Operative mortality for the entire period from 1955 through 1982 was 7.5 percent in the first 30 days following surgery. In the 217 patients who underwent 270 reoperation procedures from 1971 to 1982, the early mortality was 9.6 percent. If the reoperation attempt was in the first day following surgery, the success rate was 98 percent. If it was at a later period, the success rate at reestablishing flow and limb salvage was 95 percent.

As confirmed by previous reports, there was a very high attrition rate from coronary artery disease and cerebrovascular disease along with a significant amount of patients dying from cancer of the lung.

Table 3. Failed Aorto-Femoral Bypass

Procedure of choice
Ipsilateral graft thrombectomy
Femoral artery reconstruction
PFA—Profundaplasty
SFA[a]—End-to-end or patch
EIA—End-to-side with/without EA

[a]Femoral-popliteal bypass may be essential for limb salvage.

The most common procedure employed in this group of patients, as stated previously, was the direct approach of reestablishing inflow by way of the previously placed graft or a new abdominal aortic graft and outflow by reconstructive surgery in the distal vessels. Axillobilateral femoral bypass graft was only done in 5 patients and other extra-anatomic approaches for inflow were rare.

CONCLUSIONS

The management of aortofemoral artery bypass failure is left to the ingenuity of the vascular surgeon. We prefer to utilize the abdominal aorta for inflow and approach the problem directly (Table 3). Success in these procedures is dependent on adequate outflow into the arteries involved. In most instances, adequate outflow can be obtained by profundaplasty and endarterectomy combinations. Femoropopliteal and femorotibial bypass can also be done in conjunction with these procedures to supply more outflow.

BIBLIOGRAPHY

Bernhard VM, Ray LI, Towne JB. The reoperation of choice for aortofemoral graft occlusion. Surg 82:867, 1977.

Cohn LH, Moore WS, Hall AD. Extra-abdominal management of late aortofemoral graft thrombosis. Surg 67:775, 1970.

Crawford ES, Manning LG, Kelly TF. "Redo" surgery after operations for aneurysm and occlusion of the abdominal aorta. Surg 81:41, 1977.

Lyons JH, Weismann RE. Surgical management of late closure of aortofemoral reconstruction grafts. New Engl J Med 278:1035, 1968.

Najafi H, Dye WS, Javid H, et al. Late thrombosis affecting one limb of aortic bifurcation graft. Arch Surg 110:409, 1975.

Ray LI, O'Conner JB, Davis CC, Hall DG, Mansfield PB, Rittenhouse EA, Smith JC, Wood SJ, Sauvage LR. Axillofemoral bypass: Critical reappraisal of its role in the management of aortoiliac occlusive disease. Amer J Surg 138: 117, 1979.

5

Vasculogenic Impotence

10
Vasculogenic Impotence: An Appraisal of Diagnosis and Treatment

Ronald Virag

Between 1977 and 1982 we had the opportunity to examine one thousand patients whose main complaint was impotence. As a result of our experience, we have developed an individual methodology to help us understand the mechanism of impotence and various therapeutic techniques, both conservative and surgical. This chapter summarizes our experiences in the field of vasculogenic impotence.

NEW CONCEPTS IN THE MECHANISMS OF ERECTION

Although further work is still needed, the mechanisms of erection are now somewhat better understood, owing to recent studies incorporating (a) vascular casts obtained by injection in the branches of the penile arteries showing direct arteriovenous shunts between dorsal arteries and deep dorsal veins, which mainly communicate between the cavernous arteries and the spongy tissue [1]; (b) physiological studies of the erect penis, carried out by artificial erection (AE) [2,3] (see below), xenon washout during visual sexual stimulation (VSS) [4], and intracavernous injection of papaverine [5]; and (c) determination of the presence of a large amount of a putative neurotransmitter, vasoactive intestinal polypeptide (VIP) [6], during erection.

If we look at the four stages of erection–rest, tumescence, erection and detumescence–in the light of the new findings, it can be assumed that (1) relaxation of the smooth muscles of the cavernous tissue neurotransmitted by VIP could be the initiating phenomenon of the erectile cycle; (2) arterial delivery is proportional to the capacity of the arterial bed (modified by 1); (3) the normal arterial filling of the cavernous tissue gives rise to the intracavernous pressure until a critical level (around 75 mmHg); (4) this critical level seems to be necessary for the establishment of full rigidity of the venous outflow.

It is not yet an established fact that a permanent adrenergic tone keeps the penis from permanent erection, although in recent personal tests (unpublished data), the use of an intracavernous blocking agent (Nicergoline) was able to prolong erection for several hours by blocking the venous outflow, after we had established an erection with injection of papaverine.

How the venous outflow is blocked during erection is still an unsolved question. Any of three mechanisms could be invoked: (1) mechanical [7,21] by (a) compression of the pericavernous veins between the albuginea and Buck's fascia, (b) stretching of the terminal part of the deep dorsal vein by an external sphincter, or (c) ischiocavernous muscle contractions at the root of the crura; (2) small valves in the pericavernous veins and the deep dorsal vein, impeding the return of the blood into the glans and through the spongy veins; or (3) reflex initiated by the rise of the intracavernous pressure and under autonomic nervous system control.

Arterial filling is the principal phenomenon, and has yet to be clearly understood. It has been well established in animal studies [7] that the flow in penile arteries during erection is 20 to 50 times higher than the flow when the penis is at rest. This finding has been replicated through ultrasound studies in normal humans. Two conditions must be met for the reaction to occur: (1) good ability of the arterial bed to reply to the initiating phenomenon (this is vaso-activity), and (2) normal pressure into the arterial tree above. If these conditions are not fulfilled, adequate tumescence will not be achieved within a normal range of time, and erectile dysfunction might occur.

NEW CONCEPTS IN THE ONSET OF ERECTILE FAILURE

Until recently, most cases of impotence have been thought to be psychogenic. The first step toward establishing clear differences between the so-called "psychogenic" impotence and organic causes through the use of a dynamic methodology, nocturnal penile tumescence monitoring (NPT), was initiated by Karacan in his pioneering work [8]. In relation to the previously mentioned statement on the physiology of erection, and with a widely expanded methodology of examination of such patients (see below), the next step was to recognize the etiology of organic causes, especially when the patient presented his impotence

Table 1. The Etiology of Impotence. Results of 222 Cases Studied by a Multidisciplinary Approach

Etiology	Number of cases	Percent
Nonorganic	44	20
Organic	178	80
Arterial	118	53
Isolated	59	27
And neurologic	23	10
And venous	23	10
Neurologic and venous	13	6
Nonarterial	60	27
Venous	36	16
Neurologic	6	2.5
Venous and neurologic	12	6
Endocrine	6	2.5

Modified from P. Bouilly, Impuissance sexuelle et facteurs de risques artériels, Doctoral thesis, Paris, 1983.

as an apparently isolated symptom. It appeared [9] that in such circumstances, vascular causes were dominant (Table 1). Arteriosclerotic lesions were present in 56% of the cases in a series of 222 patients submitted to a multidisciplinary approach, including quantification of the erectile failure (see below).

When arterial lesions are present, impairment of the arterial flow to the cavernous bodies at the onset of erection will result in various degrees of erectile dysfunction when the pressure in the arterial bed is below 2/3 of the systolic pressure in the arm and intracavernous pressure (ICP) is unable to rise to the occlusion pressure (the critical level). In this case arterial impairment may be the sole cause of the impotence. When the pressure in the penile arterial bed reaches levels between 65% and 100% of the systolic pressure, occlusion pressure can be reached, but only after pronounced delay.

This has been very well documented by the study of ICP elevation and penis rigidity during injection of papaverine in the cavernous bodies [5] (Figure 1). Such cases result in impaired and/or delayed erection and the patients are exposed to all kinds of stress. For instance, the increase in time necessary to achieve an erection in a previously sexually normal male often leads to performance anxiety. This performance anxiety could be neuromediated through a rise in blood catecholamine level and cause decreased local vasoactivity.

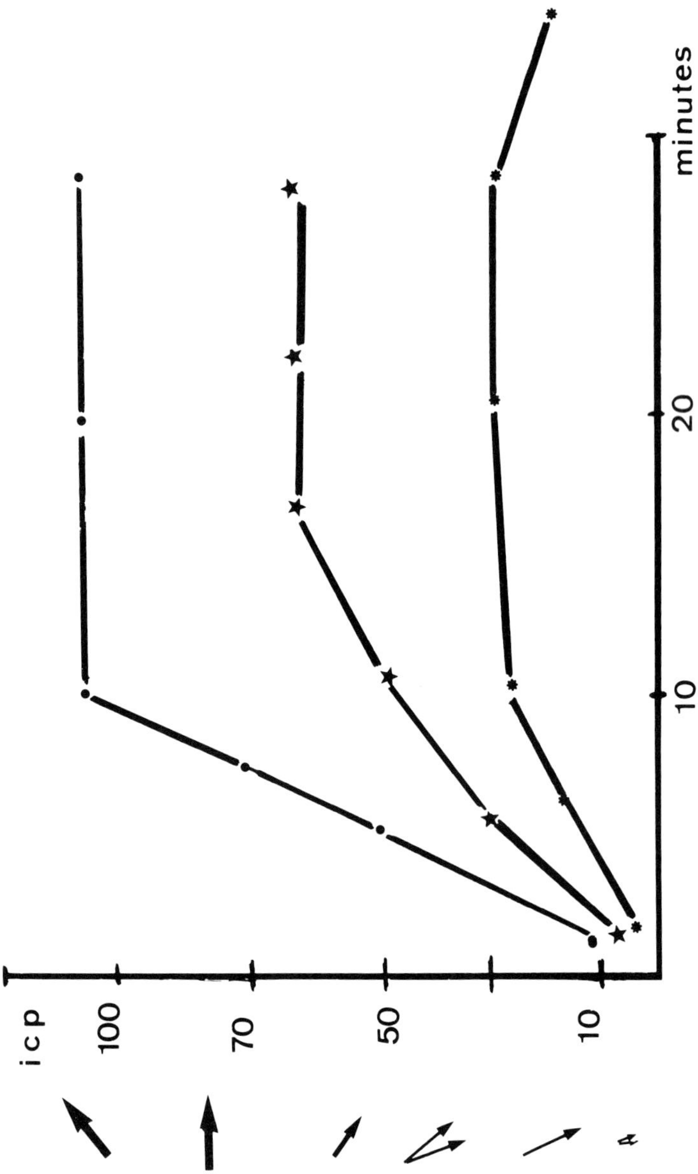

Figure 1. Intracavernous pressure (IPC) and penile rigidity (arrows) in normal erection (upper line), mild organic impotence (middle line), and severe impairment of erection (lower line).

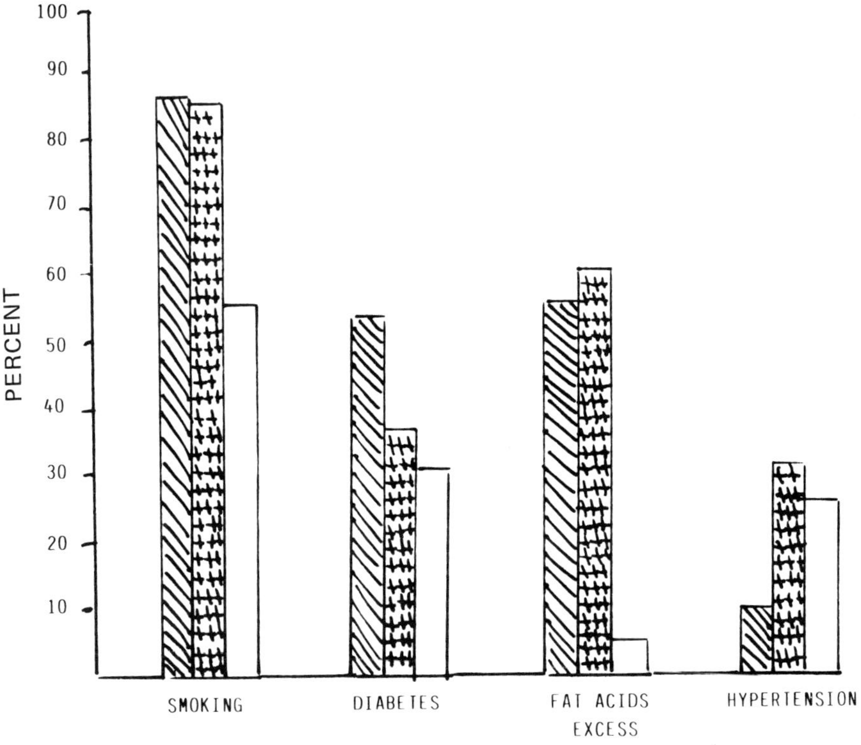

Figure 2. Percentage of the four main arterial risk factors in the normal population [white box], in a series of lower limb arteriosclerotic populations [cross-hatched box], and compared with a series of 118 impotent males with arteriographic lesions of the internal pudendal arteries [diagonal-hatched box]. Modified from P. Bouilly, Impuissance sexuelle et facteurs de risques artériels (1983).

A superficial examination of the case histories of these patients would have led to the diagnosis of psychogenic impotence.

In many cases of impotence, further support for this etiology is given by the study of the arterial risk factors in a large series (N = 440) of impotent patients [9]. Such a study has clearly shown that various degrees of organic erectile dysfunction were present in 96% of the impotent patients with two or more of the four classical main arterial risk factors (hypertension, diabetes, smoking, and high cholesterol level). In such a series, comparison of patients with organic dysfunction to those with nonorganic causes of impotence showed that statistically significant differences existed for diabetes, hypercholesterolemia, and smoking. If more than one risk factor was involved, there tended to be more severe lesions. This study supports the idea that impotence can be compared with other great vascular diseases, such as coronary heart disease, lower limb arteritis, or stroke (Figure 2).

During the first meeting of Corpus Cavernosum Revascularization (New York, 1978), Ebbehøj and Wagner [10] reported the possibility of leakages between the cavernous bodies and the spongy tissue (glans), leading to unstable or incomplete erections.

We have established the clinical features of this new pathological entity (see below) by using AE [11] and cavernosography, and relating these to NPT studies. The concept is that even if the arterial and neurologic components are normal, the erection will not remain rigid if complete closure of the venous return is not effective. Such pathology can occur when there is drainage from the cavernous bodies (for instance, in conditions such as Peyronie's disease, abnormal veins, and incompetent valves of the deep dorsal vein). Usually, this pathology in and of itself leads to partial impotence (lack of rigidity), and again leads to total impotence through physiological complications such as performance anxiety.

MULTIDISCIPLINARY APPROACH TO DIAGNOSIS OF IMPOTENCE

Table 2 summarizes the methodology of the evaluation of impotence. Here, we mention only the new trends related to vasculogenic impotence.

Doppler Studies

This field is rather well documented, but some new facts need to be emphasized.

Technical. In the flaccid penis the most valuable test is the penile blood pressure index (PBPI). It is necessary to record the systolic pressure of the central or cavernous arteries, which may be lower than that of the superficial dorsal arteries (especially in diabetic patients). In patients suspected of having lesions of the internal iliac artery, it is necessary to administer a stress test in order to recognize a pelvic steal syndrome (PSS). If, after mobilization of the buttock and the thigh muscles the PBPI falls at least 20%, there is evidence of PSS. During AE or papaverine tests (see below), the study of the Doppler curves is a valuable test of the ability of the arteries to respond to the flow changes needed for erection.

Value of the PBPI. This is a controversial topic among researchers. The critical level of normality has not been established because of the lack of objective studies. In a recent survey of 220 impotent males subjected to a complete approach, including quantitative evaluation of the erectile dysfunction and arteriography, we established that when PBPI is above 0.91 the arteriograms were considered normal. In 44 patients with clearly demonstrated

Table 2. Evaluation of Impotency—Methodology

Clinical study
Natural history of sexual life
Onset of impotence
Psychological factors
Study of erectile dysfunction
During intercourse
Outside intercourse
Morning erections
Study of ejaculation
Risk factors
Smoking
Lipid metabolism
Diabetes
Hypertension
Iatrogenic factors
Noninvasive arterial study
Doppler evaluation
Lower limbs
Four penile arteries, penile acceleration ratio (PAR)
Penile pressure index (PPI)
Plethysmography with 4 min of arterial occlusion
Somatic general evaluation
Physical study
EKG
Thoracic X-ray
Urinary
Fast glucose test
Lipid studies
Artificial erection with cavernosography
Study of intracavernous pressures (ICP)
Output to obtain (OOE) and maintain (OME) erection
Doppler during AE
Rigidity and buckling studies
Sizes of rest and erect penis
Cavernosography during AE and 15 min after infusion
Injection of intracavernous Papaverine
Measurements of penile rigidity
Penile acceleration ratio (Doppler)
Arteriography
Aortography
Selective internal iliac artery arteriograms
Neuromuscular studies
Bulbocavernous reflex latency
External popliteal sciatic latency
Hormonal evaluation
Testosterone, LH, FSH, prolactin, oestradiol
MMPI
Psychiatric evaluation
Nocturnal penile tumescence (NPI)

Modified from Virag, R, Arterial and venous hemodynamics in male impotence. In AH Bennet, ed., *Management of Male Impotence*. Baltimore, Williams and Wilkins, 1982.

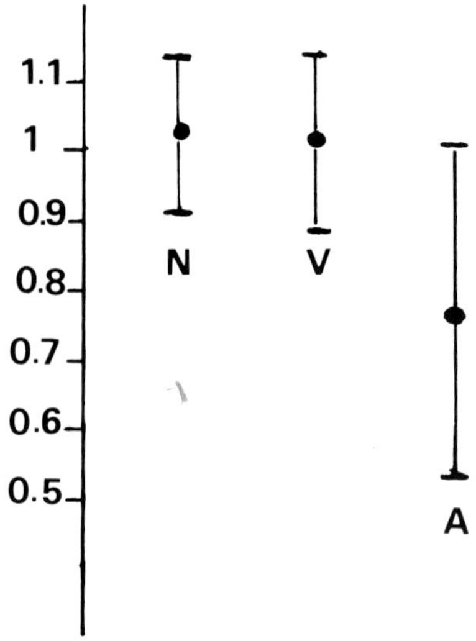

Figure 3. Mean penile blood pressure index in three series of impotency cases: nonorganic (N), n = 44; venous (V), n = 36; arterial (A), n = 118. Horizontal line figures the values of two standard derivations below and above the mean PBPI of the nonorganic series.

nonorganic impotence, the mean PBPI was 1.02 ± 0.12. This, and additional findings, are recorded in Figure 3, and are correlated with the results of arteriography (Table 3).

Postocclusive Pulse Plethysmography

This is a useful test to evaluate the vasoactivity of the penile arteries. A four-minute occlusion is maintained after registration of the basic pulse plethysmogram. After release of the cuff, the period of time and amplitude of the postischemic reactive hyperemia is registered, showing normal, delayed, diminished, or absent response. This test helps indicate impairment of arterial and/or autonomic nervous system related to the arterial response.

Arteriography

In our present practice, arteriography is performed only when there is a presumption of arterial involvement and discussion of surgery. The procedure includes aortography, using lateral views in order to see the origin of both internal iliac arteries, and bilateral selective iliac arteriograms after intracavernous

Table 3. Penile Blood Pressure Index and Results of Arteriograms

PBPI	N	Arteriographic findings		
<0.95	101	Normal	101	
0.89-0.95	15	Normal	3	14 unilateral lesions
		DUL	8	
		DUL + HUL	3	
		DBL	1	(hypoplasia)
0.85-0.89	15	HUL	1	3 unilateral lesions
		HUL + DUL	2	
		DUL	2	
		DBL	10	
0.80-0.85	22	HUL	1	3 unilateral lesions
		DUL + HUL	2	
		DBL	19	
0.75-0.80	17	HUL + DBL	1	
		HBL + DBL	4	
		DBL	12	
<0.75	52	DBL	6	
		DBL + HBL	2	
		HBL	44	

Arteriograms were classified as: Normal; distal unilateral lesions (DUL); Distal bilateral lesions (DBL); high (aortoiliac) unilateral lesions (HUL); or high bilateral lesions (HBL).

injection of 40 mg of papaverine. This modified phalloarteriography is mandatory to give a dynamic view of the pudendal arterial bed and prevents misinformation on its real status. Figure 4 shows various types of procedures in the treatment of stenosis or occlusions of the pudendal arteries and/or branches.

Intracavernous Injection of Papaverine [5]

This is a test, now routinely used, to evaluate the ability of the arterial bed to dilate. After intracavernous injection of 80 mg of papaverine, there is a strong vascular reaction, with a rise of the intracavernous pressure proportional to the arterial response. Plethysmography and Doppler studies can be performed to measure this reaction, and the results compared with PBPI and the clinical status. In normally potent or psychogenic patients, a full erection is obtained, which may last from 1 to 3 hours. When arterial lesions are present, the response to papaverine is delayed and weaker, but is always present (Figure 1). This has been used as a therapeutic tool.

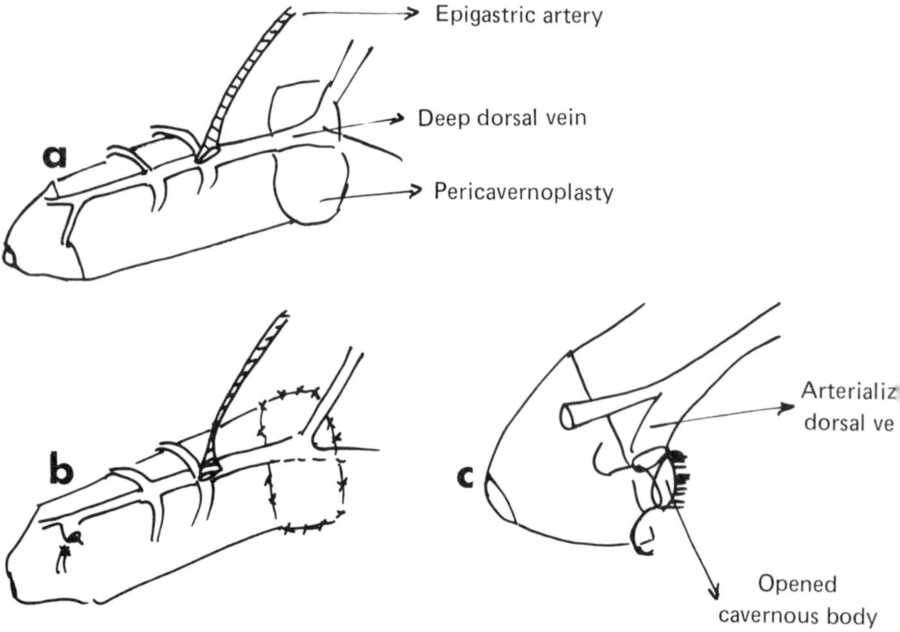

Figure 4. (a) Deep dorsal vein arterialization and pericavernoplasty. (b) Deep dorsal vein arterialization, with anastomosis to the cavernous body. A close-up of arterialized dorsal vein to cavernous body anastomosis is also shown in this figure.

Artificial Erection and Dynamic Cavernosonography [11,12]

This examination consists of an infusion of both heparinized saline and contrast medium into the cavernous bodies in order to carry out simultaneous physiologic exploration (intracavernous pressure, outflow, rigidity) and study of the morphologic changes of the cavernous bodies and the venous drainage. Comprehensive review of the results of this very important examination are published elsewhere. To summarize, the normal values of the output to obtain erection (OOE) is 130 ml/min, and the output to maintain erection (OME) is 40 ml ± 30, while the maintaining index (MI, which is OME/OOE) is 0.3 ± 0.18.

Evaluation of Penile Rigidity and Nocturnal Penile Tumescence (NPT)

We have developed a special device that is able to give a continuous measurement of penile rigidity. It has been demonstrated that penile rigidity is directly related to the ICP. This device now gives much more reliability to the NPT studies. Until the development of this methodology, the lack of parallelism between the increase of the penis's circumference and its rigidity was rather difficult to define accurately. Until the new machine was available, we used a comparative method with AE findings to calculate the NPT results, in order to obviate these problems.

Nonvascular Tests and Psychological Evaluation

Other etiologies have to be screened at the time of evaluation. Neurologic evaluation is still a problem. The question of bulbocavernous reflex latency and duration is part of our methodology, but it does not take into account the very important problem of the autonomic nervous system. This is important in assessing the patient for a revascularization procedure, as well as carefully assessing the psychological aspects, even if vasculogenic etiology is evident. As to this, all the patients are carefully screened by a MMPI study and are evaluated by a psychiatrist.

Classification

At the end of the evaluation, each impotent patient is classified as either (1) nonorganic, with or without psychiatric abnormalities; or (2) organic, with or without psychiatric abnormalities. According to the findings, the etiology may be arterial, venous, neurologic, or hormonal. Often, mixed etiologies are present, such as arterial and neurologic in diabetic patients. The presence of organic and psychologic problems in the same patient is very frequent, as suggested by a recent survey of 220 cases from our personal series (Table 1).

ARTERIAL IMPOTENCE AND ITS TREATMENT

Etiology of Arterial Impotence

The reader must consider the previously presented facts in this chapter. Etiology of arterial impotence may be summarized as follows: (1) Arteriosclerotic lesions in the main branches (aortoiliac axis with the well-known Leriche's syndrome), or in the internal pudendal arteries and branches. A special feature is represented by the isolated lesions in the cavernous arteries, or even in small branches of the cavernous tissues (especially in diabetic patients). (2) Congenital lesions, such as hypoplasia of the penile arteries may be considered, and their presence needs to be established by phalloarteriography. There are also rare occurrences of arteriovenous fistula [13]. (3) Traumatic lesions, such as pelvic bone fractures, and (4) radiation lesions occurring after radiotherapy for pelvic cancers must also be considered. (5) In some cases, there are no morphologic lesions, but vasoactivity is diminished as a result of smoking, possible drug effects, or autonomic nervous system impairment.

Hemodynamics of Arterial Lesions Related to Impotence [14]

There are three mechanisms leading to arterial impotence: (1) obstruction of the flow toward the penile arteries, (2) the steal phenomenon, and (3) decreased vasoactivity.

As mentioned previously, these causes may be associated with the establishment of impotence: An *obstruction* results in reduced pressure in the penile arteries at the onset of erection; the lower the pressure, the more severe is the symptom. The *pelvic steal* [15,16,17] results in a diversion of arterial blood from the penile area into the large muscles of the thigh and/or the leg, secondary to obstruction of the external iliac vessels and/or the muscular tributaries of the internal iliac artery. The steal may be permanent or paroxysmal at the onset of erection, or when the subject contracts his lower limb muscles during intercourse. *Decreased vasoactivity* may result in impairment of the autonomic nervous system at the onset of erection, secondary to previous failures, and lead to performance anxiety.

Whatever the etiology of any arterial lesions present, the surgeon considering cases for surgical therapy must answer several questions: Are the lesions able to produce impotence by themselves? What is the patient's psychological background? What is the general condition of the patient's arteries (cardiovascular, cardiac, lower limb), and what are the arterial risks of surgery? Does the patient need permanent treatment for hypertension?

The severity of arterial impairment is obtained by comparing the clinical status, the PBPI (after exercise), and the mean penile rigidity obtained at night after intracavernous injection of papaverine. If the patient reports complete impotence, if the PBPI is below 0.6, and penile rigidity is low, the case may be caused exclusively by arterial etiology, and can be considered severe. Many patients show partial impotence (decreased and delayed erectile capability), a PBPI between 0.75 and 0.85, and decreased penile rigidity during NPT and after intracavernous injection of papaverine. A light or mild arterial involvement may result in total impotence if the patient suffers from lack of confidence, performance anxiety, or some additional damage such as hormonal, neurologic, or psychological problems (abnormal MMPI). Such arterial lesions may be considered for semiconservative medical therapy.

Penile Hemodynamics

Through the use of AE (see above) we are able to divide the arterial lesions into two groups: (1) those needing only normal output to obtain and maintain erection, and (2) those requiring high flows to obtain and maintain erection. This division is important in the choice of treatment, especially when lesions occur in the distal arteries.

Indications for Surgical Treatment of Arterial Lesions

In the case of aortoiliac lesions with impairment of the blood supply to the lower limbs, the indications are those of the most classic vascular surgery. In cases of paroxysmal pelvic steal, it is generally admitted that reconstruction of the stealing axis would keep up the erectile function.

To summarize: If arterial blockage in the two internal iliac axes can be eliminated (through endarterectomies or bypass), the functional results are better. When procedures affecting the internal iliac artery supply are performed, we believe that microsurgery should not be conducted simultaneously. Evaluation of the PBPI after surgery is a good indication of the hemodynamic results

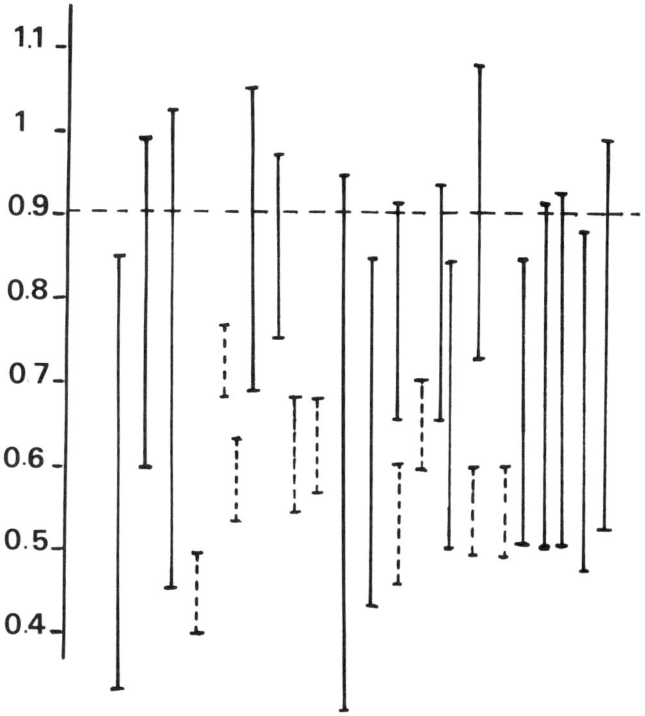

Figure 5. Evolution of the penile blood pressure index in 25 impotent patients operated on at the aortoiliac level showing 16 with a good functional result on their potency (continuous lines) and 9 without improvement (interrupted lines).

Table 4. Clinical Results of 61 Attempts at Revascularization of the Internal Iliac Arteries

Type of revascularization	N	Normal sexual life	Improved	Not improved
Unilateral	37	29%	40%	20%
Bilateral	24	58%	38%	4%
Total	61	41%	39%	20%

(Figure 5). Table 4 summarizes the results we have achieved in performing this on the aortoiliac axis, with or without lower limb reconstruction. If impotence remains unchanged after surgery, one should investigate the possible existence of remaining peripheral lesions or some additional venous or nonvascular etiology.

In patients with aortoiliac lesions for whom surgery is not recommended (because of coronary heart disease, hypertension needing major treatment), or in those patients with distal arterial lesions, mild PBPI impairment, and normal or low output during artificial erection, a semiconservative method has been recommended [5], consisting of medical therapy with oral vasoactive drugs such as Buflomedil, Naftidofluryl, and/or Nicergoline, in conjunction with periodic intracavernous injection of papaverine completed by intracavernous infusion of heparinized saline in order to produce artificial erection. These localized therapy sessions are repeated every second or third month until the erectile function is stabilized; then they are repeated every sixth month. At the same time, the patient is asked to stop smoking and to try to equilibrate any other arterial risk factors (hypertension, hypercholesterolemia, diabetes), if these are present.

When this conservative therapy has failed, or in distal arterial lesions requiring high outflow to produce AE, microsurgery is recommended. Following is a description of this surgical technique. We use the same main surgical approach described previously: deep dorsal vein arterialization [18] with various modifications according to the hemodynamic status of the penis.

VENOUS INCOMPETENCE AND SURGICAL TREATMENT

As stated earlier, so-called venous incompetence covers a new clinical entity which frequently involves young patients with primary impotence. To be considered as "pure venous incompetence," the patient must have an inability to achieve or maintain a fully rigid erection. There should be normal arterial response, but without full erection, and a very high flow needed to obtain and maintain erection. Cavernosograms taken during AE should show one or several of the following lesions: (1) abnormal communication between the cavernous tissue and the spongy tissue [20], either congenital or iatrogenic; (2) abnormal veins draining the cavernous bodies and bypassing the "big veins" [21]; (3) abnormal deep dorsal vein (phlebectasia); (4) Peyronie's disease. In a recent survey of impotence, 7 out of 14 patients had hemodynamic evidence of venous incompetence. Others have also pointed out the same underlying mechanism [23] of erectile failure in these patients. When isolated, the situation is clear. In other cases, impotence may be associated with neurologic and/or arterial lesions.

The severity of venous incompetence (VI) is given by the AE results and a dynamic cavernosogram taken after the beginning of the procedure. If the maintaining index (MI) is above 0.75 and the cavernous bodies are completely empty, as ascertained by x-ray 15 minutes after AE, the condition is severe and a complete surgical reconstruction is required. If the MI is between 0.6 and 0.7, and the cavernosogram shows that 2/3 of the cavernous body is empty, VI is mild. If the MI is about 0.5, the cavernous bodies are generally half empty, and VI is considered light.

One good indication of VI is the inability of the penis to remain rigid during AE when the pump is stopped, during a papaverine test, or during the NPT measurements. This usually matches well with the patient's anecdotal reports. Nevertheless, impotent men usually have a long history of erectile failures and are often diagnosed as having psychogenic impotence. They frequently have abnormal MMPI tests. It is obvious that they need psychological aid before and after surgical reconstruction.

Medical Therapy of Venous Incompetence

At present, there is no medical treatment available that can slow venous return. Various drugs used in peripheral venous insufficiency have not demonstrated any effect at the penis level. We have carried out experiments using intracavernous injection of Dehydrocriptine and Dehydroergotamine without any hemodynamic effect. Nicergoline, an α-blocking agent, demonstrated its ability to prolong and enhance an erection produced by a papaverine injection (administered at the same time as the Nicergoline). We usually recommend using this drug orally on patients as an auxiliary treatment when VI is present.

Surgical Treatment of Venous Incompetence

Usually, pure venous incompetence is a condition to be treated surgically. Three different operations, which can be matched, are possible: resection and/or ligature of veins, pericavernoplasty, or deep dorsal vein arterialization.

Resection or Ligature of Veins. When the dynamic cavernosogram has shown abnormal or pathologic veins, they should be ligated or resected. This is always easily done by a transversal inferior pubic approach to the roots of the cavernous bodies.

One must look carefully for abnormal venous branches rising directly from the cavernous bodies to the superficial collector. When the superficial veins are seen to be draining constantly during the dynamic cavernosograms, they ought to be ligated and largely resected. In case such ligations are performed, it is recommended to circumcise the prepuce, because of frequent postoperative edema. Treatment involving the deep dorsal vein depends on the hemodynamic results (see below). The vein is always isolated, prepared, and clamped. After clamping, an erection is sometimes obtained. In those cases, a large resection of the vein is recommended from as high as possible towards the pelvis to the first major pericavernous collector. Careful hemostasis of the small cavernous branches is mandatory. If deep dorsal vein arterialization is to be performed, the vein is only divided and prepared for anastomosis (see below).

Pericavernoplasty

For centuries, it has been known that placing a ring at the base of the penis is a way to enhance penile rigidity. Fifty years ago, Lowsley planned to make a plication of the ischiocavernous muscles. Using AE, we have observed that when VI and/or arterial insufficiency were present, the rigidity could be enhanced by compression of the bases of the cavernous bodies at an intradiastolic pressure. To perform the pericavernoplasty, we use a sizable band of reinforced silastic (Dow Corning, Inc). It is 1 mm thick, both width and length can be adapted to each patient. During the operation, erection is obtained by AE or intracavernous injection of papaverine. Approximation is now possible in order to obtain the wanted erection without strangulation. The sutures are placed all around the pubic orifice and directly on the lateral part of each cavernous body, at the edge of the spongy tissue, but not into it.

Deep Dorsal Vein Arterialization (DDVA)

DDVA was first described by Leveen [24], but later rejected by him, as a valuable operation for impotence. We have used the procedure on a new morphologic and hemodynamic basis as follows: (a) Direct revascularization of the cavernous bodies by the vein is not possible in cases with faulty valves of the pericavernous veins. (This can be studied by intraoperative retrograde venograms.) (b) DDVA is able to modify the hemodynamic conditions, especially during VI or light arterial insufficiency. (c) If a large quantity of blood is needed for the cavernous bodies, anastomosis can be performed between the extremity of the vein and the cavernous bodies (Figure 4b). (d) The amount of blood needed to be delivered can also be modulated, using as a donor graft either the epigastric artery or a saphenous graft from the leg (the thigh segment should be avoided).

Some technical points have to be emphasized. The deep dorsal vein is valvulated, and when these valvulas are patent, they have to be destroyed prior to the arterialization. In arteriosclerotic patients, the origin of the epigastric artery is frequently atheromatous, impeding its use. Anastomosis performed between the vein and the cavernous body must make a communication between the vein and the deep cavernous body.

INDICATIONS FOR TREATMENTS

Table 5 shows varous indications for the treatment of vasculogenic impotence. The indications for each procedure are the consequences of the results of the diagnostic procedures. From our experience, some rules may be established regarding these indications for medical and surgical therapy:

1. We are very careful about initiating reconstructive surgery for vasculogenic impotence, and more often recommend a penile prosthesis for patients over 60 years of age.
2. If there is unstable coronary insufficiency and/or hypertension requiring the use of several antihypertensive drugs, we most definitely avoid vascular surgery and recommend abstention or a prosthesis.
3. If there is severe neurological impairment associated with arterial and venous lesions, we discourage vascular reconstruction (except in young patients).
4. When aortoiliac and/or internal iliac arteries are obstructed, we recommend an operation on these lesions first, and try to revascularize both internal iliac arteries.
5. When arterial lesions are located in the pudendal arteries and/or branches, we always try to use semiconservative therapy prior to surgery, when AE shows normal or low maintaining index.
6. When vascular surgery is performed at the penis level, it is closely adapted to the hemodynamic findings (AE, NPT, and papaverine test).
7. Postoperative medical therapy is always mandatory, including heparin and antiplatelet drugs, vasoactive drugs, and strict control of the main arterial risk factors.

Table 5. Indications for Treatment of Vasculogenic Impotence

Etiology	Age	Penile blood pressure index (PBPI)	Maintaining index (AE)	Bulbocavernous latency	Type of procedure
Arterial I Aortoiliac level	<60	<0.75	Indifferent	Indifferent	Endarterectomy or bypass
Arterial II Internal pudendal and/or branches	All	0.75–0.85	Low or normal	Normal	Medical intracavernous injection of vasoactive drugs
Internal pudendal and/or branches	<60	<0.75	Low or normal	Normal	Deep dorsal vein arterialization (DDVA)
Internal pudendal and/or branches	<60	<0.75	High	Normal	DDVA with distal anastomosis and pericavernoplasty (See Figure 4b)
Internal pudendal and/or branches	Any	Any	High	Abnormal	Penile prosthesis
Venous	<60	>0.85	High	Normal	Surgery
			a) IM 0.4 to 0.5	⟶	Deep dorsal vein ligation and pericavernoplasty
			b) IM <0.5	⟶	DDVA and pericavernoplasty

Table 6. Results of Treatment of Vasculogenic Impotence, 1977–1982

Patient referred for impotence	1000		
Submitted to multidisciplinary approach	463		
Patients surgically treated	167		
Number of operations	176		
		Improved	Not improved
Aortoiliac reconstruction	37	67%	33%
Epigastric to cavernous body anastomosis	26	50%	50%
Deep dorsal vein arterialization	82	75%	25%
Veins ligation with or without peri-cavernoplasty	14	85%	15%
Correction of curvatures	5	80%	20%
Penile prosthesis	12		
Patients treated by intracavernous injections of vasoactive drugs	63	66%	33%

RESULTS AND COMPLICATIONS

Table 6 gives the overall results of all the cases who had a complete multidisciplinary approach. Some patients who were proposed for surgery refused the operation. Others dropped out during the postoperative survey, and one patient committed suicide while waiting for the results of the diagnosis. Some local complications were seen with operative procedures we have since abandoned. We had two severe local infections secondary to postoperative hematomas. Postoperative thrombosis of the graft is the major and most frequent vascular complication, which always is possible with such procedures as either postoperative or late complication. In this series, the overall rate was 20%. When it occurs at a late stage, the thrombosis is not always followed by a bad hemodynamic result.

On the other hand, some patients with good hemodynamic controlled results have poor or bad functional results. This underlines the very difficult point of the vascular surgery for impotence and the frequent need for psychological aid. Nevertheless, the overall satisfactory result of the series was 75% of the patients operated upon.

DISCUSSION AND CONCLUSION

Impotence is a new field in angiology [25]. Vascular surgeons have to be careful with patients with aortoiliac diseases, and try to avoid postoperative impotence for those who still have normal potency prior to reconstructive surgery; then they can start thinking about the necessity of revascularizing the internal iliac arteries in those who are impotent at the time of their aortoiliac bypass operation [14,26].

The case of isolated vasculogenic impotence is very different. It needs a multidisciplinary approach which involves the vascular laboratory with new methodologies (AE, papaverine test, penile rigidity measurements), a sleep laboratory, neuromuscular and urodynamic studies, hormonal studies, and psychological tests. The vascular surgeon may ask to be the leader of such a multidisciplinary team because of the frequency of vascular disorders, because of the necessity of considering the penis as a hemodynamic structure, and because numerous cases may be cured by vascular surgery. However, he must never forget that impotence is always a mixed psychological and organic disease. Within organic etiologies, mixed problems are frequent and have to be faced.

Since 1973 and the pioneering works of the Czech vascular surgeon, V. Michal[27], much has been accomplished. For many years, it was assumed that impotence was a function of aging by diminished sexual interest and/or hormonal dysfunction. One recent study of the arterial risk factors [9] in a series of impotent patients clearly shows the relationship among arterial involvement, aging, and impotence. Tobacco, diabetes, and hypercholesterolemia have a significant role in the onset of impotence around the age of 40. This is as significant as the prevalence of these arterial risk factors in the occurrence of coronary heart disease. The interference of psychological factors in the occurrence of impotence still plays a decisive role, but has to be reassessed in the public's mind. When impotence occurs, performance anxiety sets in and often becomes prevalent. Most sexologists or psychotherapists find an indication for psychoanalysis or behavioral therapy, forgetting the organic lesions that may be the basic factor of any apparent psychologic impotence. As stated by Karacan [28], "penile erection requires balance and coordination of the central, peripheral, somatic and autonomic nervous system as well as the cardiac, arterial, venous, endocrine and other systems. Mild anxiety, interacting with a subtle unrecognized organic defect, may upset this balance, resulting in erectile failure."

Vasculogenic impotence represents at least 65% of these unrecognized organic defects. It is the first condition that needs to be examined. After the age of 40, arterial insufficiency represents a prevalent potential etiology and has to be screened in the vascular laboratory. The value of PBPI is of paramount interest. If a man has no arterial risk factors and a PBPI above 0.91, arterial impotence may be elicited. If he has three arterial risk factors or more and claims impotence, he certainly has an organic component to his symptom. Before the age of 40, and especially when the patient has never experienced normal erections, the need for a complete multidisciplinary approach is mandatory to avoid a quick diagnosis of psychological impotence. The unstable erection syndrome with venous incompetence has to be ruled out.

In conclusion it can be said that impotence is no longer a desperate condition. Especially when vascular causes are present, it can be recognized and frequently cured.

REFERENCES

1. Wagner G, Willis EA, Bro-Rasmussen F, Nielsen MH. New theory on the mechanisms of erection involving hitherto undescribed vessels. Lancet 1982:416.
2. Virag R. Arterial and venous hemodynamics in male impotence. In AH Bennet, ed., Management of Male Impotence. Williams and Wilkins, Baltimore, 1982.
3. Michal V. Arterial disease as a cause of impotence. Clin Endocrinol Metab 11(3):725–748, 1982.
4. Wagner G, Green R. Impotence: physiological, psychological and surgical diagnosis and treatment. Plenum, New York, 1981.
5. Virag R. Intracavernous injection of papaverine for erectile failure. Lancet 1982(2):938.
6. Virag R, Ottosen B, Fahrenkrug J, Wagner G. Vasointestinal polypeptide release during penile erection in man. Lancet 1982(2):1166.
7. Dorr LD, Brody MJ. Hemodynamic mechanisms of erection in the canine penis. Amer J Physiol 213:1526–1531, 1967.
8. Williams RL, Karacan I. Sleep Disorders, Diagnosis and Treatment. John Wiley and Sons, New York, 1978.
9. Bouilly P. Impuissance sexuelle et facteurs de risques artériels. Thèse pour le Doctorat en Médecine, Paris, 1983.
10. Wagner G, Ebbehøj J, Uhrenholdt A. Infusion cavernosography in the human in the unstimulated and stimulated situation and its diagnostic value. Paper presented at the First International Conference on Vasculogenic Impotence, New York, 1978.
11. Virag R, Spencer PP, Frydman D. Artificial erection in diagnosis and treatment of impotence. Urology 24(2):157–161, 1984.
12. Perry-Spencer P. Apport de l'erection artificielle dans l'étude de l'impuissance. Thèse pour le Doctorat en Medecine, Paris, 1983.
13. Zorgniotti AW, Rossi G, (eds.), Vasculogenic Impotence. Charles C Thomas, Springfield, IL, 1978.
14. Virag R, Fryman F, Cadre N. Hémodynamique de la circulation artérielle pénienne avant et après reconstruction aorto-iliaque pour artériopathie oblitérante des membres inférieurs. Angéiologie 33:269–274, 1981.
15. Michal V, Kramar R, Pospichal J. External iliac "steal syndrome." J Cardiovasc Surg 19:255–257, 1978.

16. Metz P, Bengtsson J. Penile blood pressure. Scand J Urol Nephrol, 1981.
17. Virag R. Pelvic steal syndrome. Vasa 10:4, 1981.
18. Virag R, Zwang G, Dermange H, Legman M. Vasculogenic impotence: a review of 92 cases with 54 surgical operations. Vasc Surg 15(1):9-17, 1981.
19. Virag R. Syndrome d'erection instable par insuffisance veineuse. Diagnostic et correction chirurgicale. Journal des Maladies Vasculaires 6(2):121-124, 1981.
20. Ebbehøj J, Wagner G. Insufficient penile erection due to abnormal drainage of cavernous bodies. Urology 13(5):507-510, 1979.
21. Barbe AM. Impuissance par insuffisance erectile d'origine veineuse ou drainage veineux anormal ou prématuré des corps caverneux. Thèse pour le Doctorat en Médecine, Paris, 1981.
22. Virag R. La maladie de la Peyronie. Conditions hémodynamiques morphologiques et traitement à propos de 14 cas. To be published.
23. Metz P, Uhrenholdt A, Wagner G, Ebbehøj J. Peyronie's disease and erectile failure. J Urol 130(6):1103-1104, 1983.
24. Leveen HC, Diaz C. Treatment by corpus cavernosum revascularization. In AW Zorgniotti, G Rossi (eds.), Vasculogenic Impotence. Charles C Thomas, Springfield, IL, 1978.
25. Virag R. Angiogenic impotence: a new field in angiology. International Angiology. To be published.
26. Queral LA, Whitehouse WM, Flinn WR. Pelvic hemodynamics after aorto-iliac reconstruction. Surgery 86:799, 1979.
27. Michal V, Kramar R, Pospichal J. Arterial epigastricocavernous anastomosis for the treatment of sexual impotence. World Journal of Surgery 1: 515-519, 1977.
28. Karacan I. Psychodynamics of erectile failure in the management of male impotence. In AH Bennet, (ed.), Management of Male Impotence. Williams and Wilkins, Baltimore, 1982.

6

Renovascular and Mesenteric Vascular Disease

11
Medical Management of Renal Artery Stenosis (RAS)

Edward Meilman

I have been interested in renal artery stenosis since 1950 when I saw my first case, a young woman in her early thirties, who presented with malignant hypertension. Although her blood pressure was somewhat and briefly controlled by experimental hypotensive drugs, enough to reverse the papilledema, she underwent bilateral adrenalectomy (at the Peter Brigham Hospital in Boston), which had a brief vogue at that time. Attempts to keep her electrolytes in the normal range with adrenal steroids provoked severe hypertension. When she died, autopsy revealed extraordinary large vessel atherosclerosis and a pinpoint sized orifice to one renal artery. The pathologist, a professor at Harvard Medical School, said to me, "Well, Meilman, you've finally seen a Goldblatt kidney; you'll probably never see another one."

In only a few years clinical recognition of this formerly esoteric entity grew. Howard, at Johns Hopkins, showed that by catheterizing both ureters one could examine separately the urine from each kidney and detect the constricted side; on the renal artery constricted side, the urine was dark, concentrated (urea), and low in sodium. At that time conventional IVP films were taken at 5, 10, 15 minutes and occasionally later, when function was delayed. In 1959 [1] it was suggested that taking the first film at 3 minutes would detect deficiencies, that is, delay in appearance of contrast material, not apparent at five minutes. Later the "hypertensive IVP," starting with films at 1′, 2′, 3′ and continuing beyond 15 minutes to demonstrate delayed emptying of the renal pelvis became the rule. The appearance of contrast material in the first few minutes is a rough measure of renal blood flow so that even a one-minute delay in dye appearance on one side suggests impaired renal blood flow in that side; the late "hang-up" of dye in the renal pelvis suggests scant urine flow on that side and is the radiographic manifestation of the Howard test, obtained with more difficulty by catheterizing both ureters.

There are some simple clinical clues to the diagnosis of renal artery stenosis:

1. *A negative family history of hypertension* should alert the physician to seek a specific etiology, even though one-fourth of patients with renal artery stenosis may have a family history of hypertension. In particular, if neither parent had high blood pressure, search for a primary cause of the hypertension in that patient is likely to be rewarding.

2. *An abrupt onset.* Essential hypertension, the commonest variety, usually begins imperceptibly, often with mild labile readings. If the patient knows that blood pressure was persistently normal and on the next exam it is elevated, that is an abrupt onset. Frequently, of course, such information is not available.

3. *Other evidence of large vessel disease.* Symptoms or signs of large vessel atheroma, such as intermittent claudication of the buttocks or legs, a difference in the blood pressure of the two arms, bruits over carotid subclavian or iliac arteries, should all raise suspicion that a similar process is present in a renal artery.

4. *Bruit.* A bruit in the epigastrium, or high in the right or left upper quadrants, especially in conjunction with one or more of the above three items, is suggestive of renal artery disease. However, pancreatic disease, benign or malignant, may also produce a left upper quadrant bruit. And some normal people have bruits. Bruits heard below the epigastrium, and particularly near the umbilicus, may represent disease of the aorta, rarely the renal artery.

5. *A differential in function or size* of one kidney on the intravenous pyelogram.

Today, these clinical clues lead to angiographic studies, either via the intravenous route and image enhancement or by direct aortography with selective renal artery studies, In some instances renal vein renin studies help predict the success of surgery.

Recognizing renal artery stenosis has become less complicated than dealing with management. I shall divide the patients arbitrarily into three groups.

1. *Prepubertal.* A very rare disease, sometimes involving the intima, can cause renal stenosis. There are so few cases that I will assume that the cause is a vascular lesion causing mechanical narrowing, which should be tackled surgically.

2. *Young adult*, more often female, mostly fibromuscular dysplasia, a disease of unknown etiology. Probably most of these, even if bilateral, should be operated on—or treated with angioplasty. The oldest patient I have seen with this disorder was a 60-year-old woman.

3. *Mature and older adult*, usually atherosclerotic. Here the results of surgery suggest a role for medical management. The final role of angioplasty is still to be determined. Although a new procedure, this invasive but nonoperative modality seems very promising.

Before discussing medical management, it is necessary to review some reported results of surgical and medical management.

In 1963 Harriet Dustan et al. [2] compared operative and drug treatment in 131 patients diagnosed by angiography and followed for 1 to 6 years. Of these, 99 underwent surgery and 10 died (3 of myocardial infarction, 2 of stroke, 2 of thrombosis of remaining renal artery, and 3 of bleeding, anuria and brain hemorrhage). Of those operated, about 58% became normotensive. But in those whose high blood pressure was of less than 5 years' duration, 67% became normotensive; when the duration was over 5 years, only 43% became normal. Thus, the number of years of hypertension seemed to be an important factor. Vascular reconstruction and nephrectomy had about the same results. Neither split-function kidney studies nor fundus class correlated with good blood pressure response to surgery. Thirty-two were treated by drugs because of old age, long duration of hypertension, associated coronary or cerebral vascular disease, or azotemia. Of these, 44% achieved normal blood pressure. In a subgroup of 10 patients who were very closely followed and treated vigorously, 9 came under satisfactory control. In this study, fibromuscular and atherosclerotic patients were combined. Surprisingly younger patients did not do better than older ones.

A report from the Mayo Clinic [3] in 1965 on 54 selected patients with renal artery stenosis, or RAS (32 atherosclerotic and 22 fibromuscular), who were treated medically and followed for 20 months, indicated that 65% of 49 survivors were normotensive. But 13 had cerebral episodes, of which 5 died.

Their experience suggested that factors indicating caution with regard to surgery were: long duration of hypertension, bilateral disease, necessity for nephrectomy, associated severe cardiovascular disease, old age, and infirmities. They were reluctant to recommend surgery for renovascular disease without the presence of hypertension and the presence of arteriographic and renal function data.

In 1969 Shapiro et al. [4] reported on 115 patients with RAS of whom 43 underwent surgery. After 1-6 years 35% were dead; of the unoperated 72, 69 were followed up and 50% were dead. Surgery had not achieved a significant long-term salvage in the Shapiro study, which combined RAS from atherosclerosis and fibromuscular disease in one group.

The important report of the Cooperative Study of Renovascular Hypertension in 1975 [5] discussed the operative mortality and morbidity and helped delineate which patients would more logically be referred for operative intervention. There were 34 deaths in 577 operations on 502 patients, but the definition of operative death was most liberal and included any death due to a postoperative complication, regardless of the postoperative time interval. Looking at these 34 deaths, 28 were in patients with atherosclerotic (ATH) disease and 6 had fibromuscular (FM) disease. Thus while the ATH group comprised 59% of the patients, they accounted for 82% of the deaths. The operative mortality was 9.3% in ATH and 3.4% in FM. Those who died had three times as much angina, previous myocardial infarction, peripheral vascular and cerebrovascular disease. Renal function impairment was twice as common and left ventricular hypertrophy 1½ times as common in those who died. There was considerable variation in mortality among the different institutions in the study. In the ATH group, the presence of coronary artery disease or previous myocardial infarction increased mortality from 5.6% to 22%; even mild degrees of renal insufficiency increased mortality from 5.3% to 22%. By itself, preoperative cerebrovascular or peripheral vascular disease did not affect mortality. Both nephrectomy and arterial reconstruction had the same mortality; but combining the operation with aneurysm repair or iliac repair increased mortality to 25%. Leading causes of deaths were: uremia, hemorrhage, thromboembolism, and infection.

Reasonable conclusions from this study are that patients with coronary artery disease should have a drug trial first and surgery only if BP control is not obtained. Patients with bilateral renal impairment should try drugs.

A 1973 report from the Mayo Clinic [6] described 214 cases of RAS with 7- 14-year follow-up: of 100 operated, 84 survived and 51 were normotensive without drugs; the 84 included 26/37 (70%) ATH and 58/63 (92%) FM. The 114 who had medical treatment yielded 16 eventually to surgery. In this group, 44 had ATH and 27 died (27/44 = 61%); 70 had FM and 12 died (12/70 = 17%). Thus overall, without specific breakdown, surgery had the edge.

The advent of balloon angioplasty has been an exciting advance. Its final role is still to be determined in atherosclerotic disease. Certainly, at the moment, this nonoperative approach seems worth doing prior to surgical intervention; some patients have required a second dilatation, obviously easier than a second surgical exploration.

Assuming, for discussion, that the patient falls into an unfavorable group for surgery, such as old age, coronary disease, renal insufficiency, and multiple vascular disease, or multiple renal vascular disease makes angioplasty risky, we come to medical management.

Thus, for the surgical approach one must consider morbidity and mortality, possibility of secondary graft closure, that 30%-40% of patients may not be cured, that some diseases may be progressive, that atherosclerotic infarcts may affect the so-called normal kidney, and, finally, that life expectancy due to the patient's other vascular disease may take precedence.

The currently widely accepted drug program seems to be applicable to renal artery hypertension as well as essential hypertension. That is, diuretics, an antisympathetic-type drug (reserpine, alpha methyldopa, clonidine, beta blockers), vasodilators (hydrallazine) or a specific postsynaptic alpha blocker (prazosin), and finally a potent blocker such as guanethidine. However, since RAS is the prototypical high renin hypertension, it seems logical to start with a drug that will lower renin. Beta blockers such as propranolol will lower renin and are often effective in RAS, especially with diuretics. In this instance, either extra potassium or a potassium-sparing diuretic should be added. Low serum K in untreated patients should raise the suspicion of high aldosterone. Since primary aldosteronism is much less common than secondary, finding a low serum K suggests secondary aldosterone elevation from a high renin-angiotensin. Adding a diuretic to such a patient will certainly also lower the K, hence the advantage of combining a k-sparing diuretic.

The advent of Captopril, a specific antagonist of the enzyme (converting enzyme—CE) which converts inactive angiotensin I to the potent vasoconstrictor angiotensin II, gave a powerful tool for treating blood pressure due to RAS. Presumably Captopril works by inhibiting CE. However, it may also interfere with catecholamine metabolism and certainly prevents CE from destroying bradykinin, a potent vasodilator. Side effects that are serious include bone marrow depression (0.3%) and proteinuria (1%), these being more likely in patients with renal dysfunction. Other side effects—loss or change in taste, skin rashes and fever—are more common, especially, again, when there is renal impairment. But these are the patients in whom surgery might be vetoed.

Since diuretics and vasodilators raise renin levels, one might wonder about their advisability in RAS, yet the result, a fall in blood pressure without significant change in renal function, is what counts.

Currently other converting enzyme inhibitors which lack the SH group of Captopril, are being studied. Perhaps they will have fewer side effects.

If the gamut of hypotensive drugs is not successful in lowering blood pressure, one should consider the patient for angioplasty or surgery. Even though drugs may lower the pressure and prevent other hypertensive sequelae, they do not dilate the constricted vessel.

CONCLUSIONS

In summary, for prepubertal individuals I would always recommend surgery if technically feasible. For the young adult with FM disease, angioplasty may be the method of choice at present; if unsuccessful, I would suggest surgery in most cases, reserving drug treatment for technically difficult or failed cases. In the atherosclerotic (ATH) group, I prefer medical management; even patients with a small shrunken nonfunctioning kidney are not reliably cured by nephrectomy. Moreover, the other kidney often has unrecognized atherosclerotic vascular lesions or even infarcts studding the renal surface. These latter findings militate against a good result with surgery. As many patients in the ATH group can be controlled on medication, surgery should be tried only in the few without other compromised vascular circuits, when angiographic anatomy seems favorable for surgery and the other kidney is normal. The final role of angioplasty, attractive as it seems, remains to be established.

APPENDIX

131 Patients (DX by angio)

99 Operated

10 Died
3 MI
2 Thrombosis R.A.
3 Bleeding angina

89 Survived
58% NT

32 Drug Rx
44% NT

Dustan et al 1963 [2]. Reprinted by permission of *Circulation*.

7-14 Year Follow-up

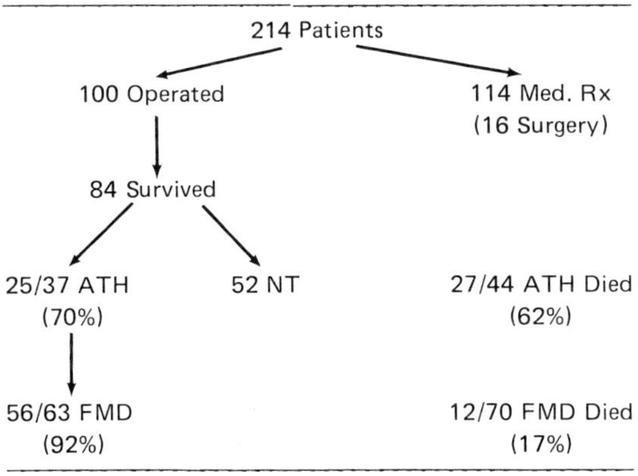

Hunt and Strong, 1973 [6]

Medical Rx

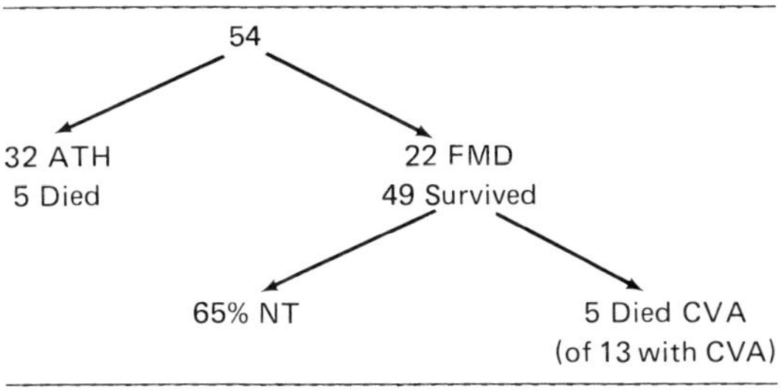

Sheps et al, 1965 [3]

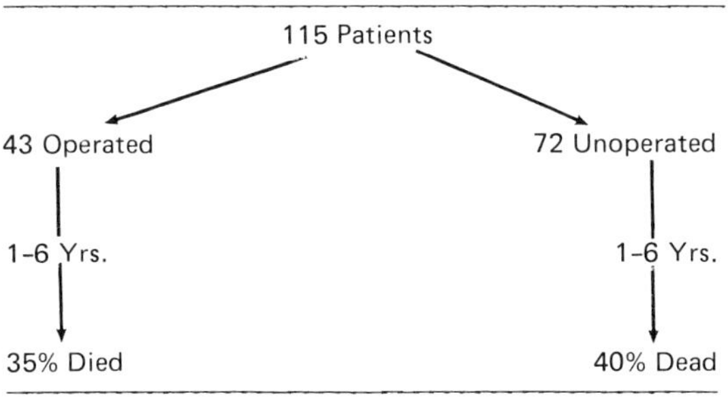

Shapiro et al, 1969 [4]. Reprinted by permission of the *Amer J Med*

REFERENCES

1. Meilman E, Azulay A, Butterly JH. Clinical diagnosis of renal artery constriction. Circulation 20:740, 1959.
2. Dustan HP, Page IH, Poutasse EF, Wilson L. An evaluation of treatment of hypertension associated with occlusive renal artery disease. Circulation 27:1018–1027, 1963.
3. Sheps SG, Osmundson PJ, Hunt JC, Shirger A, Fairbairn JF II. Hypertension and renal artery stenosis: Several observations on 54 patients treated medically. Clin Pharmacol Ther 6:700–709, 1965.
4. Shapiro AT, Perez-Stable E, Schieb ET, Bron K, Moutsos SE, Berg G, Misage JR. Renal artery stenosis and hypertension. Observations on current status of therapy from a study of 115 patients. Amer J Med 47:175–193, 1969.
5. Franklin SS, Young JD, Jr, Maxwell MH, Foster JH, Palmer JM, Cerny J, Varady PH. Cooperative study of renovascular hypertension. Operative morbidity and mortality in renovascular disease. JAMA 231:1148–1153, 1975.
6. Hunt JC, Strong CG. Renovascular hypertension. Mechanisms, natural history and treatment. Amer J Cardiol 32:562–574, 1973.

12
Surgical Management of Renovascular Disease and Chronic Intestinal Ischemia

Larry H. Hollier

Renovascular occlusive disease is the most common cause of surgically correctable hypertension. Although the advent of the B-blocking drugs has added a new dimension to the medical treatment of renovascular hypertension, there still remains a select group of patients who are best managed by renal artery reconstruction. A precise understanding of the pathophysiology of renovascular hypertension and careful selection of patients appear to be of utmost importance in the appropriate management of these patients.

Pathophysiology

No paper on renovascular occlusive disease is complete without at least a cursory discussion of the renin-angiotensin-aldosterone mechanism of hypertension.

In response to a decrease in blood pressure to the kidney, as occurs in renal artery stenosis, the juxtaglomerular cells of the kidney release the enzyme renin into the venous circulation. Although renin itself has no direct vasopressor activity, it does play a role in the development of hypertension. In the venous systemic circulation, renin acts on angiotensinogen, a glycoprotein produced by the liver, to produce angiotensin-I. This decapeptide, which likewise has no pressor activity, is changed in the lung by a converting enzyme to angiotensin-II, an octopeptide that has very powerful pressor activity [1]. Angiotensin-II produces this effect, both through its specific action of constriction of arterial wall smooth muscle causing increased peripheral resistance and by stimulating aldosterone secretion by the adrenal cortex to cause retention of sodium and water, with expansion of the extracellular fluid volume.

In view of this generally well accepted concept of renovascular hypertension, angiotensin-blocking agents and converting enzyme inhibitors have been developed to control blood pressure in these patients. Although these drugs have provided much better responses in many cases, some patients continue to be refractory and require surgical intervention to control their blood pressure or to stop the deterioration of renal function.

Diagnosis

Approximately 80 percent of patients with elevated blood pressure have essential hypertension, while only 5 percent have renovascular hypertension [2]. Since one cannot justify routine angiography in all patients with hypertension, we look for various diagnostic criteria that will help identify those patients who most likely have renovascular hypertension. We hope to avoid angiography in the majority of patients who do not have renovascular hypertension, and at the same time miss as few as possible of those patients who do have correctable lesions.

History and physical examination alone are unable to clearly delineate those patients with renovascular hypertension. However, there are some clinical characteristics that help to identify patients with renovascular hypertension when compared to patients with essential hypertension. Patients who have relatively recent onset of hypertension (especially when the hypertension accelerates rapidly), who have a negative family history of high blood pressure, and who have flank or abdominal bruits, have an increased likelihood of having renovascular hypertension. Hypertension in a young, thin, white female is more likely to be related to fibromuscular disease, while the sudden onset of high blood pressure in an elderly patient is more often related to atherosclerotic disease. However, since the overlap of physical findings, age, sex and risk factors is so great, these trends are all but useless in evaluating hypertension in an individual patient [3].

Routine blood chemistry, urine chemistry and urinalysis have not been very helpful. Serum electrolyte profile, analysis of diurnal variations in adrenal corticosteroid levels, and serum metanephrines are helpful in identifying other causes of surgically correctable hypertension, but they obviously do not identify patients with renovascular hypertension. Even plasma renin levels, when measured peripherally, have not been useful in identifying patients with renovascular hypertension. Indeed, the peripheral plasma renin activity may be high, normal or low in patients with renovascular hypertension, and only in patients with malignant high blood pressure is it invariably elevated [4].

For many years, the "hypertensive IVP," or rapid-sequence pyelogram, has been used as a screening procedure for renovascular disease. After the intravenous injection of urographic contrast medium, x-rays are taken at 1-, 2-, 3-, 4-, 5-, 10-, 15- and 30-minute intervals. Three findings are suggestive of unilateral renovascular disease: (1) one kidney smaller than the other, (2) delayed appearance of contrast in the smaller kidney, and (3) hyperconcentration of contrast medium in the smaller kidney on late films. Less than 1 percent of patients with essential hypertension have two or more of these findings present, while at least two findings are present in 45 percent of patients with unilateral renal arterial stenosis. Moreover, 17–30 percent of patients with documented renovascular hypertension have false-negative rapid sequence pyelograms. Because of this high false-negative rate, the usefulness of pyelography is somewhat limited [5].

Undoubtedly, angiography is the most accurate method of identifying renal artery stenosis. However, even angiography may be misleading unless more than simple flush aortography is done. It is most important to include selective angiography with oblique views to identify proximal renal artery stenoses which, because of the posterolateral initial course of the renal arteries, may not be seen by A-P views [6].

One must remember, however, that angiographic visualization of a stenotic renal artery does not invariably mean that this is the cause of a patient's hypertension. It appears that, if hypertensive patients are selected for surgery only on the basis of an angiographic lesion, only 50 percent will be benefited. Other tests, therefore, are necessary to determine the functional significance of an angiographically demonstrable renal artery stenosis. Of functional tests available, it would appear that lateralization of renal vein renin ratios, when positive, is highly predictive of renovascular hypertension, and correction of such a lesion is correlated with amelioration of hypertension in a large percentage of cases [7,8]. Other functional tests, such as split renal function tests, are of less predictive value and are insufficiently reliable. Renal vein renin ratios, however, when they lateralize, are predictive of good surgical results in over 90 percent of cases. However, even if the renin ratios do not lateralize, approximately 50 percent of patients will nonetheless be improved by surgical correction of the renal artery stenosis. In view of this, it is our policy to offer surgical correction to any patient with severe hypertension and significant renal artery stenosis, despite the results of renal vein renins, providing the patient is an acceptable surgical risk [7].

Surgical Treatment

In view of the recent popularity of percutaneous transluminal balloon angioplasty (PTA), it is prudent to discuss the scope of its applicability in the management of renovascular hypertension. This technique provides a relatively quick, safe and effective mechanism for relieving stenosis of renal vessels but, unfortunately, two factors decrease its utilization. First, in about 20 percent of cases it is technically impossible to achieve satisfactory dilatation of the lesion; secondly, about 20 percent of initially successful dilatations develop restenosis. Major complications occur in about 5–10 percent, and we have had one death as a result of a complication of PTA.

Perhaps the most important factor in successful PTA is the appropriate selection of patients for this procedure. Unfortunately, because of the relative simplicity of PTA, it is sometimes offered indiscriminately, to the detriment of the patient. However, unselective use of PTA for renal artery stenosis results in 30 percent immediate failure, 30 percent failure at 3 months, and good long-term results in only one-third of the patients. It is our feeling that renal artery PTA should be reserved for those patients who have a reasonable expectation of long-term good results by this technique; other patients should be offered surgical correction. We feel that renal artery PTA is the primary treatment of choice in patients with fibromuscular dysplasia of the middle-third of the renal artery and for short segment atherosclerotic lesions that are not contiguous with large aortic plaques. Fibromuscular dysplasia that extends into the branch vessels, atherosclerosis over a long segment of the renal artery, atherosclerotic plaque of the aorta that extends into the renal artery, and renal artery stenosis in a patient with a single kidney are all generally better treated by direct surgical repair. There are some patients, however, who represent such poor surgical risks that PTA may be attempted in preference to a primary surgical approach. In our experience, few patients fall into an inoperable category. It is also important to note that PTA is not without risk, and significant morbidity, as well as mortality, has been noted [9].

The effectiveness of renal artery revascularization for severe renovascular hypertension has been documented by many previous reports [10–19]. It remains our conviction that surgical revascularization of the renal artery is the preferred treatment in severe renovascular hypertension, except in those situations previously described where PTA may offer a logical alternative. It is also evident that renovascular reconstruction is of benefit in those patients who have renal artery stenosis associated with progressive renal failure [20].

Technique

Patients who are acceptable surgical risks, and who are found to have severe renovascular hypertension or progressive renal failure secondary to unilateral or bilateral renal artery stenosis, are referred for renal artery revascularization. Complete angiography of aortoiliac arteries, as well as both renal arteries, is demanded prior to any attempt at renal artery reconstruction. Careful assessment of pulmonary and cardiac risk factors is also obtained prior to surgery.

In those patients who have no significant disease of the aortoiliac arteries, we prefer to revascularize the renal arteries by use of autogenous saphenous vein grafts. If severe aortoiliac disease is present, we then prefer to reconstruct the aortoiliac segments with a bifurcated Dacron graft and then use Dacron graft for the renal artery reconstruction. By using only normal aorta or the Dacron aortic bypass graft for the origin of our renal revascularization, we are able to minimize the risk of early renal graft failure and also to decrease the late failure of the bypass that might occur because of progressive worsening of aortic atherosclerosis.

A midline approach is generally employed, since this provides wide exposure of the renal arteries, as well as the aorta. If the right renal artery is to be repaired, the right colon is reflected and the duodenum is mobilized, the aorta being approached either from the midline or laterally through the root of the right mesocolon. Isolated left renal artery repair is generally performed by exposing the aorta in the midline and exposing the left renal artery by reflecting the descending colon. When bilateral renal artery repair is planned, or when the aorta itself must be replaced, we then prefer to expose aorta and both renals by a midline approach, exposing the aorta and the proximal two-thirds of both renal arteries from the midline. In these cases we have had no trouble getting good control of the renal arteries, even when the stenotic lesions extend out to the distal third of the renal artery. The anastomosis is preferentially performed end-to-end, after spatulating the renal artery for a length of at least 1 cm. This provides for good flow with a minimum of turbulence and the least risk of late stenosis. In those patients with fibromuscular dysplasia, wherein the lesion extends beyond the level of the renal artery bifurcation, the spatulation can be extended out onto the branch vessel to provide complete repair beyond the level of stenosis. In the rare circumstance where distal branches are involved, ex vivo reconstruction may be preferred. Perfusion of the kidney is undertaken during the period of ischemia for construction of the renal artery anastomosis by using a solution of heparinized iced Collins' solution. No attempt is made to "hurry" the anastomosis, but total ischemia time is generally 15 to 20 minutes, and postoperative renal failure is very rare. Heparin (5000 units) is given intravenously prior to occlusion of the renal artery and is not reversed at the end of the procedure. Mannitol (25 gm) and Lasix (10 mgm) are generally given intravenously about 15 minutes before renal artery occlusion to have the kidney in a diuretic state prior to the onset of ischemia. After restoration of flow, a brisk urine output invariably ensues. In the early postoperative period high urinary outputs are replaced hourly in addition to regular maintenance fluids. After 12 to 18 hours, this is usually no longer necessary, and only maintenance fluids are required.

Prior to discharge of the patient after surgery, it is our policy to routinely study the patency of the graft and the integrity of the anastomosis by arteriography or digital subtraction angiography. Intravenous pyelograms, radionuclide scans and other function tests have been unreliable in determining the adequacy of the revascularization, although they have been somewhat helpful in the long-term follow-up of these patients.

CHRONIC INTESTINAL ISCHEMIA

The clinical syndrome of chronic intestinal ischemia is relatively rare and is frequently misdiagnosed because of the sublety of the symptoms. Classically, intestinal ischemia produces postprandial pain that usually starts about 30 minutes after meals. Patients soon recognize that eating causes pain and they attempt to avoid food, with a resultant loss of weight. In a recent review of this problem [21], we found 56 patients with chronic intestinal ischemia and an average weight loss of 32.5 pounds, although one patient had lost 109 pounds. The average duration of symptoms prior to diagnosis was 12.5 months, with one patient having had symptoms for 15 years.

This syndrome takes on particular importance if one recognizes that about half of the patients who present with acute intestinal infarction may give a history of symptoms of chronic intestinal ischemia; early recognition and surgical revascularization might prevent acute infarction in these patients [22].

Despite attempts to correlate gastrointestinal function tests with the ischemic syndrome, these tests have proven unreliable for diagnosis and generally serve no useful purpose. One must constantly maintain a high index of suspicion in patients who present with unexplainable abdominal pain and weight loss and, although a malignancy must first be ruled out, if no other cause is found, angiography is indicated to study the visceral vessels.

It has generally been held that one does not get the syndrome of chronic intestinal ischemia unless both the celiac and superior mesenteric arteries are occluded or severely stenotic. Indeed, many asymptomatic patients can be found incidentally to have occlusion of both of these vessels, but the extensive abdominal collaterals prevent ischemia and, therefore, symptoms do not occur, However, it would also follow that, if adequate collaterals are lacking, occlusion of even a single major vessel might result in symptoms. In our review of 56 patients with chronic intestinal ischemia, 17 of these patients had occlusion or stenosis of only one of the two major visceral arteries. This leads us to believe that, in patients with classic symptoms of chronic intestinal ischemia, if no other cause of symptoms can be found, revascularization of occluded visceral vessels may be indicated, even though only one of the two major arteries is involved. It is much more common, however, to see multiple vessel disease.

Much discussion has taken place regarding the best method of surgical repair in chronic intestinal ischemia. One might consider antegrade revascularization from the supraceliac aorta to the visceral vessels, retrograde revascularization from the infrarenal aorta, direct endarterectomy, or even patch angioplasty. Controversy also exists regarding the choice of graft material–namely, autogenous veins, Dacron or PTFE. Additionally, some authors advocate multiple vessel revascularization, while others note that revascularization of only one vessel usually provides relief of symptoms.

Our study at the Mayo Clinic showed no difference in relief of symptoms or in long-term patency, regardless of the type of graft used. Since most grafts were previously placed in retrograde fashion, we were unable to determine if antegrade grafting gave better results, although we would agree with Stoney, et al. [23] that placement of the grafts in antegrade fashion has definite theoretic advantages.

Perhaps the most important aspect of surgical revascularization relates to the long-term results. Multiple studies [21,24,25] have noted that immediate relief of symptoms can be achieved in almost all patients. However, late recurrence of symptoms becomes evident in 14–50 percent of patients [3,21, 24-27]. More specifically, it is evident that, although single-vessel revascularization may relieve symptoms immediately, the maintenance of long-term relief is related to the completeness of revascularization [21]. Whenever possible, one should attempt to revascularize all stenotic visceral vessels at the initial operative procedure. This is probably the most important principle in the surgical management of chronic intestinal ischemia.

Technique

For revascularization of multiple stenotic visceral vessels, we prefer a long midline abdominal incision. The stomach is retracted downward and to the left and the gastrohepatic omentum is opened. The crura of the diaphragm are divided between clamps and the subdiaphragmatic supraceliac aorta is exposed. A partial-occlusion clamp is then placed on the aorta at this level. If both celiac and superior mesenteric arteries are stenotic, a bifurcated graft (either Dacron or pantaloon vein [28]) is sutured to the supraceliac aorta and one limb is then anastomosed to the celiac artery or one of its branches and the other limb is brought to the superior mesenteric artery. If the inferior mesenteric artery is also stenotic, one may either patch the vessel across the stenosis or endarterectomize and reimplant the inferior mesenteric artery into the aorta. If an abdominal aortic aneurysm or aortoiliac occlusive disease necessitates infrarenal aortic replacement, we still would prefer antegrade grafting to the celiac and superior mesenteric artery as described. However, we would make certain to additionally revascularize the inferior mesenteric artery, usually by reimplanting it into the infrarenal aortic Dacron graft.

Early and appropriate diagnosis in patients with chronic intestinal ischemia and complete revascularization of all stenotic vessels should prevent the development of acute intestinal ischemia and should also provide for the long-term repair of symptoms.

APPENDIX

Surgical Revascularization. Chronic Intestinal Ischemia

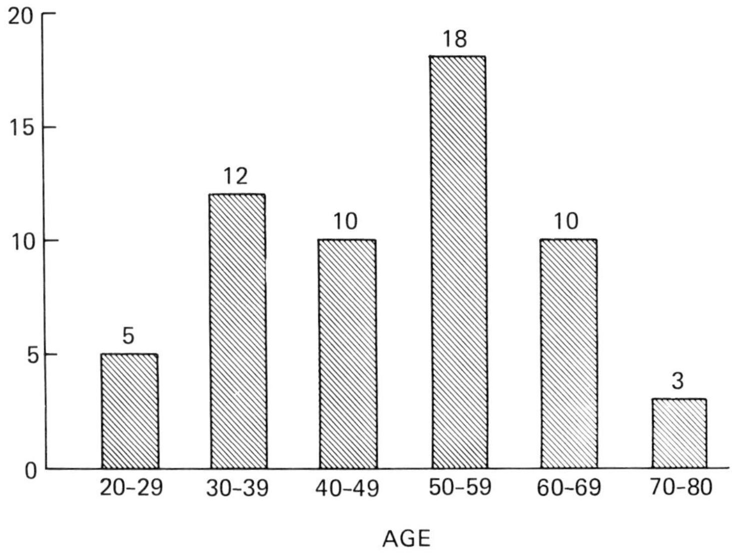

Surgical Revascularization

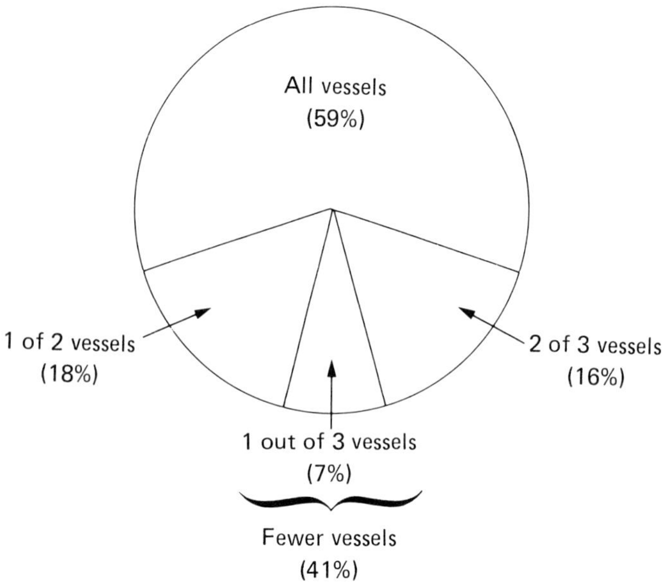

Etiology

ASO	47
Fibrous bands	5
FMD	2
Arteritis	1
Neurofibroma	1

Revascularization

	Vessels	Occlusions
Vein	37	22
Dacron	31	29
PTFE	4	25
Patch	13	15
Endart	8	25
Dilate	1	0
Reimplant	9	22

34% of patients had concomitant aortic or renal artery reconstruction.

Late Recurrence (26.5%)

Number of patients	Vessels grafted	Percent recurrence
4	1/3	50%
8	1/2	50%
7	2/3	29%
9	2/2	11%
9	3/3	11%
12	1/1	25%

Results

Early relief	96.0%
Recurrence	26.5%

6 mo.–10 yr. follow-up; mean of 38 months.

Mesenteric Ischemic Symptom—Weight Loss

Duration:	12.5 months
Range:	1 month–15 years
Weight loss:	32.5 lbs.
Range:	0–109 lbs

Symptoms of Mesenteric Artery Insufficiency

Pain	100%
Weight loss	98%
Bruit	75%
Nausea, vomiting	54%
Diarrhea	38%
Constipation	13%

Vessel Involvement

Celiac, SMA, IMA	41%
Celiac, SMA	29%
SMA, IMA	5%
Celiac, IMA	2%
Celiac	14%
SMA	9%

REFERENCES

1. Skeggs LT, Dorer FE, Kahn Jr, et al.The biochemistry of the renin-angiotensin system and its role in hypertension. Am J Med 60:737–748 (May) 1976.
2. Kaufman JJ. Diseases of the renal vessels. In WF Barker, (ed.), Peripheral Arterial Disease, pp. 303–344. Philadelphia, W. B. Saunders Co., 1975.
3. Simon N, Franklin SS, Bleifer KH, Maxwell MH. Clinical characteristics of renovascular hypertension. JAMA 220(9):1209–1218 (May) 1972.
4. Gross F. The renin-angiotensin system and hypertension. Ann Int Med 75(5):777–787 (Nov) 1971.
5. Bookstein JJ, Abrams HL, Buenger RE, et al. Radiologic aspects of renovascular hypertension: Aims and methods of radiology study group. JAMA 220(9):1218–1224 (May) 1972.
6. Dean RH, Burko H, Wilson JP, et al. Deceptive patterns of renal artery stenosis. Surgery 76(6):872–881 (Dec) 1974.
7. Couch NP, Sullivan J, Crane C. The predictive accuracy of renal vein renin activity in the surgery of renovascular hypertension. Surgery 79(1):70–76 (Jan) 1976.
8. Ernst CB, Stanley JC, Marshall FF, Fry WJ. Autogenous saphenous vein aortorenal grafts: A ten-year experience. Arch Surg 105(6):855–864 (Dec) 1972.
9. Sos TA, Sniderman KW. Percutaneous transluminal angioplasty. Sem in Roent 16(1):28–41 (Jan) 1981.
10. Foster JH, Maxwell MH, Franklin SS, et al. Renovascular occlusive disease. JAMA 231(10):1043–1048 (Mar) 1975.
11. Stanley JC, Fry WJ. Surgical treatment of renovascular hypertension. Arch Surg 112:1291–1297 (Nov) 1977.
12. Stanley JS, Fry WJ. Pediatric renal artery occlusive disease and renovascular hypertension. Arch Surg 116:669–676 (May) 1981.
13. Dean RH, Wilson JP, Burko H, Foster JH. Saphenous vein aortorenal bypass grafts: Serial arteriographic study. Ann Surg 180(r):469–478 (Oct) 1974.
14. Lye CR, String T, Wylie EJ, Stoney RJ. Aortorenal arterial autografts: Late observations. Arch Srug 110:1321–1326 (Nov) 1975.
15. Ernst CB, Stanley JC, Marshall FF, Fry WJ. Renal revascularization for arteriosclerotic renovascular hypertension: Prognostic implications of focal renal arterial vs. overt generalized arteriosclerosis. Surgery 73(6): 859–867 (June) 1973.
16. Novick AC, Straffon RA, Stewart BH, et al. Diminshed operative morbidity and mortality in renal revascularization. JAMA 246(7):749–753 (Aug) 1981.
17. Dean RH, Oates JA, Wilson JP, et al. Bilateral renal artery stenosis and renovascular hypertension. Surgery 81(1):53–62 (Jan) 1977.
18. Hunt HG, Strong CG. Renovascular hypertension. Mechanism, natural history, and treatment. Am J Cardiol 32:562–574 (Sept) 1973.

19. Belzer FO, Salvatierra O, Palubinskas, et al. Ex vivo renal artery reconstruction. Ann Surg 182(4):456–463 (Oct) 1975.
20. Zinman L, Libertino JA. Revascularization of the chronic totally occluded renal artery with restoration of renal function. J Urol 118:517–521 (Oct) 1977.
21. Hollier LH, Bernatz PE, Pairolero PC, et al. Surgical management of chronic intestinal ischemia: A reappraisal. Surgery 90(6):940–946 (Dec) 1981.
22. Bergan JJ, Dry L, Conn J, Trippel O. Intestinal ischemic syndromes. Ann Surg 169(1):120–126 (Jan) 1969.
23. Stoney RJ, Ehrenfeld WK, Wylie EJ. Revascularization methods in chronic visceral ischemia caused by atherosclerosis. Ann Surg 186(4):468–476 (Oct) 1977.
24. McCollum CH, Graham JM, DeBakey ME. Chronic mesenteric arterial insufficiency: Results of revascularization in 33 cases. So Med J 69(10): 1266–1268 (Oct) 1976.
25. Zelenock GB, Graham LM, Whitehouse WM Jr, et al. Splanchnic arteriosclerotic disease and intestinal angina. Arch Surg 115:497–501 (Apr) 1980.
26. Reul GJ Jr, Wukasch DC, Sandiford FM, et al. Surgical treatment of abdominal angina: Review of 25 patients. Surgery 75(5)682–689 (May) 1974.
27. Stoney RJ, Wulie EJ. Recognition and surgical management of visceral ischemic syndromes. Ann Surg 164(4):714–722 (Oct) 1966.
28. Hollier LH. Revascularization of the visceral artery using the pantaloon vein graft. Surg Gynecol Obstet 155:415–416 (Sept) 1982.

7

Vascular Injuries

13
Management of Vascular Injuries

Malcolm O. Perry

INCIDENCE AND ETIOLOGY

Most arterial injuries are the result of penetrating trauma caused by stabbing or gunshot wounds, but some of the more difficult problems are encountered in patients who have sustained blunt trauma [14]. Over half of the injuries in my series were caused by gunshot wounds, and most of the others by stab wounds; blunt trauma was the etiology in only 9% [19]. The peripheral arteries are the most frequently injured, as illustrated in Table 1. The vessels in the extremities are more vulnerable, probably because the arteries are longer and more superficially placed.

Although blunt trauma is a less common cause of arterial injuries than penetrating wounds, such injuries occur with sufficient frequency to be of great concern, especially since their management is often more difficult than the treatment of a simple stab wound or localized gunshot wound [4,9]. In the report by Reynolds and his associates, 46 of 191 arterial injuries were caused by blunt trauma, and of these 13 involved the popliteal artery; the brachial and superficial femoral arteries were injured 6 times each [14]. Killeen examined the records of 1300 patients who had sustained blunt trauma to the abdomen; only in 1 patient was the abdominal aorta injured, but Thal and Dajee et al have reported several cases of blunt trauma with injuries of the abdominal aorta [3,7, 19]. Some of these were thought to be related to the use of automobile seatbelts.

Table 1. Arterial Injuries, Distribution

Extremity	501
Aorta	31
Visceral	37
Cervical	96
Total	665

Connolly estimates that the incidence of arterial injury associated with long bone fracture ranges between 0.6 and 3%; Steer reported only 10 arterial injuries in 655 patients who had fractures or dislocations of the long bones [2,21]. These are extremely serious injuries, however, as emphasized by Lefrak [9]. He followed up 152 patients who had knee dislocations, and found that of the 42 people with popliteal artery injuries, 24 subsequently required amputation. In Snyder's series of 83 popliteal artery injuries 22 of the cases were caused by blunt trauma [18]. Blunt trauma is an uncommon cause of injuries of arteries in the upper extremity. In Flint's 146 cases, only 3% were caused by blunt trauma, and Reul reported that 14% of the arterial wounds of the upper extremity were the result of nonpenetrating injuries [5,13].

MECHANISMS AND TYPES OF INJURY

Major vessels may be injured by direct blows sustained in falls or motor vehicle accidents, but more commonly these wounds are caused by acts of violence. With penetration trauma the artery may be contused, lacerated, transected, or only punctured. The damage produced by knives or low-velocity missiles is usually confined to the wound tract and the adjacent structures, but with high-velocity wounds there may be extensive damage because of the cavitation effect produced by such a missile [12]. Moreover, as the blast cavity collapses there is a powerful suction effect which can draw into the wound surface structures such as dirt, pieces of clothing or bits of skin. These wounds, like those caused by close-range shotgun blasts, often are very difficult to manage because of the extensive destruction of the neurovascular structures and the surrounding soft tissue.

Special problems are encountered when shotgun woulds are treated (see Figure 1). Although the muzzle velocity of shotgun pellets is of a magnitude similar to that produced by the familiar .22 caliber rifle bullet (approximately 1200 feet per second), the dispersion of a large number of pellets from a close-range blast causes serious and widespread damage. The plastic wadding and fillers

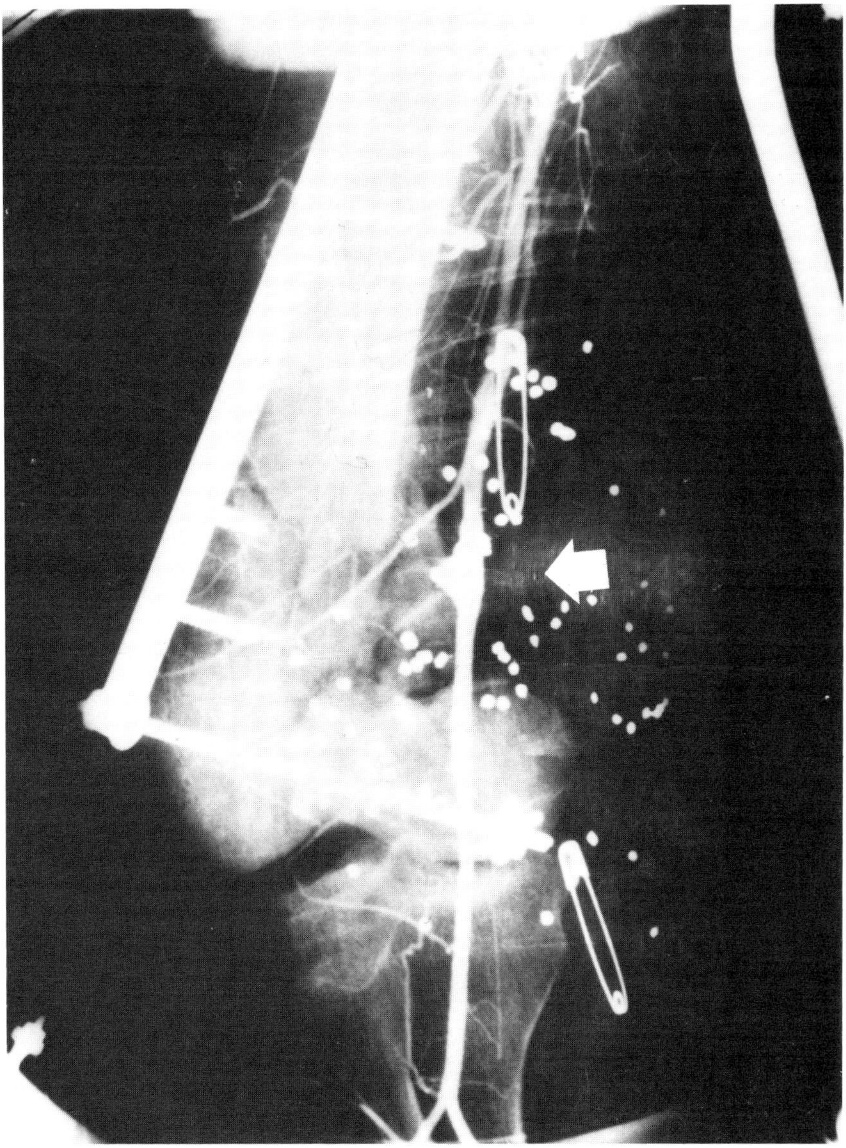

Figure 1. Shotgun injury. From M.O. Perry, *The Management of Acute Vascular Injuries*, Williams and Wilkins, © 1981. Reprinted by permission of the publisher.

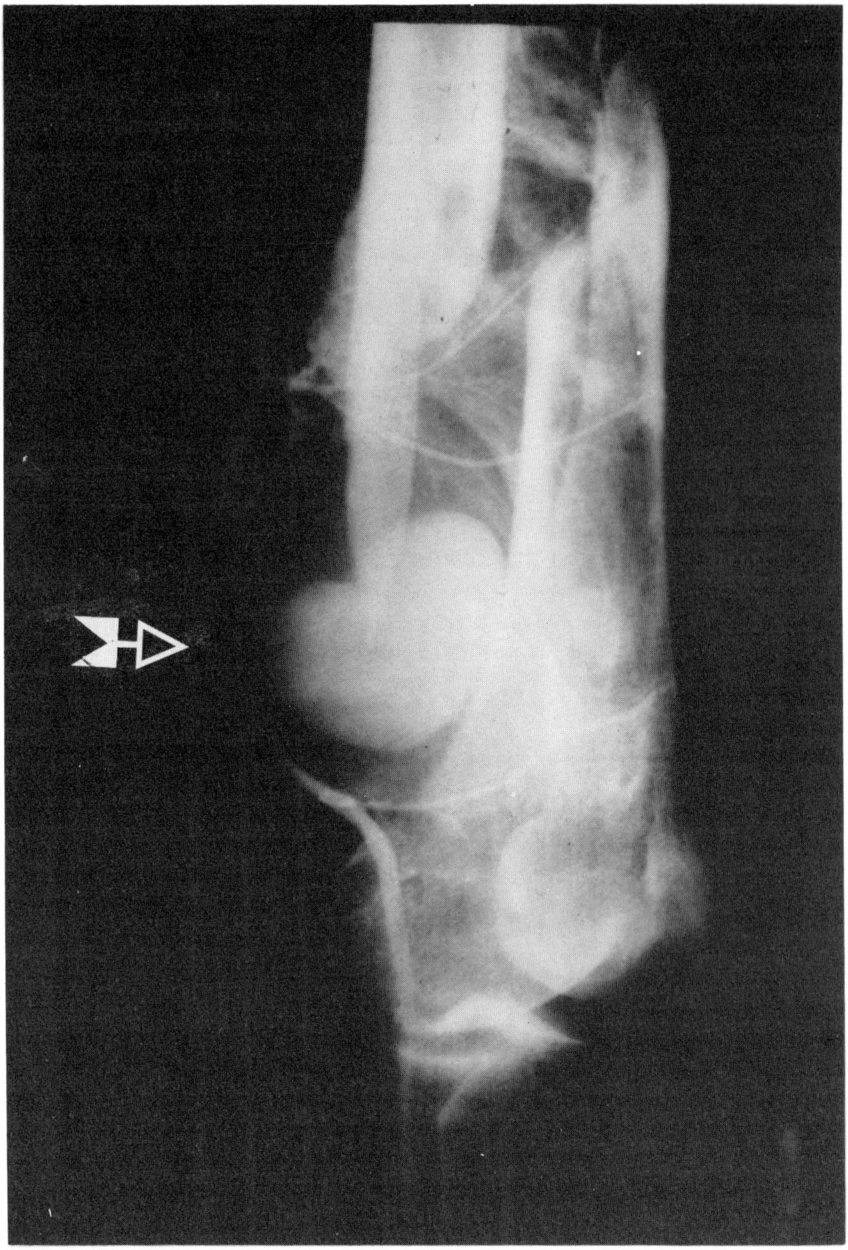

Figure 2. Femur fracture. From M. O. Perry, *The Management of Acute Vascular Injuries*, Williams and Wilkins, © 1981. Reprinted by permission of the publisher.

used in modern shotshell ammunition are less troublesome than the old fiber inserts, but bits of clothing and surface materials may be carried into these wounds, and thus they often are heavily contaminated.

Vascular injuries caused by blunt trauma have increased in frequency and seriousness as automobile freeway traffic grows. Motor vehicle accidents are a major cause of vascular trauma, and the accident victims commonly have multiple injuries. There may be direct vessel trauma, but often the vascular wounds are the result of fractures [2,4]. This is likely to occur where major vessels are adjacent to the long bones, and especially near joints where the vessels are relatively fixed and particularly vulnerable to shear forces. Even if the vessel is not injured directly by the blow, the bony fragments from a fracture may lacerate the artery or the pieces of bone may become secondary missiles and even damage remote vascular structures. The bending and sudden break of large, heavy bones such as the femur or tibia releases tremendous forces, and the damage to soft tissue and neurovascular structures is often extensive. The effects can be similar to those produced by the cavitation associated with high-velocity bullets, and after the bones fall back into near normal position the magnitude of the injuring forces may not be appreciated and the severity of damage is likely to be underestimated [9]. (See Figure 2.)

Fracture dislocations at the knee are especially likely to produce serious vascular injuries, as described by Lefrak and Dart [4,9]. The popliteal arteries are particularly vulnerable to these forces because they are relatively fixed proximally by the adductor muscles of the thigh and distally by the soleus muscle. The collateral arteries making up the genicular system are small and relatively fragile, and with dislocations or fractures they are easily torn. In the course of evaluating a patient involved in a motor vehicle accident, it is very easy to miss an unstable knee, especially when the patient has more dramatic injuries which take precedence during resuscitation. In such patients a contused artery which was initially patent is likely to clot if hypotension persists or if treatment is delayed. In these situations propagation of the clot can produce severe and intractable ischemia of the lower extremity.

CLINICAL FEATURES

Injuries of large arteries usually can be identified readily because of severe hemorrhage, but less extensive wounds may not be so evident. Ischemia distal to the area of the arterial injury may not be present, especially if there are intervening collateral vessels which supply adequate flow, and if the patient is not hypotensive. Except for injuries of the common femoral and popliteal arteries this is the usual picture; ischemia is not commonly seen in patients with injuries

Table 2. Arterial Injuries, Clinical Features

Diminshed or absent pulse
Major hemorrhage with hypotension
Large or expanding hematoma
Bruit at or distal to injury
Anatomically related neurological defect
Proximity of injury to major vessel

of the superficial, profunda femoral or brachial arteries. If ischemia is present it is an important finding, but its absence does not preclude a significant vascular wound [18,19].

In most patients with arterial injuries, the signs and symptoms listed in Table 2 usually establish the diagnosis without delay. Most of these patients will have deficiencies in the distal pulses. The pulse wave is a pressure wave, however, and reaches velocities up to 10 meters per second. It can be transmitted beyond intimal flaps, through limited areas of soft, fresh clot, and via the collateral circulation to the distal extremity [12]. The flow wave has a velocity of approximately 40 cm per second, and is distinct from the pulse wave. The physical examination must take this discrepancy into account. With anatomical provisions for flow through the collaterals, and with some injuries limited only to vessel wall damage or to secondary vessels in the extremities, it is not surprising that distal pulses have been found to be relatively normal in between 10% and 20% of patients with operatively proven arterial injuries [19].

Patients who have a deficit in distal pulses, a large hematoma, persistent hemorrhage or ischemia are very likely to have a serious vascular wound, and the diagnosis is easy to establish in these situations. It is more difficult when the patient has multiple injuries, or when the vascular wound is the result of blunt trauma, and there is widespread damage to bones and soft tissue. This makes the clinical examination more complicated, and if there is an associated nerve injury neuromuscular function may be quite difficult to assess.

When arterial injuries are associated with fractures of the long bones, or dislocations of the knee or elbow, ischemia is a common finding. In fact, in the 22 cases of blunt trauma from Snyder's series of popliteal artery injuries only one patient presented without ischemia, and overall 60% of the 83 patients had ischemia, regardless of the etiology [18]. One of the major problems in the assessment of these patients is the tendency of the examiners to assign the ischemia to external compression, spasm, or other factors rather than arterial occlusion. This misconception can result in untoward delays in establishing the diagnosis, and in initiating proper therapy, and thus may permit propagation of a clot which can unfavorably alter the situation.

Patients with wounds of large intra-abdominal vessels often have only the presence of a penetrating wound, hypotension and perhaps abdominal distension to indicate the seriousness of the problem. Usually there is little difficulty in establishing the diagnosis, but occasionally the wound may be small and benign in appearance, and there may be doubt as to whether a major injury exists. This is particularly likely in people with small stab wounds that pass between the ribs. In most cases, bleeding, or other intracavitary wounds suggest the need for immediate operation.

Radiographic examination of the chest and abdomen may disclose free air, displacement of viscera, and intraperitoneal fluid. In many cases, these studies are of little help, however, and surgical exploration is needed.

ADJUNCTIVE DIAGNOSTIC PROCEDURES

The detection of Doppler signals and the measurement of distal arterial systolic blood pressure by the Doppler or any of a variety of plethysmographic techniques are very helpful, but the specificity of these tests is limited by the same hemodynamic features which govern the pulse wave and blood flow [12]. It is common to note subtle abnormalities in these measurements when examining patients with vascular injuries, but relatively normal values are also seen, thus compromising the reliability of these methods for excluding vascular wounds. This may be a particular problem in the patient who has multiple injuries and who also has hypotension from other causes.

Arteriography may be especially useful in the evaluation of vascular wounds when a patient presents with equivocal signs, and the wound tract is in proximity to major vascular structures [20]. (See Table 3.) In a study of 143 patients with penetrating wounds of the extremities, high grade biplane arteriography was found to be very reliable in detecting the presence of major arterial injuries [17]. Arteriograms are not infallible, however, and may be especially misleading in attempting to evaluate injuries to the great vessels around the thoracic outlet, the shoulder girdle and the hip. It is difficult to obtain good biplane projections in these areas, and it requires many views to avoid overlapping the vessel images.

Table 3. Indications for Arteriography

Blunt trauma, fractures
Penetrating injuries, chest
Cervical injuries—base of skull
Assessment multiple pellet wounds
Injuries forearm, leg

Small puncture wounds and tangential wounds of the arteries can be missed in these situations if there is no extravasation of contrast material. Although arteriography is usually reliable, false negatives do occur, and the arteriogram must be used in concert with the clinical evaluation and the other functional tests.

When firm indications for operation are present arteriograms may be unnecessary, and untoward delay is undesirable. In fact, if the patient is unstable, further evaluation is best performed in the operating room. Such patients should not be sent to the x-ray suite unattended, where they may experience cardiovascular collapse. If there is some doubt as to the distribution and the nature of the injuries, an arteriogram can be performed in the operating room during preparation for surgery or even during the operative procedure, if the question arises after the exploration has begun.

The Seldinger arteriographic technique is very popular because many areas of the arterial tree can be inspected via a single arterial entry, but direct arterial puncture continues to be useful in many cases. This is especially true in the extremities when one wishes to evaluate the femoral-popliteal system after the patient is in the operating room. The common femoral artery can be punctured directly with an 18 gauge arteriogram needle. Approximately 30 ml of iothalamate is injected and the films exposed just as the infusion is finished. This will produce satisfactory pictures of the femoral, popliteal and tibial system, and can be of great assistance both in diagnosis and in planning the operative procedure.

PRIORITIES AND RESUSCITATION

The management of trauma patients is often a stern test of the discipline and training of the responsible surgeon. The patient with multiple injuries presents dramatically: bleeding, pale, short of breath, and often with a low blood pressure. A successful resuscitation requires that certain priorities be established, and specific plans of treatment formulated. (See Table 4.) Once control of the airway has been secured, the vital signs assessed, and the overall evaluation completed, the priorities can be set. All of the injuries should be identified, and if external bleeding is present, it usually can be controlled with

Table 4. Priorities in Management

Airway, bleeding, resuscitation
Venous access upper and lower extremities
Stabilize fractures
Serious associated injuries—head, chest

direct finger pressure, pressure dressing, or pressure on proximal vascular structures. Tourniquets are rarely if ever needed; if they are misapplied they are likely to increase the blood loss. No attempt should be made to blindly clamp bleeding vessels located deep in the wound, because this is very likely to cause further nerve or vascular damage, and moreover, it is usually ineffective. In some instances the MAST suit (G Suit) has been used successfully to control bleeding, and assist in raising arterial blood pressure while definitive surgery is begun, but of course this may not be possible with lower extremity wounds.

The trauma patient often has impressive fluid and blood requirements, and adequate venous access lines are needed. Large catheters are placed into uninjured upper and lower extremity veins, and carefully secured. During the selection of veins for fluid resuscitation the possibility of an injury to the inferior vena cava should be considered, and the lines should be placed to insure that the solution can reach the general circulation; it may be necessary to occlude the vein proximal to the line to control bleeding.

One of these lines is committed only for fluid replacement; it is not used for drug administration or anesthetic manipulations. If hemorrhage is severe the rate of blood replacement will have to be rapid and continuous. There may be a need for the use of venous autografts for reconstruction, and thus it is often prudent to preserve the saphenous or cephalic veins for use as arterial grafts.

In the majority of trauma patients the combination of a balanced electrolyte solution such as lactated Ringer's and whole blood is chosen for resuscitation. As described by Shires et al, trauma and shock induce internal shifts of extracellular fluid, which are best treated by appropriate electrolyte infusions [17]. Blood loss is replaced with blood, but it is wise not to overtransfuse, especially if cardiac disease is present, or if the patient has had cardiopulmonary trauma.

Rheologic and oxygen transport studies suggest that a whole blood hematocrit of approximately 30% is optimum, and that further increases of hemoglobin are unneeded and may increase blood viscosity unnecessarily. There are little convincing data suggesting that the infusion of colloid solutions at this stage is of any additional value, and some studies suggest that giving such solutions may be harmful, and increase the likelihood of fluid overload [16,22].

PREPARATION FOR SURGERY

Fractures should be stabilized to prevent further damage to neurovascular and muscular structures, and splints, semirigid dressings, skeletal pins and traction are usually employed. The ultimate plan of repair must be considered while these devices are being put in place, and many surgeons prefer some form of external fixation as a final solution to fracture treatment, but this may not always be possible [21]. Other studies have reported little difference in the infection rate, ultimate healing or complications seen in patients who had either internal or external bone fixation, but the consensus of opinion favors the use of external methods whenever possible [2]. The extent of soft-tissue damage, the adequacy of debridement and the treatment of associated wounds appear to play an important role in the results obtained in these situations, and it is difficult to assign responsibility for a specific complication to a single factor such as the method of bone fixation.

In patients with vascular injuries caused by fractures it is usually preferable to repair the major vessels first, and then to fix the bone, but this may not always be feasible. If the limb is to be shortened and the repair can be completed without untoward delay it is often easier to complete the orthopedic repairs and the debridement, and then to reestablish blood flow, but if distal ischemia is present the vascular repairs must take precedence. Injuries of the popliteal artery which also involve the collateral circulation are associated with reduced distal blood flow, and ischemia is often a problem. Temporary inlying shunts can be introduced into the popliteal artery and vein to restore flow while extensive orthopedic maneuvers are being completed [19]. Regardless of the priority that is established for the repair of the vessels and the orthopedic maneuvers, the vascular surgeon should remain in attendance during these reconstructive efforts in order to insure that the arterial and venous repairs remain patent while the other injuries are being treated.

When multiple wounds are present, and especially if fractures and other injuries are to be treated, several incisions may be needed. If these are poorly placed the intervening tissue may be devitalized, important collateral vessels may be divided unnecessarily and the final skin cover may be difficult to arrange. In some cases orthopedic and vascular repairs can be performed through common approaches, and secondary surgical trauma can be minimized. This is especially important when vascular insufficiency may become a problem or when the patient has multiple wounds, or in the older patient who has established atherosclerotic disease with limited collateral potential. When a vascular injury is associated with extensive soft tissue damage, as seen in avulsive wounds and close-range shotgun blasts, wide debridement will be required. In such situations it may be necessary to relocate the reconstructed artery to restore blood flow to the distal extremity, and exploratory incisions should keep these areas clean. In other cases remote subcutaneous bypasses may be needed prior to completion of debridement in order to prevent contamination of the selected areas and to restore blood flow. Meticulous care in opening and handling these incisions is essential if secondary infections of these grafts are to be avoided.

Prophylactic antibiotic administration is considered appropriate in many trauma cases, and antibiotics are widely used in elective vascular surgery, although the practice is not supported by unequivocal data [12,14]. It is generally agreed that if antibiotics are to be employed tissue and blood levels of the drug must be obtained preoperatively if the regimen is to be effective. Since wound contamination with trauma is likely, such drugs may be of help in reducing the incidence of infection, especially when separate incisions are to be made for other procedures, such as subcutaneous or remote bypass grafting. Semisynthetic penicillin or cefazolin are often recommended in these situations, and are usually begun just before surgery, and stopped on the first or second postoperative day.

Careful closure of such wounds is always required; the tissue should be handled gently, debridement should be adequate and closure should be performed without foreign bodies, dead space, hematomas or tension. A separate closure of fascial layers is desirable in order to interpose a tissue barrier between the repaired vessel and the skin in the event that superficial infection intervenes. Skin incisions in the groin seem to be more vulnerable to infection, and therefore it is especially important to close the femoral sheath and fascia separately from the skin and subcutaneous tissues. Drains are not commonly employed in vascular operations, but they may be used in selected cases to prevent the local accumulation of blood and serum. There is little rationale in inserting drains for control of infection because this complication is usually delayed, and the drains ordinarily will not be left in place for longer than 24 hours.

The majority of vascular repairs do not require limb splinting because the vessels are repaired without tension, and due regard to joint motion is a part of the operative planning. Associated fractures may force changes in this policy, but the splinting must be tailored to the specific situation encountered. When splints are applied, the risk of compressing vascular repairs with circumferential dressings must be kept in mind. If limb swelling is a threat, such dressings are best avoided.

Early exercise is recommended after a vascular repair in the extremities if there are no contraindications because of bone or soft tissue wounds. If ambulation is not possible a rigorous program of sequential leg exercises is advised to reduce venous stasis and to minimize muscle and joint dysfunction. Ambulation should be encouraged as pain permits, and in most cases walking is not limited by the type of vascular repair performed.

METHODS OF REPAIR

The repair of vascular wounds should be performed in the operating room under general anesthesia in most situations. Control of bleeding is usually obtained with direct digital pressure or pressure dressings. An unstable patient is taken immediately to the operating room, where preoperative preparations are completed. The patient is placed in the supine position, and in most cases vertical incisions are employed, since they can be extended in either direction, and they are parallel to the associated nerves and veins, which should be preserved during the operation.

The extremities are draped to permit proximal and distal extension, and if there are injuries near the shoulder girdle or the hip, the abdomen and chest are also prepared in case it becomes necessary to open the body cavities to obtain proximal control of the vessels.

With injuries in the root of the neck below the sixth cervical vertebra (C6), it is often prudent to open the chest through a middle sternotomy incision at the beginning of the operation, and obtain control of the innominate, common carotid and subclavian vessels if it is thought that injuries of one of the great vessels exist [5,13]. If the wounds are in the supraclavicular area of the neck above C6, local extrathoracic incisions are satisfactory for exposure and repair, although it may be necessary in some cases to remove the medial half of the clavicle in order to expose the second portion of the subclavian artery. Injuries of the first portion of the subclavian artery require thoracotomy.

The abdomen is explored through a midline incision from xiphoid to pubis. A thorough exploration is performed first, then priorities of repair are set, and organs with more susceptibility to hypoxia revascularized first.

Exposure and control of the common femoral artery is usually quite direct and requires only a vertical incision in the femoral triangle, but if there is a large, obscuring hematoma it may be advisable to approach the external iliac artery through a muscle-splitting incision parallel to the inguinal ligament, and then the surgeon can place a tape or vascular clamp on the external iliac artery before the hematoma in the groin is entered. With injuries in the extremities distal to the femoral canal, exposure and control is usually straightforward and can be obtained through the standard vertical incisions. If there is a great deal of deformity of the distal extremity because of multiple wounds, fractures or shotgun blasts, it may be helpful to place an orthopedic tourniquet over the proximal portion of the thigh, and if difficulty is encountered in obtaining adequate control, inflation of the tourniquet will limit the bleeding.

Once the vessel is isolated, the method of repair will be dictated by the type of injury. Since most of the injuries are lacerations or transections, resection and anastomosis are usually favored. In the femoral, brachial and popliteal arteries sufficient mobilization allows resection of a 1 or 2 cm segment or artery and a direct end-to-end anastomosis. If that is not the case, interposition of an autogenous graft, usually the greater saphenous vein taken from the ankle, is preferred. It is not often possible in arteries of this size to obtain a satisfactory tangential repair of a laceration without narrowing the vessel, so resection and anastomosis or interposition grafting is recommended in most cases.

The selection of the suture material is largely the choice of the operating surgeon, but there is an increasing tendency by many surgeons to use the synthetic materials (such as Dacron, teflon or polypropylene) since these sutures have a great deal of tensile strength, and they are less reactive than the natural fibers. Continuous simple sutures are generally employed in vascular surgical operations and are satisfactory for use in large vessels, but in arteries of 4 mm or less diameter it is preferable to use interrupted simple sutures. This is particularly important in young patients, and in children in whom vessels can be expected to grow, but it is also useful in many other patients, since at the time of repair the vessel frequently is somewhat smaller than it will be following restoration of adequate blood pressure.

ANTICOAGULATION

Most vascular surgeons utilize systemic heparinization during the repair of small arteries, and a few surgeons also administer low-molecular-weight dextran during and after the operation. There are few data to support one method over the other, but most surgeons will use some form of anticoagulation when performing small vessel repair, although they do not continue the drug beyond a few days postoperatively [1,6,14,18].

Interoperative heparin is used in a great number of vascular operations and it is given in an almost endless variety of regimens. In most patients who have only a single isolated vascular injury the intravenous administration of 3500 to 5000 USP units of heparin will give satisfactory protection during the time of the repair. If the patient has multiple injuries, or if there are associated wounds of the brain, retina, or spinal cord, it is probably best to irrigate locally with a solution containing 100 units of heparin per 10 milliliters of saline. This infusion will usually retard local thrombosis and permit completion of the vascular repair. Despite the use of anticoagulation, routine Fogarty catheter exploration of the vessels proximal and distal to the injury is an important adjunctive maneuver since the presence of backbleeding is no guarantee that distal thrombosis has not occurred. The blood may be returned to the operative area via intervening collateral systems. Following the arterial repair there is usually no indication to continue full systemic anticoagulation during the post-operative period.

ASSESSMENT OF REPAIR

Clinical evaluation of the patency of a vascular repair is usually straightforward, and basically consists of observing arterial flow past the repaired area, palpation of distal pulses, and inspection of the distal extremity.

Because of the hemodynamic features controlling arterial blood flow, it is apparent that adequacy of the distal flow may not be insured by the presence of a pulse, as described in the section on diagnosis, but it is unusual for an arterial repair followed by the immediate reappearance of distal pulses to fail. More commonly, the surgeon may find that after what appears to be a satisfactory arterial repair, the distal pulses are weak or not present, and the question then becomes where is the occlusion. In most cases if pulses are not immediately reestablished there is an intraluminal obstruction, usually a distal clot, and unless this can be located and extracted easily an operative arteriogram is needed. In patients who have multiple injuries and who remain hypotensive, distal pulses and Doppler signals may be absent even in the presence of an adequate repair. This is especially true if the body core temperature is reduced and if resuscitation is not yet complete. In these situations, an operative arteriogram is needed regardless of the findings and many vascular surgeons routinely perform such studies in every case.

Regardless of the method that is chosen to evaluate the vascular reconstruction, a basic examination of function remains the most important. It has been repeatedly observed that even patients with normal distal pulses can have significant ischemic problems because of small vessel obstruction. Therefore, testing for the perception of light touch and evaluating the adequacy of muscular function are important maneuvers in the postoperative period. If a patient has disturbances in light touch and motor function, especially of the intrinsic muscles of the extremity, further studies are required, and this usually means that an arteriogram is needed. The noninvasive techniques for assessing blood flow cannot be depended upon to adequately examine the situation. The skin and subcutaneous tissues may survive a degree of ischemia which will prove to be lethal to underlying muscles and nerves, and careful evaluation of neuromuscular function is mandatory regardless of pulses, arterial pressure, skin color or warmth [12].

ADJUNCTIVE METHODS

Management of Spasm

Arterial spasm is often seen in patients with vascular trauma, and in rare cases may be responsible for stasis and thrombosis. In most situations when spasm is thought to be the cause of poor distal flow following a vascular repair, arteriography almost invariably reveals clots. If there is some question as to distal patency, an operative arteriogram will usually reveal the vessels to be open; there may be irregular areas of narrowing, but smooth patency of the intimal surface is seen. In these situations, the spasm will resolve over the ensuing hours, Doppler signals will become stronger, blood pressure will rise, and subsequently pulses become palpable.

Table 5. Indications for Fasciotomy

Combined arterial and venous injury
Massive soft tissue damage
Delay between wounding and definitive repair
Prolonged hypotension
Swelling of extremity

In rare cases, as reported by Kinmouth, spasm can be relentless and it may be necessary to employ other methods of treatment [8]. Mechanical or hydraulic dilation appear to be most effective, but a number of drugs have been recommended. A 2.5% solution of papaverine applied directly to the artery may be useful. Additionally, 10-15 mg of papaverine can be injected into the artery. Other drugs have been recommended, but there is no consensus of opinion as to their usefulness [19]. Most of these patients will respond quite satisfactorily to local dilatation, and patience.

Fasciotomy

Patman and his associates recommend that fasciotomy be considered for the conditions listed in Table 5 [11]. It is clear that if fasciotomy is to be performed, it should be accomplished before irreversible muscle and nerve damage occurs. Recent studies by Matsen have done much to clarify the indications for fasciotomy, but these studies must be used in concert with the clinical findings [10]. Matsen has demonstrated when the compartmental pressure exceeds 45 mm of mercury, cell damage is likely to occur unless decompression is done. If fasciotomy is performed on the basis of these pressure measurements, or because of hypesthesia in the forefoot, and before obvious swelling has occurred, the results are quite good. When fasciotomy is delayed until the extremity is massively swollen, or until there have been prolonged disturbances in neuromuscular function, fasciotomy is likely to be of less benefit; muscle debridement is often necessary, and long-term disability may be severe.

The techniques of decompression as described by Patman have been widely used. The anterior compartment of the leg, bounded by relatively rigid fascial sheaths, is more vulnerable than the others and it is most often involved. When swelling is minimal or absent, adequate fasciotomy can be performed through limited skin incisions, which then can be closed primarily. If this is not possible, or if there is significant swelling of the skin and subcutaneous tissue, wide dermotomy may be required. Long incisions are necessary in these limbs to decompress all the muscle compartments. In some cases, resection of 8-10 cm of the shaft of the fibula may be needed to insure adequate decompression of the deep muscle compartments. Such incisions should be carefully protected from contamination, and it is best to close them early, either secondarily with sutures or tape, or by applying skin grafts. Such open wounds are a potential portal of entry for infection and early cover is needed to minimize this risk.

In managing wounds of the popliteal, femoral and tibial arteries, it is common for fasciotomies to be performed in conjunction with the exploratory incisions; this is almost invariably the case when simultaneous popliteal and tibial injury exists. If there is any question as to the adequacy of the fasciotomy created as the result of the exploratory incision, it is a simple matter to extend the fasciotomy distally prior to skin closure.

VEIN INJURIES

Although there continues to be some controversy about the importance of repairing venous injuries, the data presented by Rich and his colleagues strongly support simultaneous repair of the popliteal or common femoral veins when there are combined injuries [15]. In fact, in Rich's study of over 200 popliteal vein injuries, when repair was undertaken thromboembolic events occurred in only 13%. In contrast, over half of the patients who had ligation of the popliteal vein ultimately had thromboembolic complications.

Moreover, several authors believe simultaneous repair of the popliteal vein enhances patency rates of a popliteal artery repair [14,18,19]. In most situations resection of the damaged vein and end-to-end anastomosis is used, and although long-term patency varies among the reported series, venous insufficiency is less, and limb salvage appears better with primary repair of both vessels.

Wounds of the inferior vena cava and other major abdominal veins are serious and often lethal injuries. Although aggressive operative management of the problems has reduced the mortality rate in IVC injuries to 11% when only the lower vena cava is damaged, multiple venous injuries are common. Moreover, in caval wounds at or above the renal veins, a mortality rate of over 50% is seen, reflecting the magnitude of the hemorrhage, and the difficulty in obtaining control.

In patients who have sustained penetrating abdominal trauma, retroperitoneal hematomas which are above the brim of the pelvis, and centrally placed over the great vessels should be explored, and the major vessels repaired. In contrast, the pelvic hematoma from a fractured pelvis is best left undisturbed, unless there are specific indications to enter it to repair known injuries of other organs or major vessels.

REFERENCES

1. Bergentz SE, Hansson LO, Norback B. Surgical management of complications of arterial puncture. Ann Surg 164:1021–1025, 1966.
2. Connolly J. Management of fractures associated with arterial injuries. Amer J Surg 120:331–334, 1977.
3. Dajee H, Richardson ITN, Iype MO. Seatbelt aorta: acute dissection and thrombosis of the abdominal aorta. Surg 85:263–267, 1979.
4. Dart CH, Braitman HE. Popliteal artery injury following fracture or dislocation at the knee. Arch Surg 112:969–973, 1977.
5. Flint LM, Snyder WH, Perry MO, Shires GT. Management of major vascular injuries in the base of the neck. Arch Surg 106:407–413, 1973.
6. Karmody AM, Lempert N, Jarmolych J. The pathology of postcatheterization brachial artery occlusion. J Surg Res 20:601–606, 1976.
7. Killeen DA. Injuries of the SMA vessels secondary to non-penetrating abdominal trauma. Ann Surg 30:306, 1964.
8. Kinmouth JB. Physiology and relief of traumatic arterial spasm. Br Med J 1:59–65, 1952.
9. Lefrac EA. Knee dislocation, Arch Surg 111:1021–1024, 1976.
10. Matsen F. Compartmental syndromes. Hosp Prac 15:113–117, 1980.
11. Patman RD. Fasciotomy: indications and techniques. In RR Rutherford (ed.), Vascular Surgery, Chapter 50. Philadelphia, W. B. Saunders and Co., 1979.
12. Perry MO. Acute vascular insufficiency. In RR Rutherford (ed.), Vascular Surgery, Chapter 46. Philadelphia, W. B. Saunders and Co., 1977.
13. Reul GJ, Beall AC, Jordon G, Mattox KL. The early operative management of injuries to the great vessels. Surg 74:862–873, 1973.
14. Reynolds RR, McDowell HA, Deithelm AG. The surgical treatment of arterial injuries in the civilian population. Ann Surg 189:700–707, 1979.
15. Rich N, Spencer F. Venous injuries. In Vascular Trauma, Chapter 8. Philadelphia. W. B. Saunders and Co., 1978.
16. Sher MH. Principles in the management of arterial injuries associated with fracture dislocations. Ann Surg 182:630–635, 1975.
17. Shires GT, Canizaro PE, Carrico CJ. Shock. In SI Schwartz (ed.), Principles of Surgery, Chapter 4. New York, McGraw-Hill Co., 1979.
18. Snyder WH, Thal ER, Bridges RA, Fry WJ, Perry MO. The validity of normal arteriography in penetrating trauma. Arch Surg 113:424, 1978.
19. Snyder WH, Watkins WL, Whidden LL, Bono GE. Civilian popliteal artery trauma: an eleven year experience with eighty three injuries. Surg 85:101–108, 1979.
20. Thal ER, Perry MO. Peripheral and abdominal vascular injuries. In RR Rutherford (ed.), Vascular Surgery, Chapter 48. Philadelphia, W. B. Saunders and Co., 1977.

21. Thal ER, Snyder WH, Hays RJ, Perry MO. Management of carotid artery injuries. Surg 76:955-962, 1974.
22. Weaver DW, Ledserwood AM, Lucas CE, et al. Pulmonary effects of albumin resuscitation for severe hypovolemic shock. Arch Surg 113:387, 1978.

8

Transluminal Angioplasty

14
Transluminal Angioplasty: History and Current State

Charles T. Dotter

Nearly two decades have passed since the first trial of transluminal angioplasty and the birth of interventional angioplasty [1]. Fortunately, the effort was successful. Transluminal angioplasty has weathered general skepticism to emerge as an accepted, successful method for treating arteriosclerotic ischemia–nuclear weapons notwithstanding, the worst threat to man's health at this time. Based on the number of dilating catheters sold last year, the assumption that one in ten served as a successful alternative to aortofemoral bypass grafting, angioplasty may have saved 500 lives and $200,000,000!

Clearly, where transluminal angioplasty can be done with equal or greater safety, it is now the procedure of choice for the relief of atherosclerotic obstruction. For this statement to be valid, the results of angioplasty should approximate those of surgery. That they are became a matter of record in 1982, when immediate and long-term success rates were collected from 12 major centers (Table 1). These results are comparable to those of vascular surgery, despite the fact that transluminal angioplasty is often done on "salvage" patients whose disease or general medical condition contraindicates surgery. Unlike vascular surgery, transluminal angioplasty is a relatively new technique, and many of

Table 1. Transluminal Angioplasty: Collective Summary of Results, May 1982

	No. treated	Percent immediate success	Percent long-term success	Complications	No. deaths
Femoropopliteal	2,337	87%	69%–5 yrs.	2%	3
Iliac	1,725	93%	84%–3 yrs.	1.2%	1
Renal	792	95%[a] 91%[b]	78%–2 yrs. 57%–4 yrs.	2.1%	0
Total	4,854			<2%	4

[a]Fibromuscular dysplasia
[b]Arteriosclerosis

those performing it have not yet had time to gain optimal technical skills. If transluminal angioplasty fails, it rarely precludes or prejudices the outcome of a subsequent surgical effort; when the dilating catheter succeeds—as it does in 80-90%—it obviates the need for the scalpel.

Transluminal angioplasty was initially confined to treating larger arteries of the pelvis and legs. With Grüntzig's development in 1976 of an improved balloon dilating catheter [2], angioplasty became feasible in smaller, less directly accessible arteries, including renal and coronary ones. There followed a near-explosive increase in interest and use of the technique. From 1964 through 1973, 15 scientific reports on transluminal angioplasty were published; from 1974 through 1982, at least 700 reports have appeared. The titles of these reports indicate that an important accelerant was the previously lacking enthusiasm of cardiologists.

The first patient ever treated by percutaneous transluminal angioplasty was an 83-year-old lady with gangrene who refused amputation, thereby providing an opportunity to try it. A localized 95% stenosis in her popliteal artery was easily dilated, her gangrene healed spontaneously, and her leg stayed on until she died of untreated coronary narrowing nearly three years later. The first iliac dilation (and the first use of a balloon catheter for angioplasty) was done in 1965. Follow-up angiography over 14 years later revealed continuing patency; clinically, it is still open 18 years after the initial procedure! Details of the recorded history of transluminal angioplasty are available through its extensive bibliography [3]. So much for the past; the future is even more exciting.

Some day we will find medical means for preventing or relieving atherosclerotic disease. Until then, transluminal angioplasty will play an important role. Future improvements will result from the experiences and innovations of others. Selective clot lysis will play a supporting role, utilizing streptokinase or urokinase. With the aid of a three-dimensional computer-enhanced image guidance and future special purpose catheters, we may learn how to do percutaneous transluminal embolectomy and endarterectomy; perhaps even heart valve replacement.

REFERENCES

1. Dotter CT, Judkins MP. Transluminal treatment of arteriosclerotic obstruction: Description of a new technique and a preliminary report of its application. Circulation 30:654–670, 1964.
2. Grüntzig A. Die perkutane Rekanalisation chronischer arterieller Verschlusse (Dotter-Prinzip) mit einem neuen doppellumigen Dilatationskatheter. Rofo 124(1):80–86, Jan 1974.

3. Dotter CT, Ruble EJ. Transluminal angioplasty, a comprehensive, chronological bibliography, 1964–1982. Proceedings of second symposium on percutaneous transluminal angioplasty, Nürnberg, May 1982. Ed, Zeitler, E. Springer-Verlag, Berlin, 1983.

15
Percutaneous Transluminal Angioplasty (PTA) for Limb Salvage in Severe Leg Ischemia

Ernst Schneider

This chapter gives primary and six months results after PTA for limb salvage in 173 patients (61 men, 112 women, mean age 75 years, 51% diabetics) with ischemic rest pain with or without gangrene. The patients were selected by clinical, noninvasive and angiographic criteria: rest pain depending on reclining position without (stage III) or with ischemic acral necrosis (stage IV) after long-lasting claudication, severely pathological or no pulse tracing from the toes, systolic pressure (Doppler) below 60 mmHg in the ankle arteries, and angiographically proved multilevel occlusive disease with occlusion of at least two calf arteries. The main parameter for successful therapy was primary limb salvage and the preservation of the threatened extremities over at least six months. In 137 patients (79%) out of the whole group of 173 and in 112 (77%) of 146 with complete 6-month follow-up, PTA was primarily successful; that means that at least one hemodynamically important arterial segment could be reopened, resulting in a clinical improvement and a decrease of the arm-ankle pressure gradient of 20 mmHg or more. In fact, PTA could reopen an average of 1.6 occluded segments/patient of the angiographically verified 2.5 occluded levels/patient. In 34 patients, the procedure failed. In 16 of them, surgical revascularization was possible; whereas in 18, primary amputation could not be avoided. Six months later, 17 successfully treated legs had to be amputated too. During the follow-up period of six months, 22 patients (15%) died, 124 were alive, 99 (80%) with preserved and 25 (20%) with amputated legs. PTA alone saved 82, PTA combined with surgery 2 more, and surgery alone 15 after primary failure of PTA of these 99 legs. Seven deaths were probably directly related to major amputation.

Thus, PTA is an efficient, less invasive therapeutic procedure, which should be considered whenever an amputation of an ischemic leg seems inevitable, especially in high-risk patients for extensive vascular surgery.

PRIMARY RESULTS AFTER PERCUTANEOUS TRANSLUMINAL ANGIOPLASTY (PTA) COMBINED WITH LOCAL FIBRINOLYSIS (LTL) IN LEG ARTERY OCCLUSION

In 71 patients with leg artery occlusion (34 men, 37 women, mean age 70 years), 76 LTL combined with PTA and 4 LTL alone were performed. Twenty-nine patients had typical intermittent claudication (stage II), whereas 42 suffered from ischemic rest pain with or without acral necrosis (stage III and IV). The mean age of occlusion was 36 days (1 day–5 months). Eighty occluded arterial segments were treated: 3 iliac, 66 femoropopliteal, and 11 crural occlusions. The mean occlusion length was 11.8 cm (1–30 cm). In 13 cases streptokinase (SK) and in 67 urokinase (UK) was injected through the end hole of an angiographic catheter into the occluding thrombus or embolus in a mean dosage of 1,000U SK or 15,000U UK/cm occlusion length. Once the thrombotic part of an occlusion is lysed, the atherosclerotic stenosis can be dilated by PTA in the same session. Seventy occlusions (87.5%) of 80 could be reopened by this procedure, followed by clinical and hemodynamically assessed improvement. In 10 cases (12.5%), the procedure failed due to incomplete LTL and impossible passage through the occlusion in 4 patients, 2 early reocclusions and 4 emboli which underwent a partial lysis only. From the whole group, 10 patients needed surgery: 4 embolectomies, 3 bypasses, 1 patch angioplasty and 3 amputations at calf level (one after femorocrural Dardik bypass). As local complications, 2 hematomas and 2 false aneurysms with spontaneous healing are to be mentioned. One sudden death five days after a combined treatment and a cerebral infarction in another patient 3 days later were not directly related to the procedure. Thus, the LTL combined with PTA represents an efficient therapeutic modality to reopen even longer acute and subacute artery occlusions by dissolution of the thrombus and dilatation of the underlying atherosclerotic stenosis in the same session. We prefer UK to SK because the lack of antigenic properties permits repeated local thrombolysis in the same patient.

16
A Surgeon's Viewpoint of Balloon Angioplasty

Marko Turina

Percutaneous transluminal angioplasty (PTA) of coronary artery stenosis was introduced by Grüntzig in Zurich in 1977. The procedure quickly gained universal acceptance, and the number of coronary dilatations increased steadily until 1980 when 84 PTAs were performed, reflecting a large proportion of external referrals. Since then the number has decreased and in 1982 only 37 procedures were done in Zurich. This represents a total incidence of 3.6% of all coronary angiographies performed by 4 referring institutions.

Our present indication for PTA is a short (less than 1 year) history of angina in a patient with single-vessel disease, having a short concentric noncalcified stenosis. Early success rate is approximately 70%, defined as increase in diameter and reduction in pressure gradient. In 20% of successful PTAs a recurrence of stenosis occurs within 6–12 months. These patients are subjected to redilatation; if the vessel cannot be dilated or restenosis occurs, operation is performed. Serious complications occurred in 6/37 patients subjected to PTA in 1982 (16%). Immediate coronary artery bypass grafting (CABG) was performed without mortality or significant morbidity. Myocardial infarction could be prevented in all cases revascularized within 4 hours after occlusion, although some enzyme washout (CK-MB) was observed. In the last 2 years, the complication rate was much higher when PTA was performed urgently in unstable angina as opposed to elective procedure (29% vs. 5%). Intraoperative dilatations are performed in selected patients during CABG, when a distal lesion is encountered in a proximally stenosed vessel; intraoperative angiographic control is considered mandatory. Stenosed CABG are not dilated; the only exception is a late (more than 3-5 years) atheromatous change in bypass vein which might be amenable to PTA. The overall impact of PTA on practice of coronary surgery in Zurich has been minimal. The number of CABG procedures increased steadily throughout the period, the incidence of patients receiving single and double CABG remained constant, and the number of distal anastomosis in patients receiving CABG—reflecting the extent of coronary artery disease—remained exactly the same.

In summary, percutaneous dilatation and coronary surgery are complementary therapeutic interventions, each tailored to a specific subset of patients with coronary artery disease.

9

Arteriosclerotic Peripheral Vascular Disease

17
The Natural History of Atherosclerotic Disease as Deduced from Observations on the Carotid Plaque

Anthony M. Imparato

Concepts regarding the basic nature of atherosclerotic plaque have varied. Among these concepts are that it is a reaction to lipid material deposited within the arterial wall; a reaction to incrustation of platelet and fibrin on the intimal surface, with subsequent fibrous organization being a neoplastic-like process; or that it represents a reaction to hemodynamic trauma. The performance of carotid endarterectomy in numerous patients presenting with a variety of cerebrovascular insufficiency syndromes has permitted the removal and inspection of carotid bifurcation plaques at various stages of development (Figure 1).

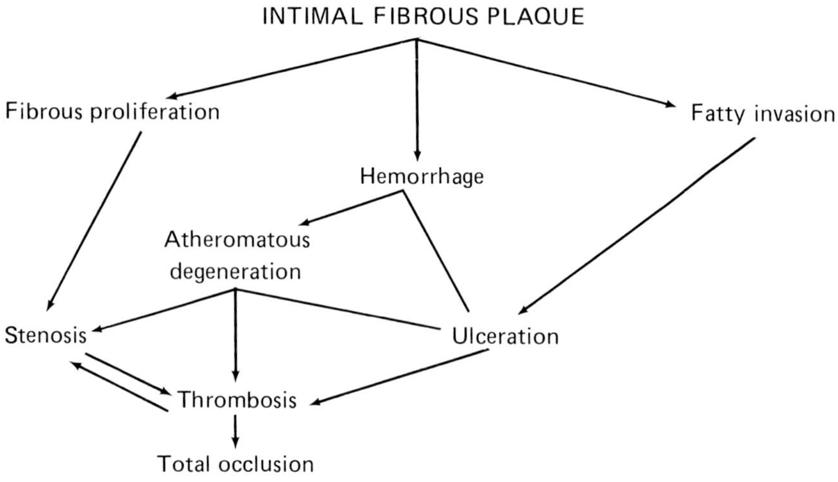

Figure 1. The evolution of carotid bifurcation plaque and the mechanisms by which symptoms are produced.

VARIETIES OF CAROTID PLAQUES

Simple Fibrous Intimal Plaque

What appears to be the earliest reaction at the carotid bifurcation associated with symptoms is the simple fibrointimal plaque which involves the carotid bulb, the proximal external carotid artery, and the proximal internal carotid artery, rarely extending beyond the proximal 2 to 3 cm of the origin of the internal carotid artery. The surface is pearly white with no gross breaks in continuity of the luminal lining which, on both light and electron microscopy, appears to be composed of flattened cells, while the thickening is due to layers of fibroblasts.

A lesion identical with the fibrointimal plaque is reproducible in the experimental laboratory by employing a number of techniques that damage the arterial wall. We have employed hemodynamic models to explain various flow disorders except those such as balloon catheter trauma, which has the additional feature of platelet adhesion as one of the primary phases. The hemodynamic models evolve through almost simultaneous occurrence of three phenomena: fragmentation of the internal elastic lamella, migration and differentiation of smooth muscle cells which acquire the morphology of fibroblasts, and the beginning of endothelial cell separation.

Fibrointimal Plaque with Intramural Hemorrhage

The fibrointimal plaque is next encountered in association with intramural hemorrhage that occurs under the fibrous cap, without ulceration of the surface, and may be associated with increased vascularity of the fibrous portions of the plaque. The hemorrhage may be acute or may show evidence of having occurred in stages with breakdown of red cells and the development of cholesterol clefts.

An apparent progression of the intramural hemorrhage is to fracture of the luminal lining with the development of a frank ulcer which conceivably might be the source of emboli.

The Fibrointimal Plaque with Localized Collections of Atheromatous Debris

Localized collections of atheromatous debris occur either as such or in association with hemorrhage of various ages. There appears to be a gradual transition from fresh intraplaque hemorrhage to atheromatous debris passing through the phase of breakdown of the hemorrhage, the appearance of cholesterol clefts, and finally the appearance of frank amorphous debris. These collections of atheromatous debris occur at the same site as the intraplaque hemorrhage, namely at the very origin of the internal carotid artery. I have never seen such a hemorrhage involving the external carotid artery. Rarely is the common carotid below the bulb involved. A break may occur in the luminal lining of the localized collection of atheromatous debris resulting in ulceration.

Ulcerations of Fibrointimal Plaques

Frank ulceration with total dissolution of the luminal lining, either into a hemorrhage or a collection of atheromatous debris, or into the medial or deeper layers, can be encountered. When hemorrhage and atheromatous debris are deep to such areas of ulceration, the mechanism appears clear. An instance in which the ulceration is shallow, or in which there are pits which are lined with fibrin, fresh or old thrombus, or flattened cells, the mechanism of ulceration may not be clear.

Thrombosis

The end stage of the atherosclerotic process appears to be thrombosis with total occlusion of the vessel. Thrombosis may occur in combination with mechanisms which markedly narrow the lumen of the vessel. In one-third of operated patients intraplaque hemorrhage is grossly visible and does produce marked stenosis, which may proceed to thombosis. In other instances, collections of atheromatous debris are associated with stenosis and subsequent thrombosis. In some instances, relatively shallow breaks in the intimal surface appear to result in thrombosis. Stasis and thrombosis with propagation of thrombus to the intracranial portion of the internal carotid artery may occur in association with stenotic lesions at the carotid siphon.

The Role of Platelets

It has not been possible to demonstrate that platelets are deposited in areas where embolization to the intracranial carotid might have occurred. Most frequently, areas of ulceration contain either granular yellow particles or breakdown products of intramural hemorrhage. Least frequently encountered is laminated thrombus in the bottom of pitted areas of the fibrous plaque.

18
Popliteal and Tibial Artery Revascularization

John B. Chang

Femoral-popliteal and femoral-tibial artery bypasses have been demonstrated to be effective [1,2,3,4]. The greater saphenous vein has proven to be the prime choice for graft material [5,6,7]. With femoral-popliteal artery bypasses and further distal revascularization procedures, the results are far superior to the expected outcome in comparable patients undergoing primary amputation [1,8,9]. Combined disease in the aortoiliac artery system can be treated prior to or subsequently to the femoral-popliteal or tibial artery revascularization [10,11]. When multiple levels of occlusion prohibit the conventional technique of femoral-popliteal artery bypass or femoral-tibial artery bypass, such patients can be benefited by utilizing multiple or sequential bypass technique[11,12,13,14,15,16]. Composite graft has been disappointing [14]. However, in selected cases of small vessel revascularization, I have used composite graft, as I describe in detail. Noninvasive vascular studies in follow-up have been practical in recognizing an anatomically patent graft with significant hemodynamic deterioration. With this type of approach, proper treatment, including reoperation, permits salvage of the majority of these patent grafts prior to ultimate failure from thrombosis [18]. Secondary femoral-popliteal artery construction has been popular in major medical centers. Also, one series of cases provided justification for an aggressive approach toward secondary femoral-popliteal reconstruction with acceptable operative mortality [19]. Vigorous attempts at revision of failed grafts may prevent or constructively delay amputation [20]. Therefore, the risk of jeopardizing the knee joint should not be considered a major contraindication to limb salvage procedures, especially if a femoral-popliteal bypass is contemplated [22]. However, the potential adverse effect on the final amputation level should be included among considerations when making a final determination for revascularization [21]. A bypass procedure, where an attempt was made to use a potentially inadequate greater saphenous vein, has been managed with in situ vein bypass technique. The merits and criticisms of this procedure have been well described [23,24,25].

Arteriosclerosis is a multisegmental disease often involving vital organs. However, the attrition rate of patients having initial success with their operations is strikingly high. It appears unlikely that revascularization of severely ischemic limbs contributes substantially to improved longevity, but the quality of survival in a patient is undoubtedly enhanced by preservation of a useful and comfortable limb [27].

Using PTFE graft, available data appear to be encouraging, particularly if the distal anastomosis is at above-knee level [1,26]. In addition to noninvasive vascular studies and conventional angiographic technique, digital subtraction angiography (DSA) has been used for preoperative evaluation and follow-up studies after bypass procedures, particularly where a patient may require further surgical procedures. For small vessel bypasses, the technique of intra-arterial digital angiography has been helpful in providing detailed information on distal runoff down to the foot [28].

METHODS AND MATERIALS

The study is based on my personal experience with 550 cases of popliteal and tibial artery bypasses. Conventional femoral-popliteal artery bypasses with autogenous greater saphenous vein grafts were performed in 195 cases. Femoral-tibial artery bypasses with autogenous greater saphenous vein grafts were performed in 85 cases. In 30 cases, femoral-popliteal-tibial artery bypasses with autogenous greater saphenous vein grafts were performed. Popliteal-tibial artery bypass grafts were performed with greater saphenous vein grafts in 30 cases. One hundred fifty cases were femoral-popliteal bypasses with PTFE grafts. In 20 cases, femoral-tibial artery bypasses were done with PTFE. Femoral-popliteal bypasses were done with biograft, utilizing human umbilical veins in 20 cases.

The remainder consisted of composite grafts employing arm and leg veins. Others utilized bank veins, arm veins and superficial femoral veins as graft materials. I followed up all patients from six months to eight years postoperatively. Follow-up evaluation was done by my clinical evaluation, noninvasive vascular studies and, in selected cases, with DSA studies and/or angiographic confirmation.

PREOPERATIVE EVALUATION

All patients who required revascularization had ischemic rest pain with or without organic ischemic change such as gangrene and/or ischemic ulcers. Mere claudication was not considered an indication for revascularization in this series. Preoperative evaluation included complete vascular examination incorporating noninvasive vascular studies to investigate other underlying vascular problems, such as carotid artery disease, occlusive aortic-iliac artery disease, or aneurysmal disease. In many cases, DSA technique was used on an outpatient basis for preoperative angiographic studies. If the DSA was not compatible with the clinical evaluation and hemodynamic studies, then conventional angiography was performed on an inpatient basis.

For distal small vessel disease in some earlier cases of our series, distal runoff was examined down to the foot by delayed pictures taken after the postischemic period. In some recent cases, distal runoff was studied with intra-arterial injection technique of digital angiography. It is important to visualize the distal runoff down to the foot, no matter what technique one uses, either conventional angiography or intra-arterial DSA. Figure 1 shows this example. Figures 1A, 1B and 1C show conventional angiographic technique indicating occlusive disease in the bilateral superficial femoral arteries with distal runoff at the popliteal artery on the left side. However, the symptomatic right side with gangrene has no distal runoff, either in the popliteal or tibial segment. But in the delayed films, Figures 1D and 1E show the distal runoff down to the foot through the anterior tibial artery (arrows). A similar situation is shown on Figures 2A, 2B and 2C. Figures 2A and 2B illustrate a conventional arteriogram showing a patent iliofemoral artery system down to the common femoral level. Severe arteriosclerotic disease was noted throughout the superficial femoral artery down to the knee level, where complete occlusion occurred without distal runoff. Delayed films, shown on Figure 2C, disclose no reconstructible tibial artery runoff. However, at the foot, dorsalis pedis and distal posterior arteries are visualized.

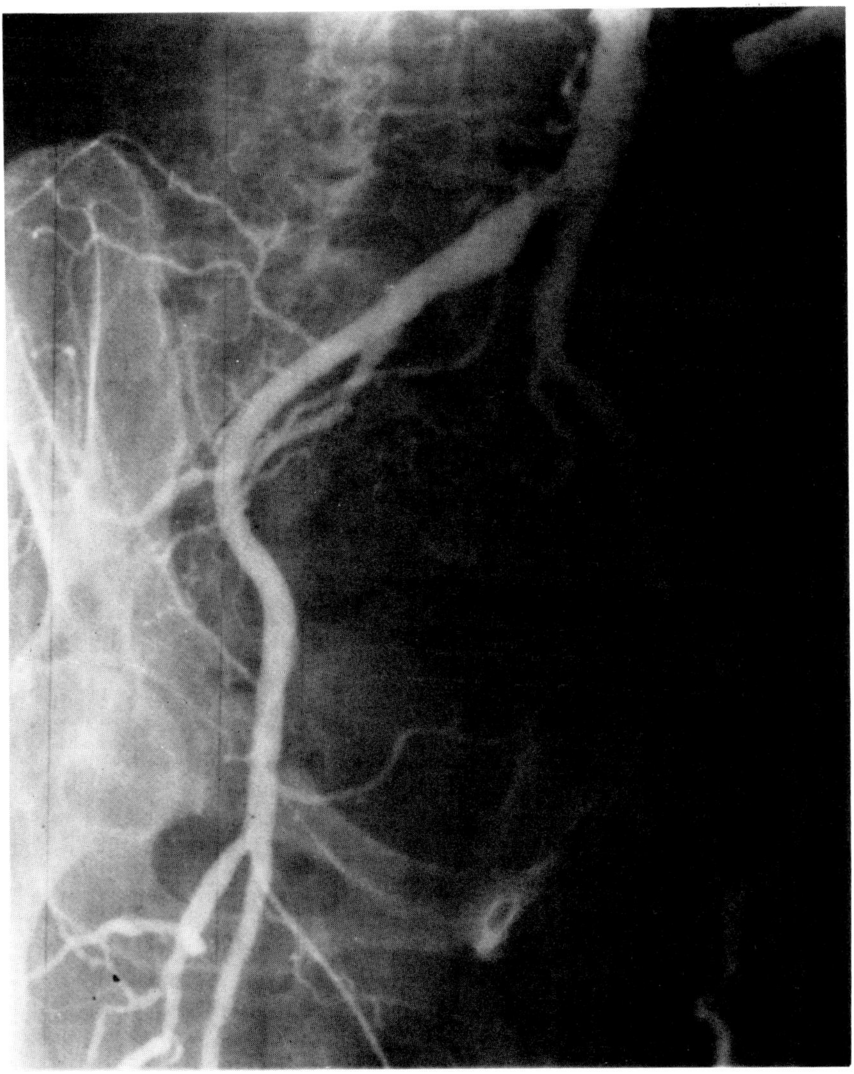

Figure 1a. Patient with intermittent claudication of both legs and ischemic rest pain in right foot. Angiography shows a patent aortoiliac artery system.

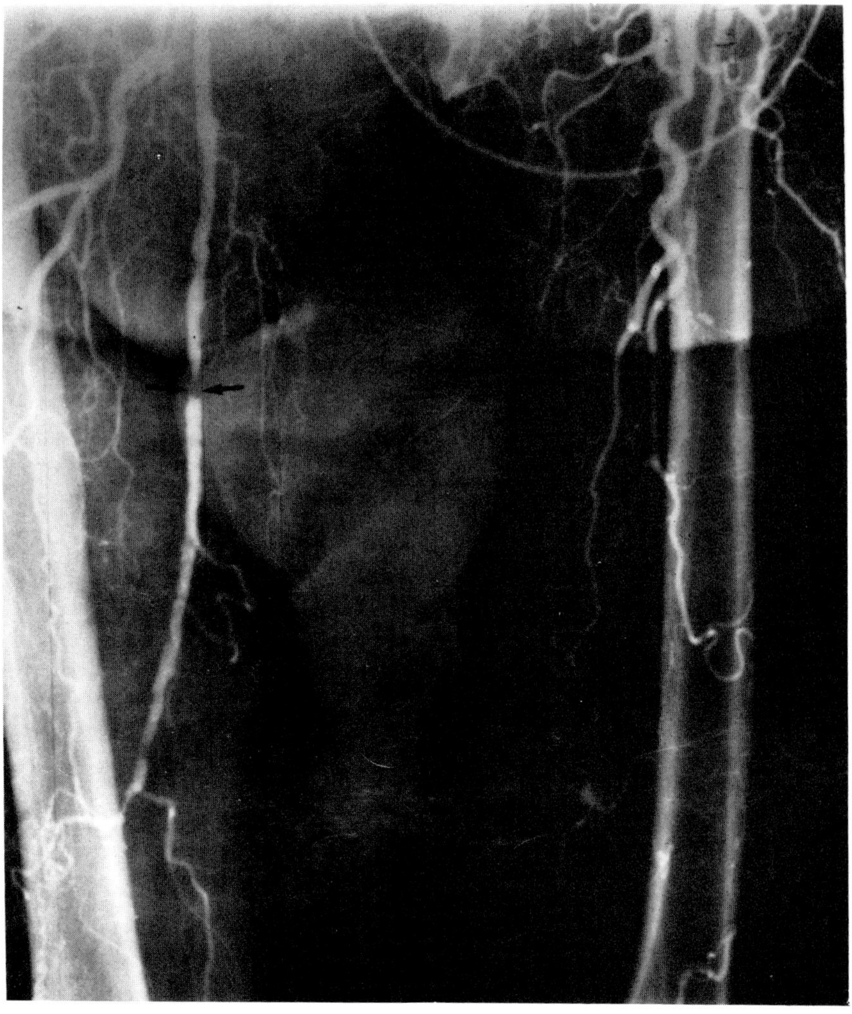

Figure 1b. Complete occlusion of left superficial femoral artery system as well as right distal superficial femoral artery with complete occlusion proximally (arrows).

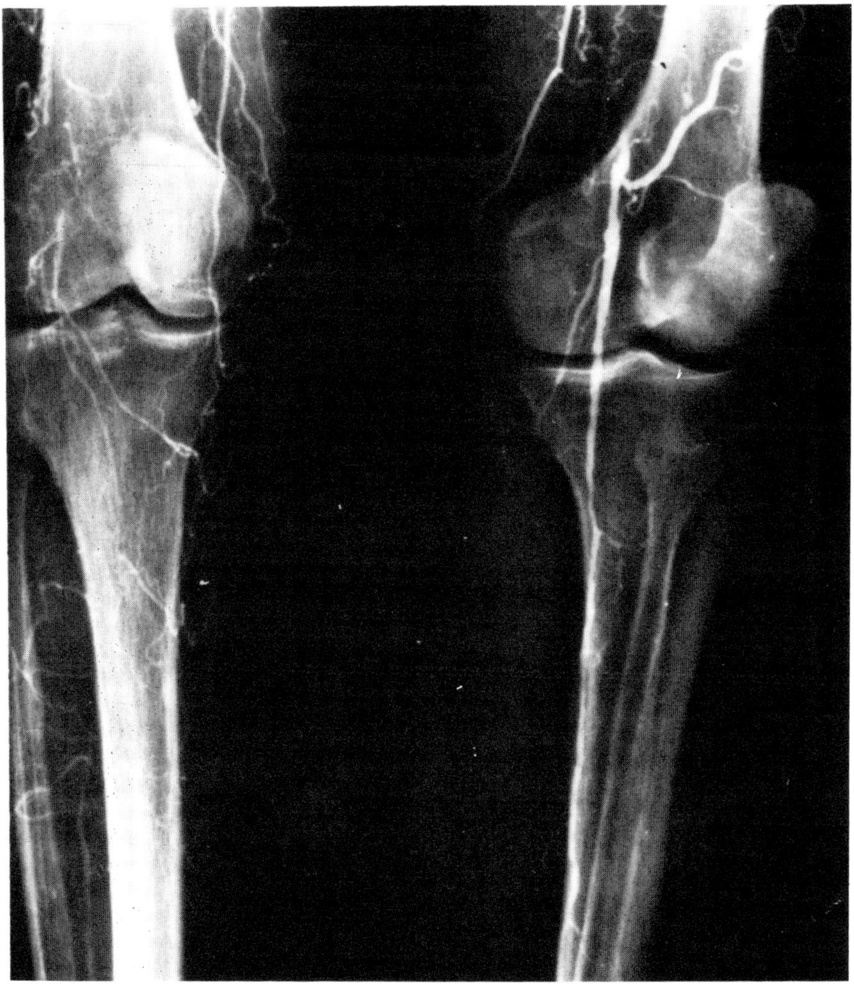

Figure 1c. Distal runoff on the left side shows through the left popliteal artery system. However, on the right leg there was no distal runoff.

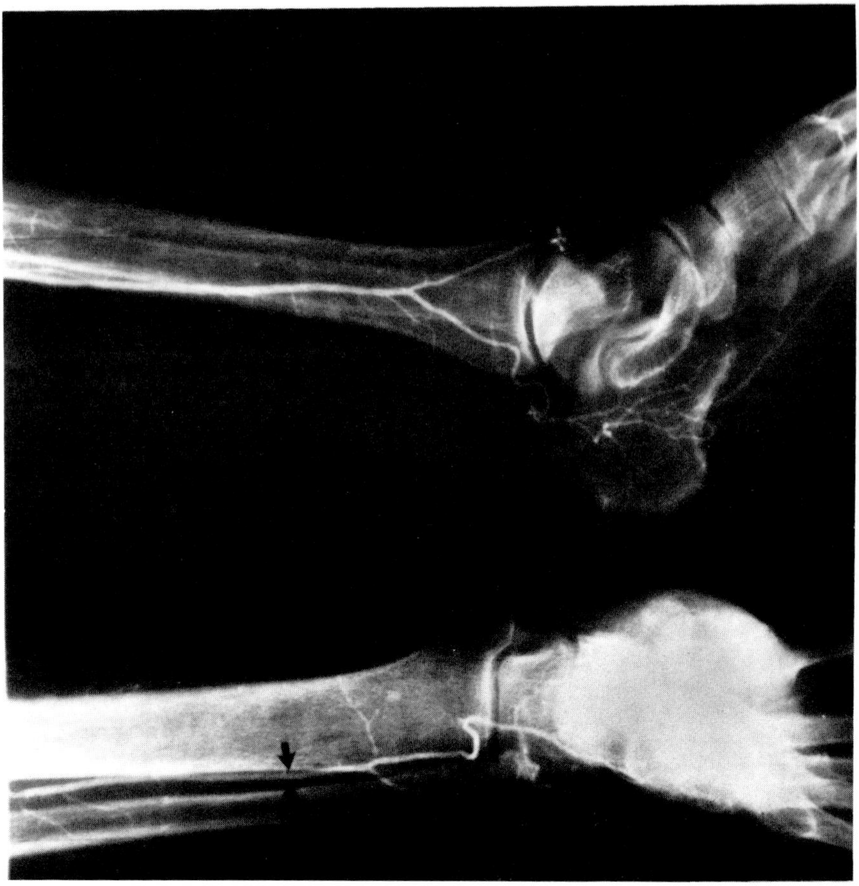

d

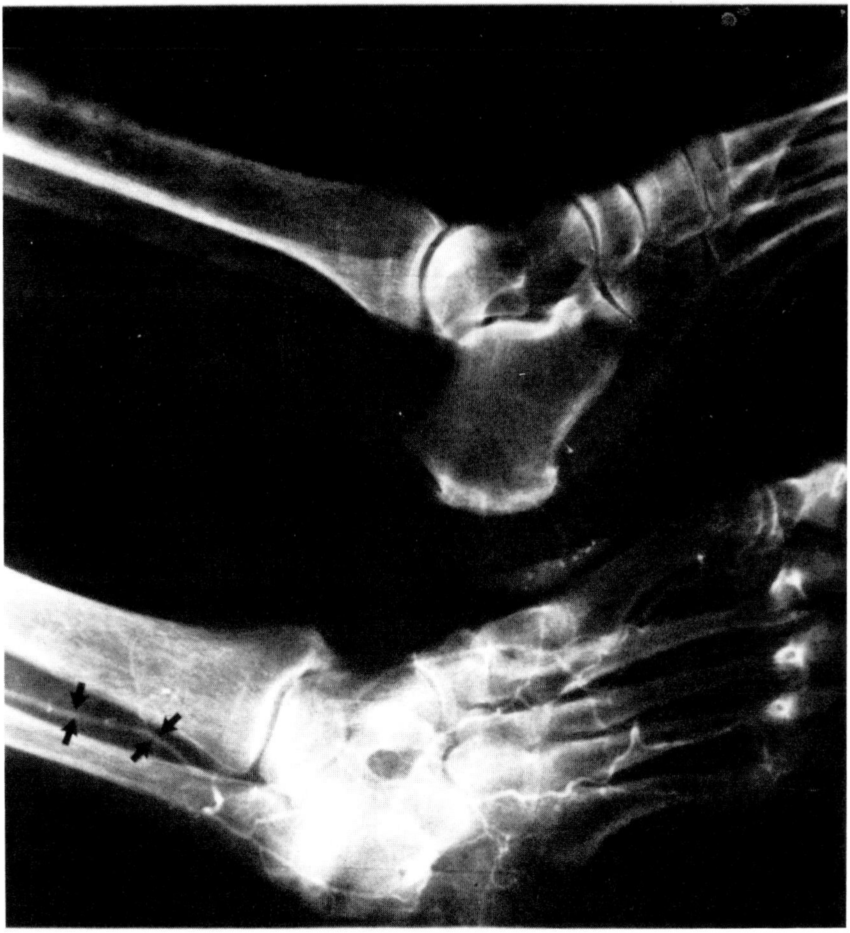

e

Figure 1d, 1e. Delayed films show distal runoff to the foot through anterior tibial artery (arrows).

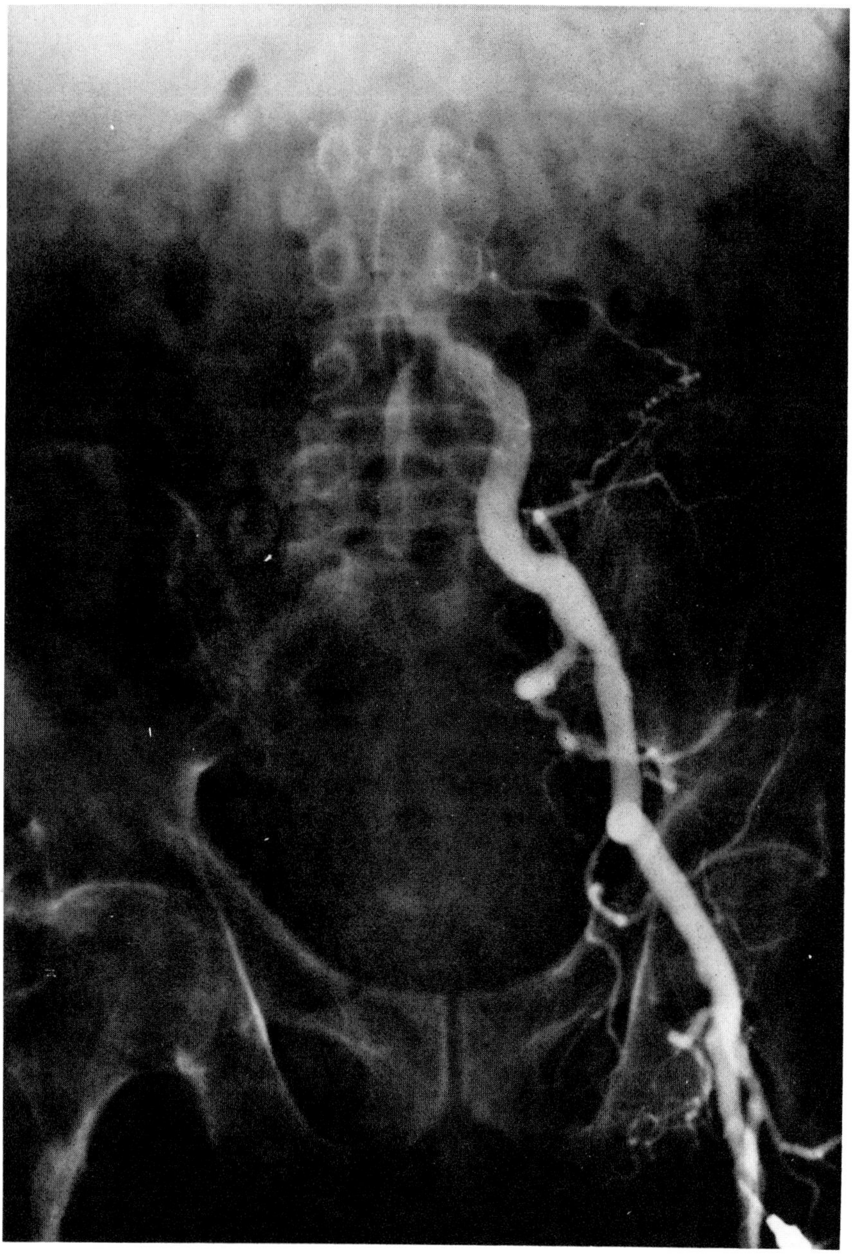

Figure 2a. Conventional angiographic film showing patent iliac artery system.

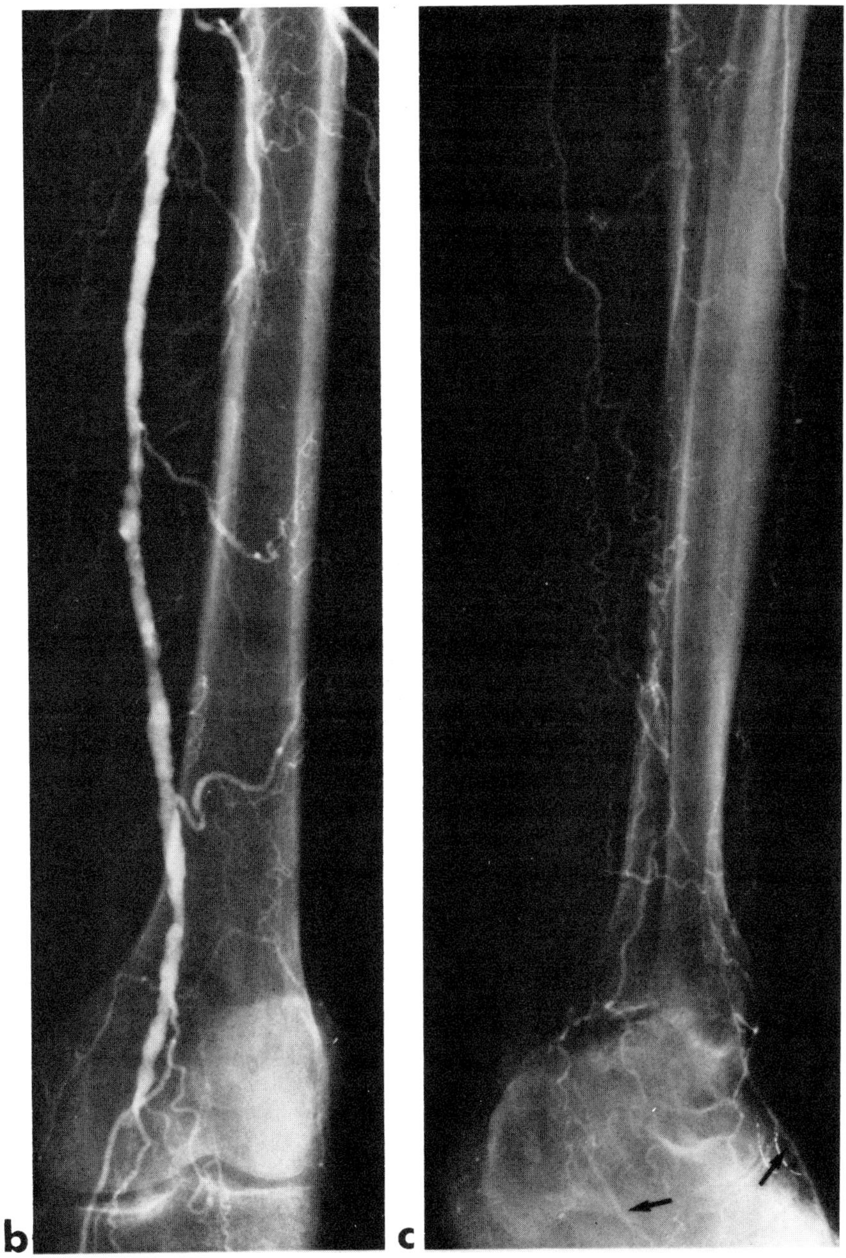

Figure 2. **(b)** Extensive arteriosclerotic change through the superficial artery with complete occlusion at the popliteal artery. **(c)** On the delayed film, the dorsalis pedis artery and distal posterior tibial arteries are shown (arrows), to which small vessel bypass was possible.

SURGICAL TECHNIQUES

Femoral-Popliteal Artery Bypass

This is a conventional and most commonly practiced bypass technique. It was my belief and intention to utilize autogenous greater saphenous vein as the graft material. If this was not available, arm vein was considered an alternative choice in a reasonably good-risk patient in a fairly young age group, if the distal runoff was poor. If arm vein was not available, in selected cases bank vein or a segment of superficial vein was used. In a poor-risk patient with no available veins, PTFE graft was used. In some recent cases, biograft with umbilical vein was employed. If graft material is used for bypass, it is important that proximal artery be selected properly. If the superficial femoral artery and deep femoral artery are not adequate, the common femoral artery should be used. If the common femoral artery has extensive disease and therefore is not suitable for a graft, we do not hesitate to go on to the further proximal iliac artery system for the proximal anastomosis.

The size of the PTFE graft was selected on the basis of the distal runoff, the size of the receiving artery, and the donor artery. The most common size of the PTFE was 8 mm, but PTFE has been used ranging in size from 6- to 10-mm Gore-tex graft with no statistical difference in this series. If the distal runoff was good with decent artery at above-knee for femoral-popliteal or iliopopliteal artery bypass, 8- or 10-mm Gore-tex grafts were used. The tunnel was usually made along Hunter's canal, rather than subcutaneously, with the technique described previously [1]. Patients with occlusive disease in the superficial femoral and tibial arteries with limited runoff at the remaining popliteal segment, complicated by thrombotic disease in the remaining distal runoff, were treated with intraoperative thrombectomy, intraoperative utilization of streptokinase, and then femoral-popliteal artery bypass, as illustrated in Figure 3. As shown in Figure 4, in long-term follow-up after extra-anatomic bypass, if the proximal artery on the donor side has further progressive disease or distal arterial disease, the recipient limb becomes ischemic again. In this particular situation, the femoral-femoral artery bypass graft was converted into an axillofemoral artery bypass and then to a femoral-popliteal artery bypass. In many instances, by converting the bypass procedure and reestablishing pulsatile flow, distal bypass was not necessary. In patients with severe arterial insufficiency in both legs with ischemic change and angiographic findings of occlusive ipsilateral iliac artery disease and occlusive disease in the bilateral superficial femoral artery system, the problem can be managed by doing an extra-anatomic bypass from the contralateral patent iliofemoral artery system and then a femoral-popliteal artery bypass on the donor side, as described in Figure 5. In this situation, on the left side, a distal bypass is normally not needed.

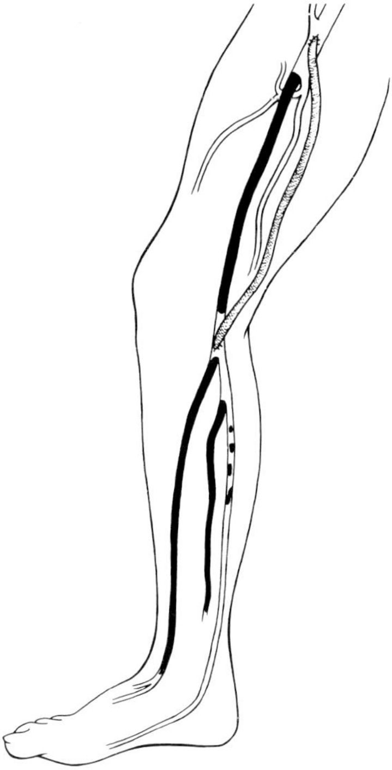

Figure 3. Patient who had chronic arterial insufficiency with acute exacerbation due to thrombosis of the remaining tibial artery. The posterior tibial artery had multiple thromboses. These were removed, and local streptokinase was given. In addition, a femoral–popliteal artery bypass was done.

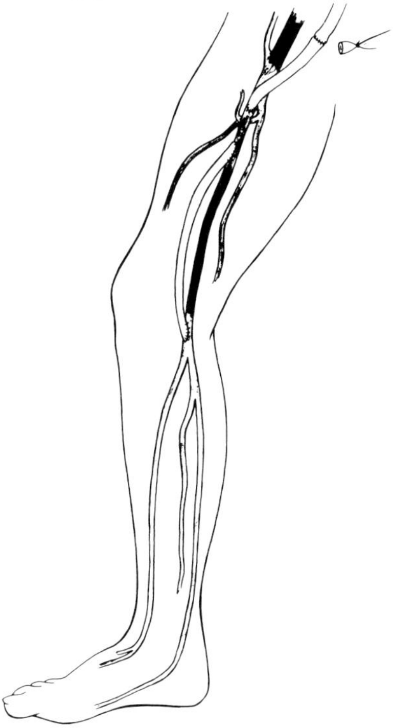

Figure 4. This patient had femoral–femoral artery bypass and right femoral–popliteal artery bypass six years prior to the onset of further arterial insufficiency with hemodynamic deterioration due to progressive disease of the left iliac artery system. Subsequently, the femoral–femoral artery bypass graft was thrombosed. This was managed by adding new inflow from the right axillary artery into the segment of the left femoral–right femoral artery bypass graft, converting it into an axillo–femoral artery bypass. This additional inflow was able to give pulsatile flow into the patent right femoral–popliteal artery bypass graft, and the limb was saved.

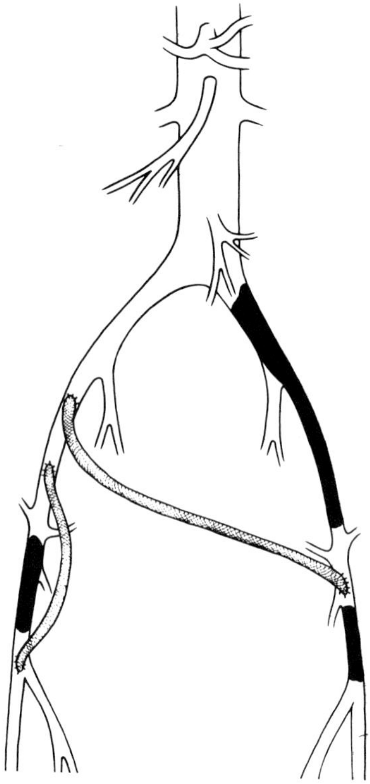

Figure 5. Patient with severe arterial insufficiency in both legs due to occlusive disease in the bilateral superficial arteries and left iliac artery system. This was managed by doing extra-anatomic bypass from the right external iliac artery to the left femoral artery, then an additional distal bypass to the right popliteal artery. This patient did not need further bypass on the receiving side (left).

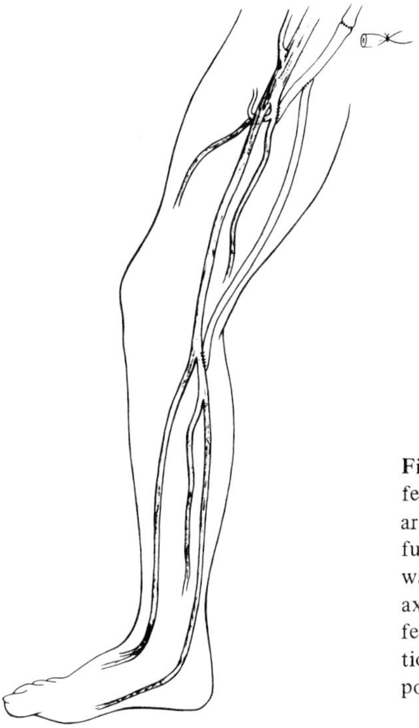

Figure 6. This patient had left femoral–right femoral bypass five years prior to a new onset of arterial insufficiency and graft thrombosis due to further deterioration on the donor side artery. This was managed by adding inflow bypass from axillary artery into the right side graft from left femoral–right femoral artery bypass. Then, additional bypass was given from the graft into the popliteal artery.

The patient with extensive distal disease with an occluded femoral-femoral artery bypass graft can be treated by converting it into another type of extra-anatomic bypass such as an axillofemoral artery bypass. If the distal runoff is poor because of extensive distal disease, the graft can be extended distally to the popliteal artery, as illustrated in Figure 6. When the patient develops increased ischemic change on a receiving limb with a functional femoral-femoral artery bypass graft, more study has to be done in the follow-up period to investigate further progression of arteriosclerotic occlusive disease in the femoral or popliteal artery system. The patient in Figure 7 had a functional femoral-femoral artery bypass graft with further progression of the arteriosclerotic disease, resulting in extensive occlusive disease of the superficial femoral artery and the proximal deep femoral artery. There was runoff at the popliteal-tibial artery system. This patient, having ischemic change four years after a femoral-femoral artery bypass graft, had the problem solved by a sequential bypass extending from the common femoral artery down to the deep femoral artery and then to the popliteal artery, as illustrated in Figure 7.

In patients with occlusive disease involving the entire femoral artery system down to the popliteal and tibial arteries, many times the deep femoral arteries are also diseased with occlusion. An example of this problem is illustrated in Figure 8. In this case the entire superficial femoral, popliteal, and anterior tibial arteries were occluded, as were the common femoral artery and the proximal parts of the deep femoral arteries. The peroneal artery had multiple stenotic lesions. The posterior tibial artery had arteriosclerotic change, but this was the only distal runoff to the foot. In this situation, endarterectomy can be done in the popliteal-tibial artery segment with transluminal angioplasty of the peroneal artery. Then the deep femoral artery can be revascularized by an external iliac artery-deep femoral artery bypass using PTFE, 8 or 10 mm, depending on the size of the profunda femoral artery. In this case, cephalic vein was used because there was no available saphenous vein system, due to previous surgeries. The cephalic vein graft was anastomosed to the distal profunda femoral artery distal to the ilio-deep femoral artery bypass graft anastomosis. Then distal anastomosis was made on the long segment of endarterectomized popliteal-tibial artery as an onlay patch anastomosis (Figure 8).

Femoral-Tibial Artery Bypass

The best choice of graft for femoral-tibial artery bypass is the autogenous greater saphenous vein. However, in many instances, the greater saphenous vein is not available. For that reason many different techniques and graft material have been utilized. For the conventional femoral-tibial artery bypass graft, the graft is usually passed through a subcutaneous tunnel. In a femoral-popliteal-anterior tibial artery sequential bypass, the graft is normally brought through a tunnel made along Hunter's canal down to the popliteal fossa. Then a

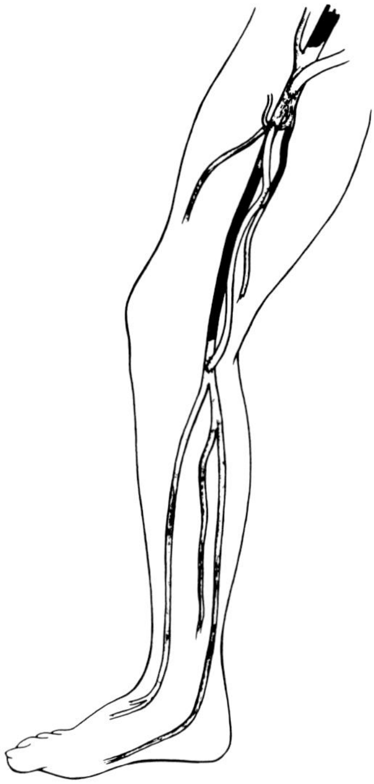

Figure 7. Patient, who has a functioning femoral–femoral artery bypass graft, has further deterioration at four years postoperatively due to further distal occlusive disease in the superficial femoral artery. Also, long segment of proximal profunda femoral artery is occluded. This was treated with sequential bypass from common femoral artery to distal profunda femoral artery in side-to-side fashion and then to the popliteal artery in end-to-side fashion.

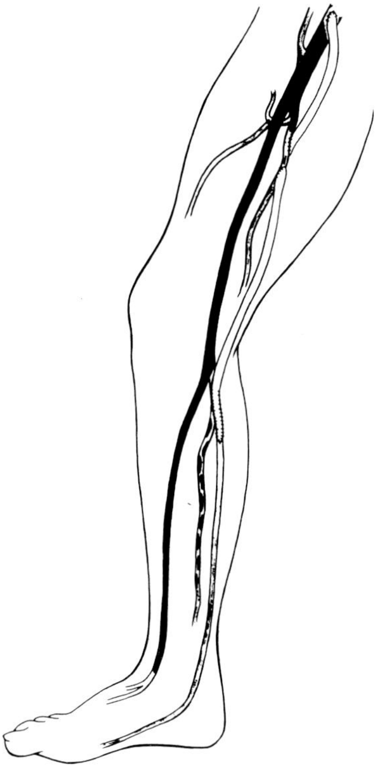

Figure 8. Patient with extensive occlusive disease involving entire common femoral, superficial, and anterior tibial artery system. The proximal profunda femoral artery was also occluded. This was managed by external iliac artery to deep femoral artery bypass with a graft. Then transluminal dilatation of the peroneal artery with endarterectomy of the popliteal–peroneal trunk was done. Then additional bypass was done from the distal profunda femoral artery down to the popliteal–tibial trunk by doing long anastomosis over the endarterectomized segment of the popliteal–tibial artery and to the posterior tibial artery. In this case cephalic vein was used as a graft, because the patient had no available saphenous vein systems (because of previous operations). I prefer proximal anastomosis of the autogenous vein to the artery rather than to the graft itself. As shown, segment of profunda femoral artery acts as a bridge between the synthetic graft and the cephalic vein bypass graft.

side-to-side anastomosis is made between the side of the graft and the side of the popliteal artery. The graft is then brought through an opening made at the interosseous membrane to the anterior lateral aspect of the leg to the level of the exposed anterior tibial artery.

Angioplasty

With femoral–popliteal or tibial artery bypasses, it often has been necessary to do an additional procedure such as endarterectomy, angioplasty, or transluminal balloon dilatation. The patient in Figure 9A had extensive occlusive disease involving the entire superficial femoral artery, the anterior tibial artery,

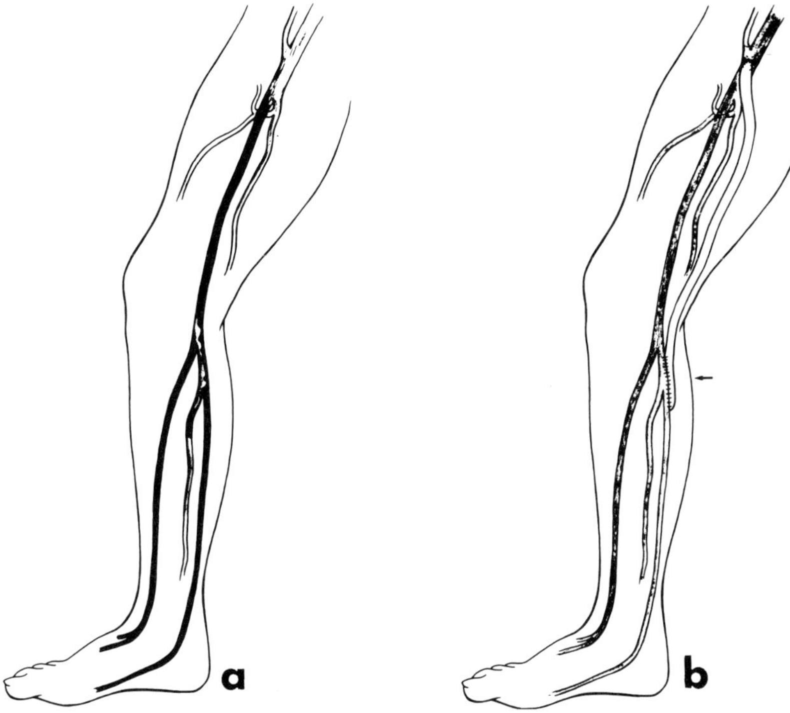

Figure 9. **(a)** Patient with extensive occlusive disease involving the entire superficial femoral artery and anterior tibial artery as well as posterior tibial artery. Small segment of popliteal artery has multiple stenotic lesions as well as proximal portion of the peroneal artery. The distal runoff, however, was through the peroneal artery to the foot. **(b)** The problem in Figure 9a was solved by doing extensive endarterectomy of the popliteal–peroneal trunk and transluminal dilatation of the peroneal artery. Then the femoral–popliteal artery bypass was done. The distal anastomosis was made as an onlay patch anastomosis to the long segment of endarterectomized popliteal–peroneal trunk (arrow).

and the posterior tibial artery. A small segment of the popliteal artery had multiple areas of stenosis. The only runoff to the foot was through the peroneal artery, which also had multiple stenoses. This problem was managed by doing endarterectomy of the popliteal segment and the peroneal trunk in addition to transluminal balloon dilatation of the peroneal artery. Then a distal anastomosis was made with angioplasty (onlay patch anastomosis), as shown in Figure 9B (arrows). In long-term follow-up, the greater saphenous vein graft may be found to be stenotic due to subsequent phlebosclerosis. If the graft is narrow in the segmental area, it can be repaired without having to do an entire bypass again.

The patient in Figure 10 had stenosis at the functioning popliteal–dorsalis pedis artery bypass graft. This was treated satisfactorily by doing angioplasty with a vein (arrow). If the popliteal–tibial artery segment has extensive occlusive disease, endarterectomy can be carried out from the popliteal artery down to the peroneal trunk, or even to the peroneal or posterior tibial artery. Then a distal anastomosis is made over this long arteriotomy. The patient in Figure 11 had an endarterectomy of the popliteal peroneal trunk, and distal anastomosis was done over this arteriotomy, as shown.

Femoral–Popliteal–Tibial Artery Sequential Bypass

In patients with multiple occlusive diseases involving the femoral, popliteal or tibial artery system, management can be accomplished, but it represents a surgical challenge. Instead of bypassing to an isolated popliteal segment, sequential bypass can be performed by extending the distal anastomosis to the available distal tibial artery. The patient in Figure 12 had extensive occlusive disease involving the entire superficial artery as well as the anterior wall of the common femoral artery. There was a small popliteal segment with extensive occlusive disease in the proximal tibial arteries. However, the profunda system appeared to be intact with a good pulse. The problem was solved by doing deep femoral artery-popliteal segment-posterior tibial artery sequential bypass with an autogenous greater saphenous vein graft. In a similar situation with more extensive disease involving the common femoral artery as well as the proximal portion of the deep femoral artery, the patient in Figure 13 also had complete occlusion of the superficial femoral artery as well as of the popliteal-proximal tibial artery system. This was treated with a bypass operation designed on the same principle of multiple sequential revascularization. As shown in Figure 13, external iliac artery-deep femoral artery-peroneal artery-posterior tibial artery sequential bypass was done with autogenous greater saphenous vein graft.

Another variety of a similar principle is shown in Figure 14. In this situation, iliac artery-posterior tibial artery-anterior tibial artery sequential bypass was done with an autogenous greater saphenous vein graft. Depending on the anatomical and pathological situation, the distal portion of the sequential

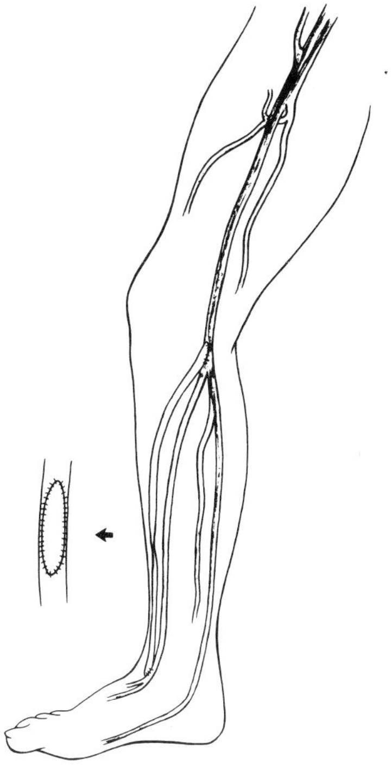

Figure 10. Stenosis at the midportion of functioning greater saphenous vein graft of popliteal–dorsalis pedis artery bypass. This was managed with angioplastic technique utilizing vein patch graft (arrow).

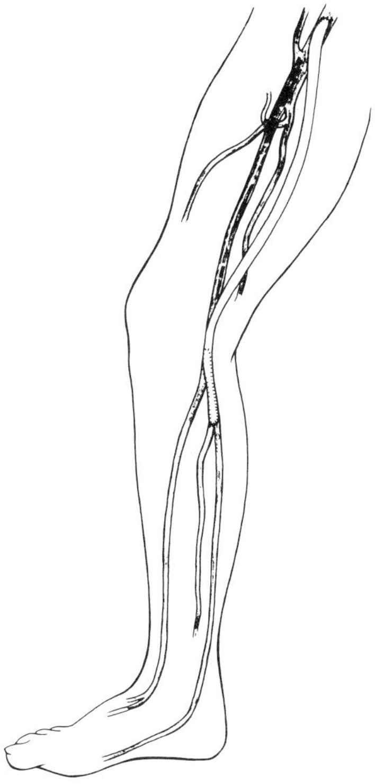

Figure 11. Patient with extensive occlusive disease in the superficial femoral artery–popliteal artery system, with extension to the proximal tibial arteries. This was treated with extensive endarterectomy and onlay patch graft by anastomosing the distal vein graft into the long segment of the endarterectomized artery.

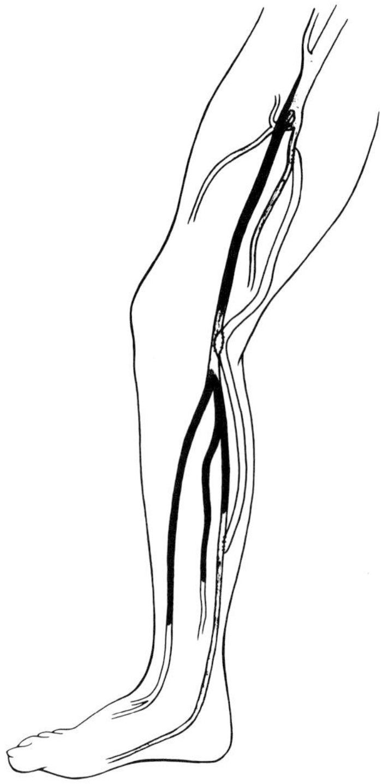

Figure 12. Patient with extensive occlusive disease involving superficial femoral artery with calcification on the common femoral artery. A small segment of popliteal artery is open, in addition to one distal runoff through the distal posterior tibial artery. This was managed by doing sequential bypass from profunda femoral artery to the popliteal artery segment in side-to-side fashion and then to the distal posterior tibial artery in end-to-side fashion.

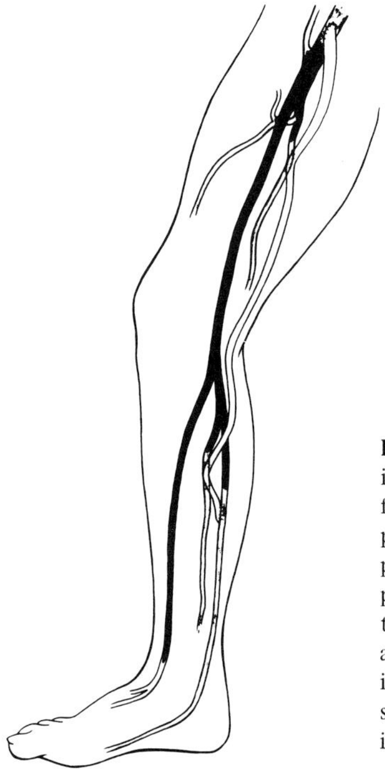

Figure 13. Patient with extensive occlusive disease involving the common femoral artery, superficial femoral artery, deep femoral artery at the proximal portion, entire anterior tibial artery, and popliteal–peroneal trunk including proximal portion of peroneal artery and posterior tibial artery. Sequential bypass was carried out from external iliac artery down to the distal profunda femoral artery in side-to-side fashion, peroneal artery in side-to-side fashion, and then to the posterior tibial artery in end-to-side fashion.

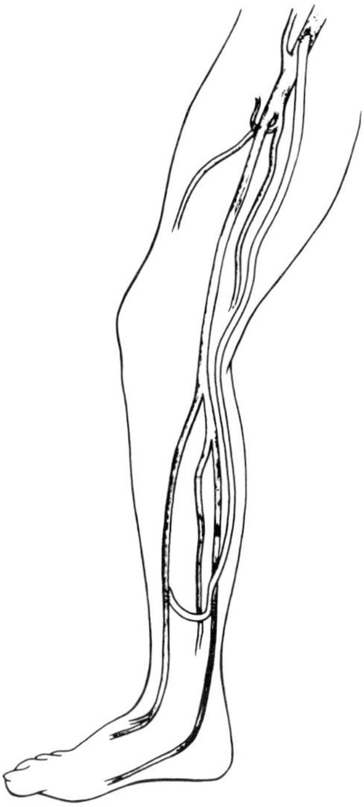

Figure 14. Another alternative of sequential bypass from external iliac artery down to posterior tibial artery in side-to-side fashion and then to anterior tibial artery in end-to-side fashion.

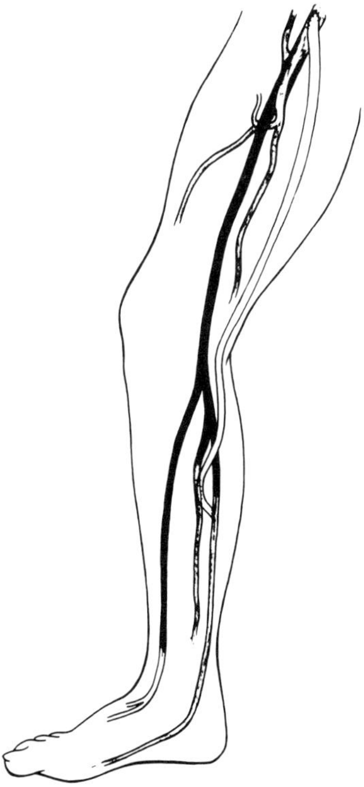

Figure 15. Patient with extensive occlusive disease involving common, superficial, and popliteal–tibial artery system with calcification extending into the profunda femoral artery. This was managed by doing sequential bypass from the external iliac artery down to the peroneal artery in side-to-side fashion and then to the posterior tibial artery in end-to-side fashion.

anastomosis can be varied. One example is shown in Figure 15. In this situation the graft was brought down to the peroneal artery in side-to-side fashion and then to the posterior tibial artery in end-to-side fashion.

Popliteal–Distal Tibial Artery Bypass

Many patients with distal tibial artery disease, giving ischemic change and gangrene to the foot, often have a patent superficial femoral artery down to the popliteal artery system. Major occlusive disease occurs at the popliteal–tibial artery junction or proximal tibial arteries. Sometimes this obstructive disease is extensive throughout the tibial artery system down to the ankle or proximal foot; this is more common in diabetic individuals.

This variety of problems is now challenged by small vessel bypasses and microsurgical technique. The principle of multiple revascularization is important also in this small vessel revascularization. In a distal anterior tibial artery of dorsalis pedis artery bypass, the proximal anastomosis can be done at the popliteal fossa. The graft is then brought through an opening made at the interosseous membrane, down to the anterior lateral aspect of the leg subcutaneously to the exposed level of the anterior tibial artery or dorsalis pedis artery. As shown in Figure 16, popliteal-tibial revascularization is done by sequential anastomosis to the posterior tibial artery in side-to-side fashion and then to the anterior tibial artery in end-to-side fashion. When the autogenous saphenous vein is not available in its entirety for bypass procedure in multiple fashion, additional vein can be obtained from the arm. The most commonly used arm vein is the cephalic vein.

The patient in Figure 17 required sequential bypass to the distal posterior tibial artery as well as to the dorsalis pedis artery, but there was a limited length of available greater saphenous vein; therefore, the cephalic vein was used in addition. In this situation, the cephalic vein was laid between the distal posterior tibial artery and the dorsalis pedis artery. Then the greater saphenous vein was brought down from the popliteal anastomosis to the cephalic vein in T shape.

For proper blood flow, care should be taken that the cephalic vein of the T graft has no interfering valve. Utilizing a similar principle, the patient in Figure 18 was treated by popliteal artery–dorsalis pedis artery bypass with an autogenous greater saphenous vein graft. Then the arm vein was used to extend to the posterior tibial artery, as shown. The popliteal artery–dorsalis pedis artery bypass graft was brought through an opening at the interosseous membrane and then subcutaneously along the anterior lateral aspect of the leg down to the dorsalis pedis artery (Figure 18). In a similar situation, if the vein graft is available in its entire length, the bypass can be done in a sequential manner, as illustrated in Figure 19.

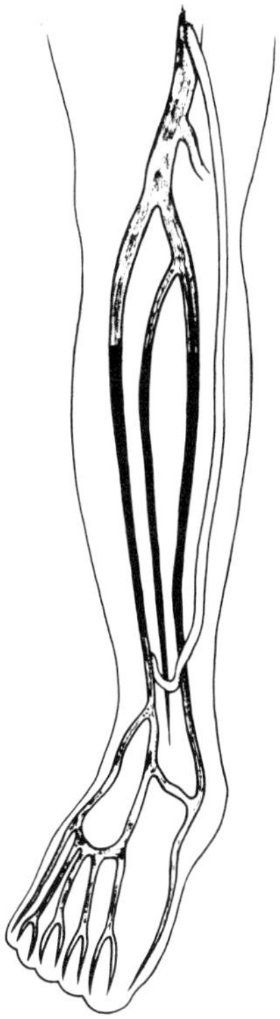

Figure 16. Patient with patent popliteal artery and extensive occlusive disease in all tibial arteries. Delayed angiographic film shows distal runoff on the foot through distal posterior tibial artery and dorsalis pedis artery to the foot. This was managed with popliteal artery–posterior tibial artery in side-to-side fashion and then to the anterior tibial artery in end-to-side fashion.

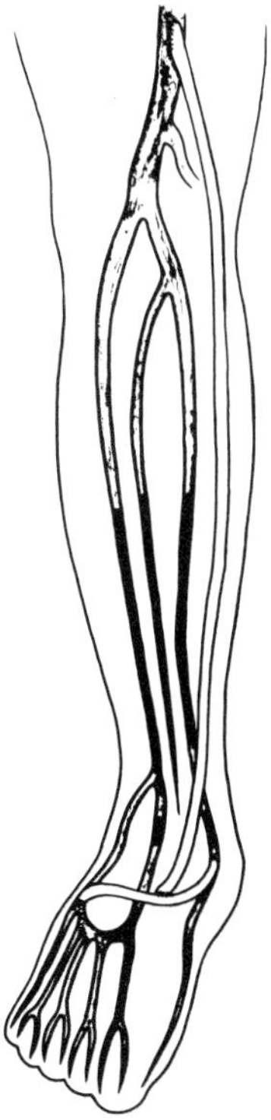

Figure 17. Patient with patent femoral–popliteal artery system with complete occlusion of tibial arteries. Distal runoff to the foot was through the dorsalis pedis artery and distal posterior tibial artery. The patient also had a limited length of available saphenous vein; therefore, a segment of cephalic vein was used. The cephalic vein was anastomosed to the dorsalis pedis artery and then to the distal posterior tibial artery, as shown. Then the saphenous vein graft was anastomosed into the cephalic vein in T shape. Care should be taken to be certain that the arm vein has no interfering valve in the segment.

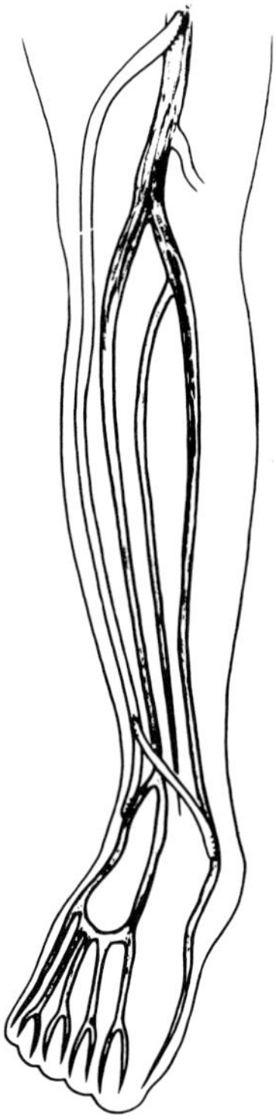

Figure 18. Popliteal–dorsalis pedis artery bypass with saphenous vein graft. Then bypass was extended to the distal posterior tibial artery using cephalic vein.

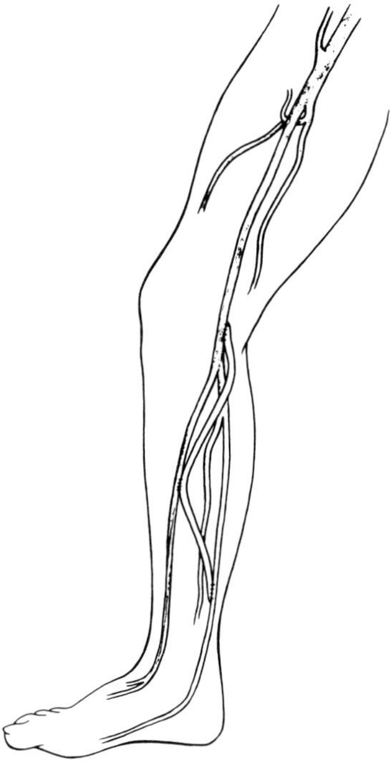

Figure 19. Patient with extensive obstructive disease at the tibial arteries with distal runoff through the anterior tibial artery and distal posterior tibial artery. Sequential bypass was done from the popliteal artery to the anterior tibial artery in side-to-side fashion. Then the graft was brought out to the distal posterior tibial artery in end-to-side fashion. In this situation the vein graft was brought through an opening at the interosseous membrane down to the anterior tibial artery. Then the vein was closed over the tibia to the posterior tibial artery distally.

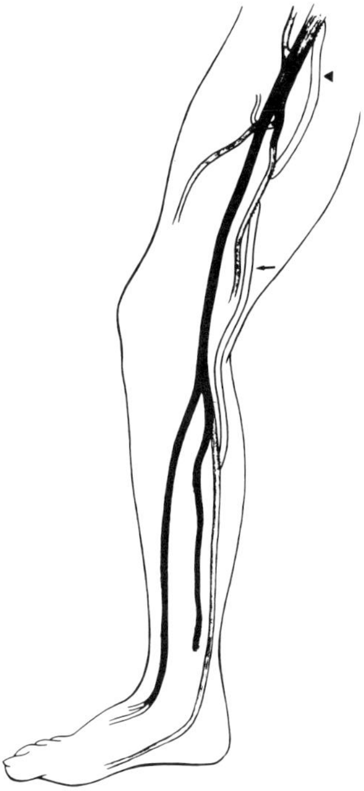

Figure 20. Patient with extensive disease in the femoral arteries involving the superficial femoral artery as well as the profunda femoral artery. Distal runoff is only through the posterior tibial artery. Because of no available saphenous vein, this problem was solved by doing external iliac artery to the deep femoral artery bypass with PTFE (triangular arrow). Then cephalic vein was used from the distal deep femoral artery to the posterior tibial artery bypass (arrow).

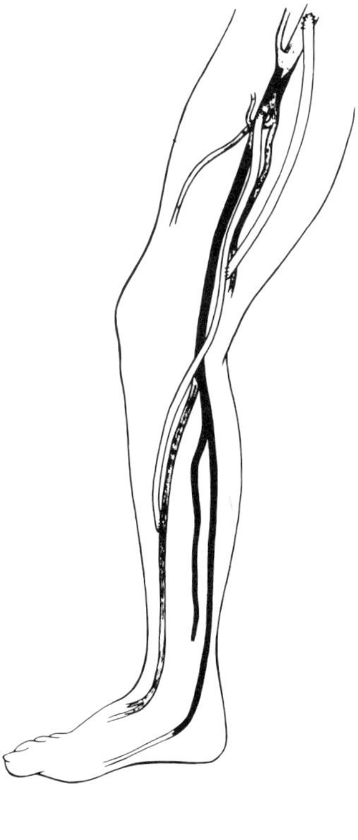

Figure 21. Patient who has functioning saphenous vein graft to the anterior tibial artery developed further ischemic symptoms with increased hemodynamic deterioration four years postoperatively, due to proximal disease at the common femoral artery. This was managed by adding PTFE graft from the external iliac artery to the functioning vein graft.

Composite Graft

When a careful search for an autogenous vein graft fails to provide proper or sufficient vein graft, a composite graft has been used. The composite graft in femoral-popliteal position has not been superior graft material, as discussed. However, in small vessel bypass, the composite graft may have a place. Long-term behavior of the composite graft in small vessel bypasses has been under investigation in my series. The patient in Figure 20 had extensive occlusive disease involving the entire superficial femoral artery as well as the popliteal, anterior tibial, and peroneal artery systems. This patient was further complicated with occlusive disease in the long segment of the profunda femoral artery. This problem was managed by doing external iliac artery-profunda femoral artery bypass with PTFE. Then cephalic vein was used for distal profunda femoral artery-posterior tibial artery bypass. A segment of profunda femoral artery was used as a bridge between the synthetic graft and the cephalic vein graft instead of making a direct anastomosis. This technique also protects the proximal graft to the profunda femoral artery.

In patients with a functioning femoral-tibial artery bypass vein graft with hemodynamic deterioration due to proximal disease, the principle of composite graft technique was used, as shown in Figure 21. PTFE graft was extended from the external iliac artery down to the functioning vein graft of the femoral-tibial artery bypass (Figure 21).

RESULTS

I have followed all the patients, with noninvasive vascular studies and clinical evaluation being the main methods. However, in cases of ischemic change or clinical and hemodynamic suspicion of impending graft failure, DSA or conventional angiography has been performed. The results are summarized in Table 1.

CONCLUSIONS

1. The long-term patency rate of femoral-popliteal or femoral-tibial artery byass with autogenous vein graft has been acceptable.
2. For patients with obstructive disease in multiple areas, there are many alternative approaches for revascularization by utilizing the principle of sequential bypass technique.
3. For patients with small vessel disease, distal small vessel bypasses have been encouraging, utilizing distal tibial arteries.

Table 1. Long-Term Results of Popliteal and Tibial Revascularization

1. *Femoral-popliteal bypass with autogenous greater saphenous vein graft.* The long-term patency at the fifth year was 84% and at the eighth year, 70% (see Figure 22).
2. *Femoral-tibial artery bypass with autogenous greater saphenous vein graft.* The long-term patency rate at the fifth year was 68% and at the eighth year, 60% (see Figure 23).
3. *Femoral-popliteal artery bypass with PTFE.* The five-year patency rate was 75%, if the distal anastomosis was made at above-knee level (see Figure 24). However, the patency rate was 60% when distal anastomosis of the PTFE graft was made at below-knee level (see Figure 25). The major factors for this are thought to be the condition of distal runoff, and partially the fact that the graft was across the knee joint.
4. *Femoral-tibial artery bypass with PTFE graft.* The long-term patency rate of this position was not satisfactory (see Figure 26).
5. *Femoral-popliteal-tibial artery sequential bypass with autogenous greater saphenous vein graft.* This group of patients, facing major limb loss with extensive occlusive disease in multiple areas, shows an encouraging long-term patency rate. The long-term patency rate at the fifth year was 70% (see Figure 27).
6. *Popliteal-distal tibial artery bypass with autogenous vein graft.* The patency rate of this position has been encouraging. It was 70% at the third year and 65% at the fifth year (see Figure 28).
7. *Femoral-popliteal artery bypass with biograft (human umbilical vein graft).* Limited experience with this graft has shown no major advantage over PTFE graft (see Figure 29).

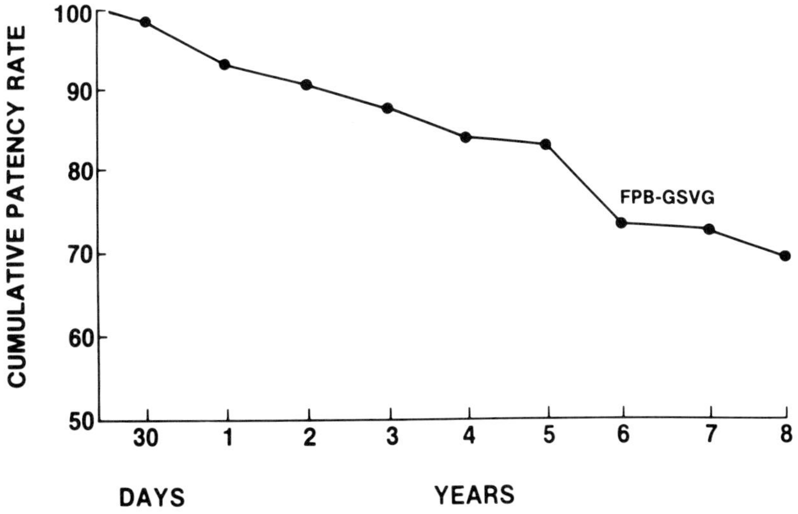

Figure 22. Comparative patency in saphenous vein grafts (femoral–popliteal bypass).

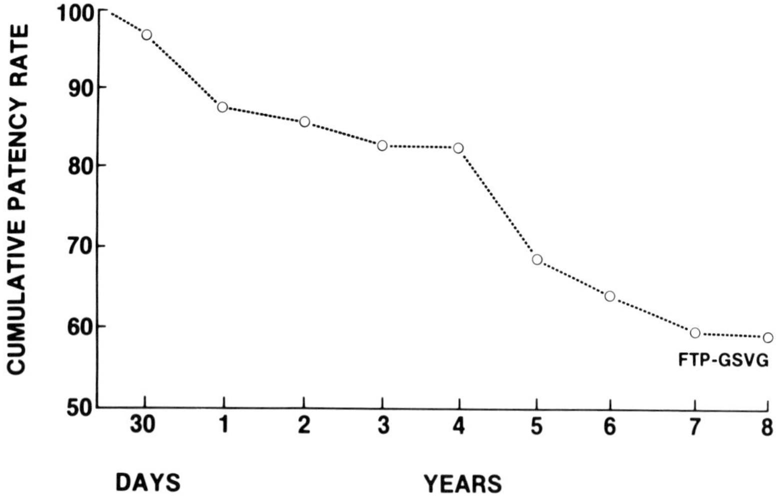

Figure 23. Comparative patency in saphenous vein grafts (femoral–tibial artery bypass).

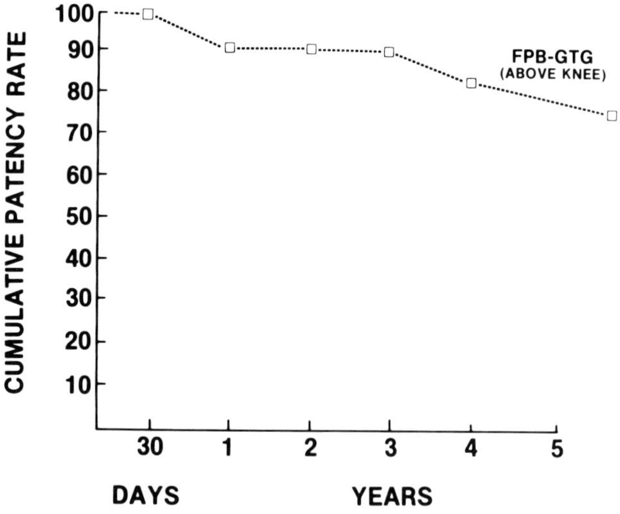

Figure 24. Patency rate of Gore-tex grafts (femoral–tibial artery bypass, above knee).

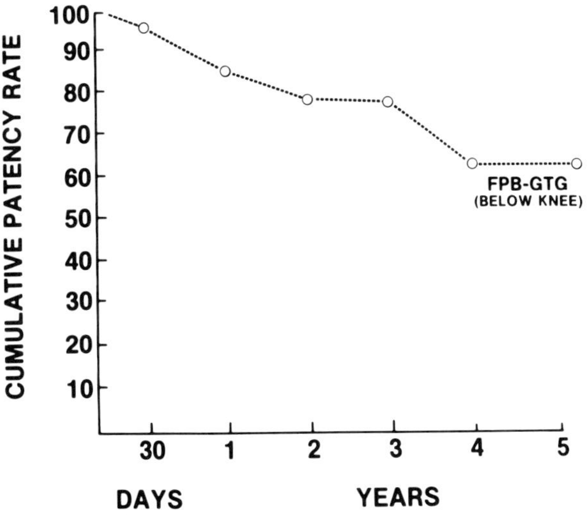

Figure 25. Patency rate of Gore-tex grafts (femoral–tibial artery bypass, below knee).

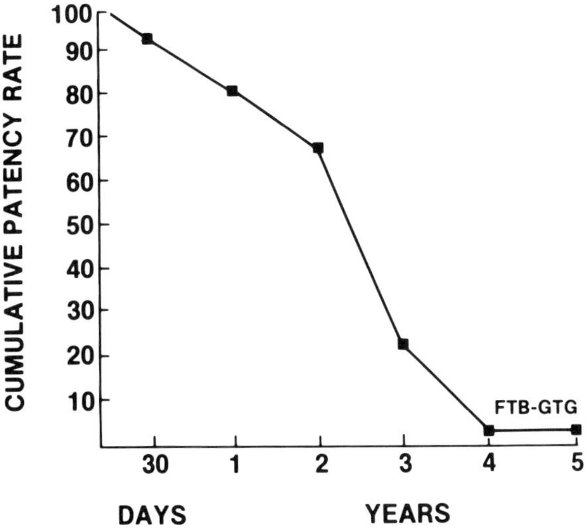

Figure 26. Patency rate of Gore-tex grafts (femoral–tibial artery bypass with PTFE graft).

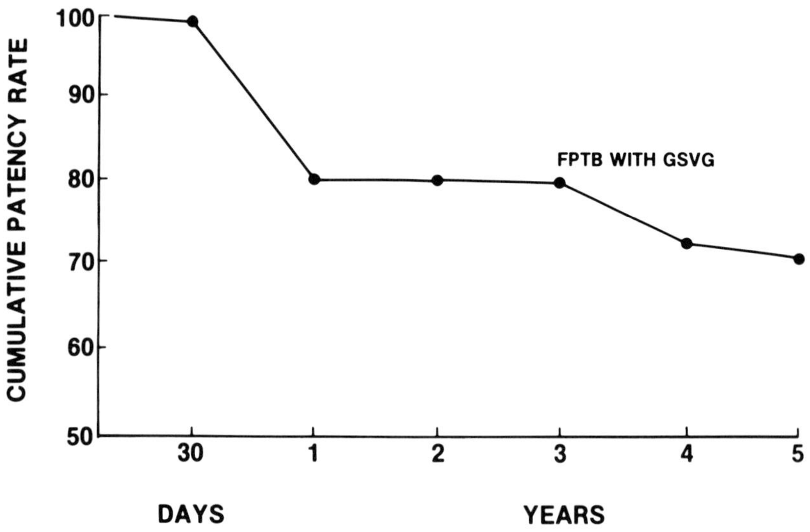

Figure 27. Patency rates of GSVG bypasses (femoral-popliteal-tibial artery sequential bypass).

a

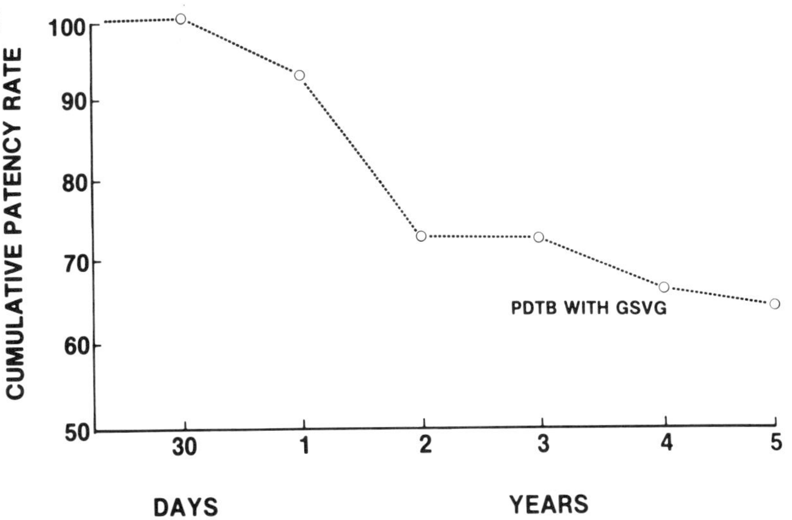

b

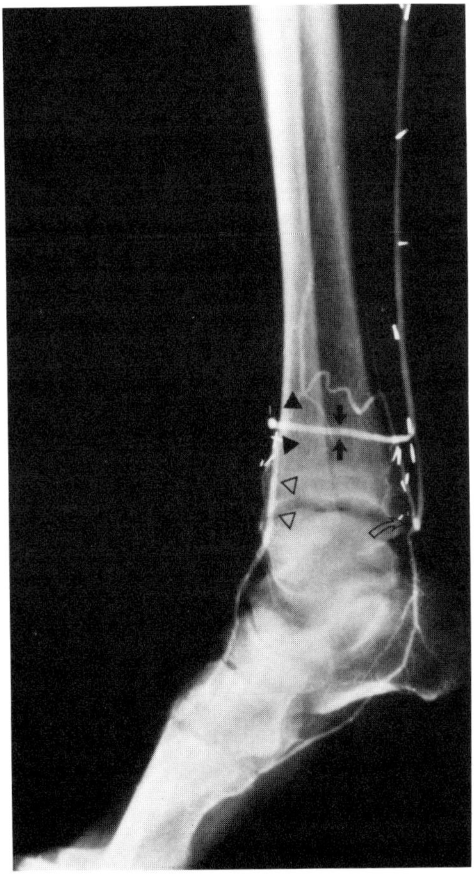

Figure 28. (a) Patency rates of GSVG bypasses (popliteal–distal tibial artery bypass). (b) This angiographic film shows patent saphenous vein graft to the distal popliteal artery (open arrow) and jump graft from the saphenous vein graft into the dorsal pedis artery (arrows and triangular arrows). Distal dorsalis pedis artery is well visualized through the graft (open triangular arrows).

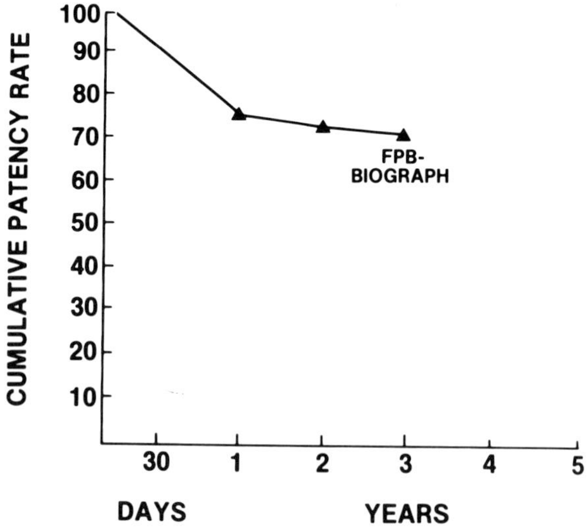

Figure 29. Patency rate of Gore-tex grafts (femoral–popliteal artery bypass with biograft).

4. Femoral–popliteal bypasses with PTFE have been acceptable up to five years. Therefore, in the high-risk group with no readily available greater saphenous vein graft, PTFE can be an alternative choice of graft, in the author's experience.
5. Femoral–tibial artery bypasses with PTFE or other synthetic material have been discouraging.
6. Adequate preoperative evaluation and proper angiographic studies down to the foot may give further indication for small vessel bypass or sequential bypass rather than simple femoral–tibial artery bypass graft in selected cases for longevity of the bypass result. For patients who are undergoing popliteal or tibial artery revascularization, it is important that the proximal arterial system be checked. If there is proximal disease in the aortoiliac artery system, this has to be treated properly [10].
7. In long-term follow-up, it is our policy to put all patients on an antiplatelet agent, unless medically contraindicated.
8. In postoperative follow-up evaluation, patients are examined on a regular basis with necessary noninvasive vascular studies. If there is clinical suspicion of impending graft failure with change on hemodynamic studies, such patients are to be studied with DSA technique or conventional angiography. If angiographic study shows a patent graft without evidence of distal disease, most likely the problem lies in the proximal arterial system. With this information, proper management can be obtained. Conventional angiographic films on a patient (Figure 29) shows a patent

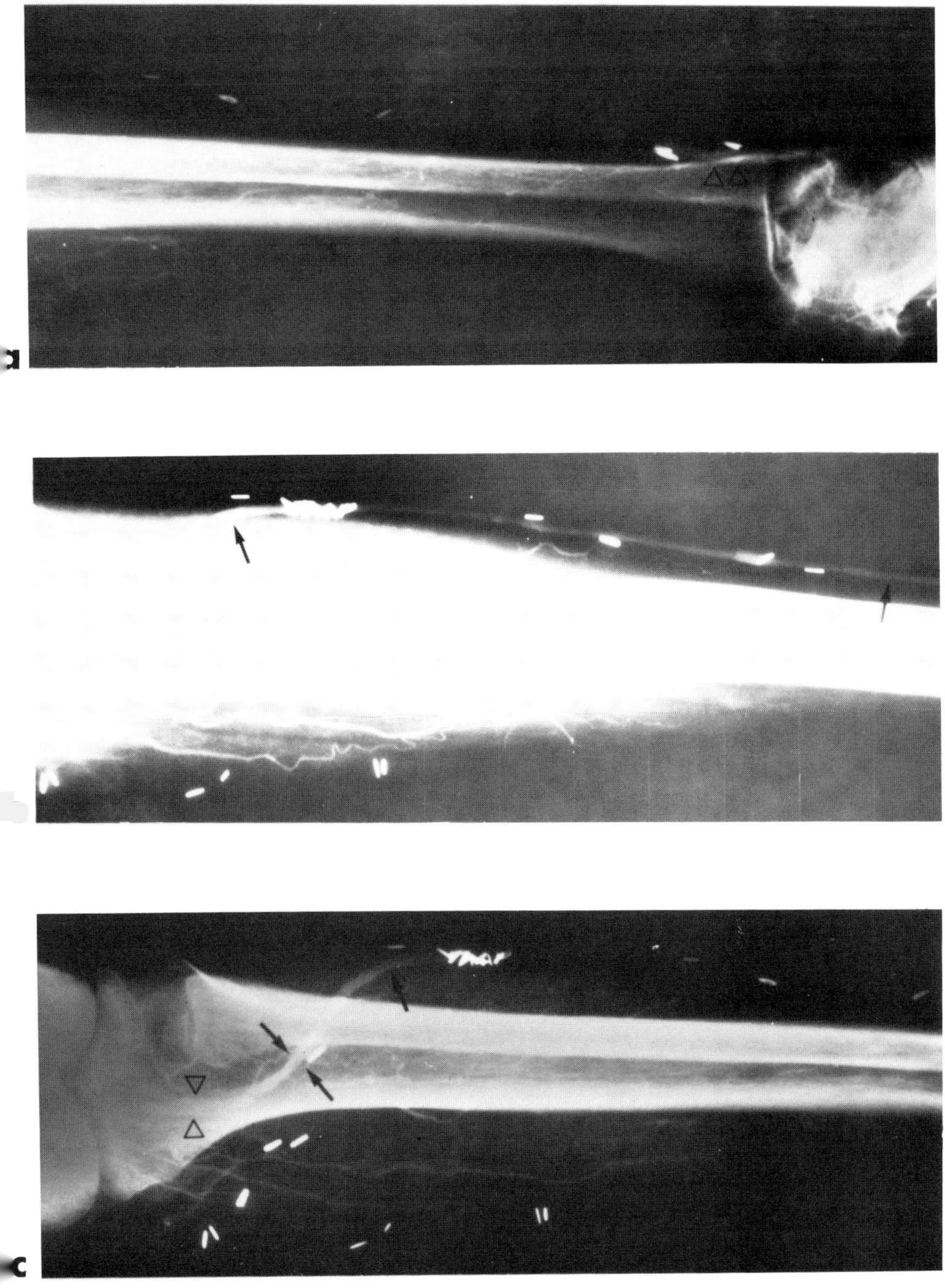

Figure 30. **(a)** Angiogram showing patent popliteal anterior tibial artery bypass graft. Proximal anastomosis at the triangular arrow. Patent vein graft is shown, as indicated by arrows. **(b)** Patent vein graft to the dorsalis pedis artery from the popliteal artery (arrows). **(c)** Distal anastomosis of the popliteal–dorsalis pedis artery bypass (triangular arrows).

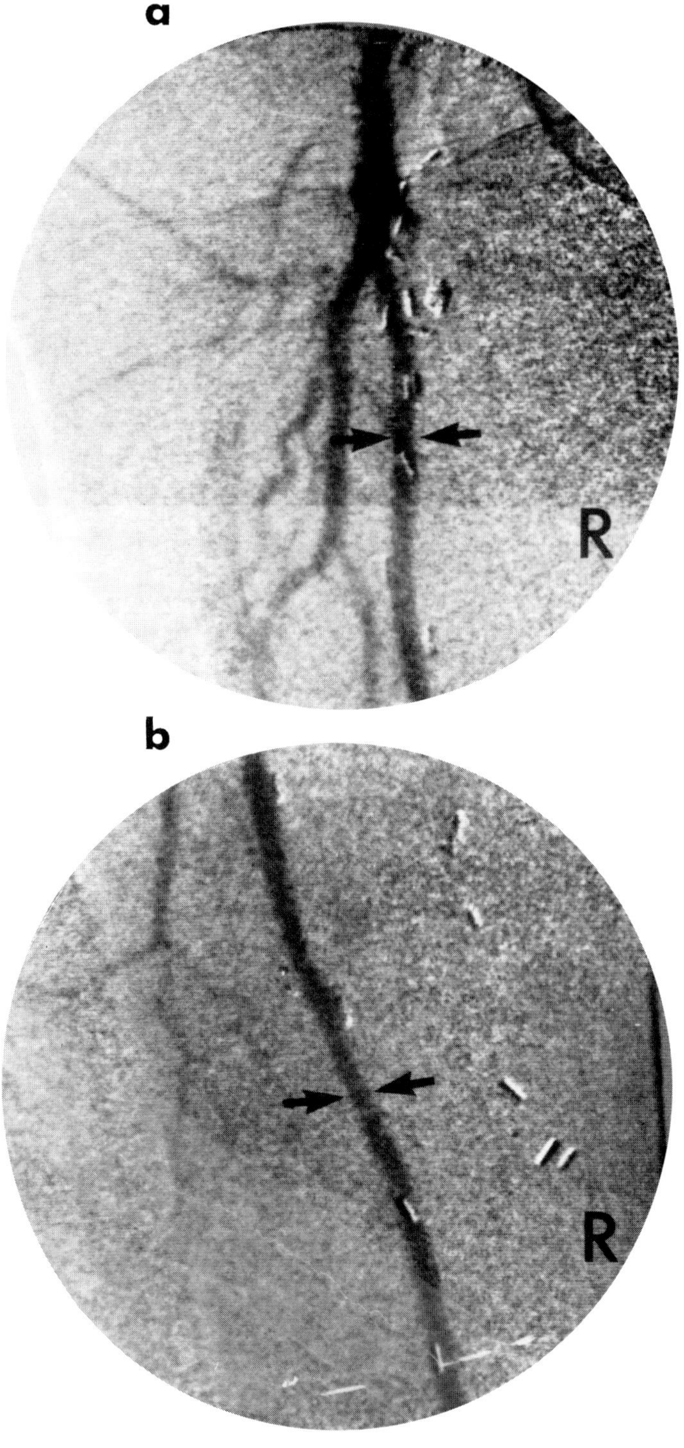
a
R
b
R

c

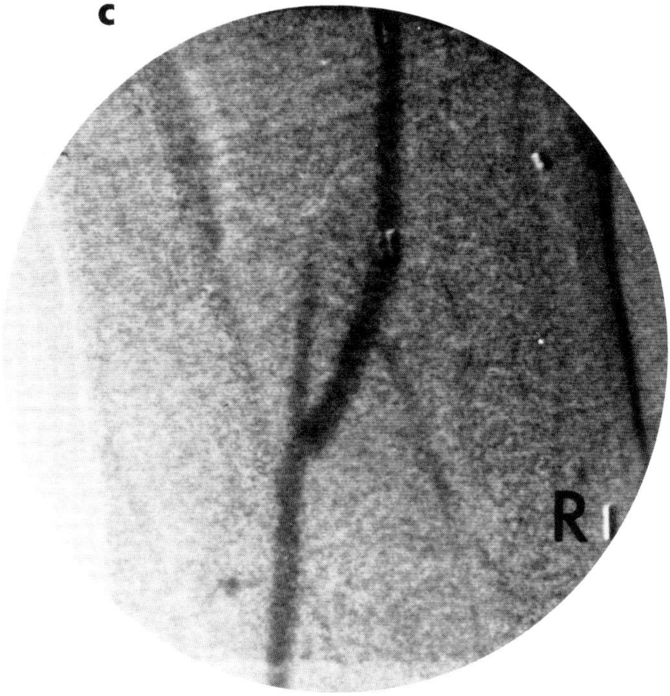

Figure 31. **(a)** DSA film showing patent graft at the femoral region (arrows). **(b)** DSA film showing integrity of vein graft at midportion. **(c)** DSA film showing patent vein graft and distal anastomosis.

graft of popliteal-anterior tibial artery bypass with autogenous vein graft (Figure 30). Similar information can be obtained with DSA technique, as shown on Figure 31. The DSA study shows a patent graft. With this technique, combined with intra-arterial injection, the integrity of the graft material can be examined as well as the proximal and distal arterial systems. Figure 31B shows integrity of the graft (arrows).

REFERENCES

1. Chang JB. Femoropopliteal and femorotibial arterial bypasses for limb salvage. Vasc Surg 15:4, 1981.
2. DeWeese JA, Rob CG. Autogenous venous grafts ten years later. Surg 82:6, 1977.

3. Dhall DP, Mavor GE. Long-term behavior of reversed saphenous vein grafts for advanced femoro-popliteal disease. Surg Gynecol Obstet 146:241, 1978.
4. O'Donnell JA, Brener BJ, Brief DK, et al. Realistic expectation for patients having lower extremity bypass surgery for limb salvage. Arch Surg 112: 1356, 1977.
5. Edwards WH, Mulherin JL, Jr. The role of graft material in femorotibial bypass. Ann Surg 191:6, 1980.
6. Sonnenfeld T, Cronestrand R. The advantages of the great saphenous vein as a femoropopliteal graft. Scand J Thor Cardiovasc Surg 14, 1980.
7. Kacoyanis G, Whittemore AD, et al. Femorotibial and femoroperoneal bypass vein grafts. Arch Surg 116, 1981.
8. Reichle F, Martinson M, Rankin K. Infrapopliteal arterial reconstruction in the severely ischemic lower extremity. Ann Surg 191:1, 1980.
9. Raviola C, Nichter L, et al. Femoropopliteal tibial bypass: What price failure. Am J Surg 144, 1982.
10. Chang JB. Surgical treatment of aorto-iliac artery disease. Angiology 32:2, 1981.
11. Martinez BD, Hertzer NR, Beven EG. Influence of distal arterial occlusive disease on prognosis following aortobifemoral bypass. Surg 88:6, 1980.
12. Jarrett F, Berkoff HA, et al. Femorotibial bypass grafts with sequential technique. Arch Surg 116, 1981.
13. Rainey JB, Smith RC, Jenkins AMcL. Sequential grafts for limb salvage in the presence of widespread occlusive vascular disease. Ann R C Surg Engl 64, 1982.
14. Jarrett F, Berkoff HA, Crummy AB. Sequential femorotibial bypass: Clinical results. Canadian J Surg 23:1, 1980.
15. Rosenfeld JC, Savarese RP, et al. Sequential femoropopliteal and femorotibial bypasses. Arch Surg 116, 1981.
16. Burdick JF, O'Mara C, et al. The multiple sequential distal bypass graft: Improving nature's alternatives. Surg 89:5, 1981.
17. LaSalle AJ, Brewster DC, et al. Femoropopliteal composite bypass grafts: Current status. Surgery 92:1, 1982.
18. O'Mara, CS, Flinn WR, et al. Recognition and surgical management of patent but hemodynamically failed arterial grafts. Ann Surg 193:4, 1981.
19. Whittemore AD, Clowes AW, et al Secondary femoropopliteal reconstruction. Ann Surg 193:1, 1981.
20. Wooster DL, Provan JL. Fate of the limb after failed femoropopliteal reconstruction. Canadian J Surg 25:4, 1982.
21. Kazmers M, Satiani B, Evans WE. Amputation level following unsuccessful distal limb salvage operations. Surg 8:6, 1980.
22. Samson RH, Gupta SK, et al. Level of amputation after failure of limb salvage procedures. Surg Gynecol Obstet 154, 1982.
23. Connolly JE, Kwaan JHM. In situ saphenous vein bypasses. Arch Surg 117, 1982.
24. Gruss JD, Bartels D, et al. Arterial reconstruction for distal disease of the lower extremities by the in situ vein graft technique. J Cardiovasc Surg 23, 1982.

25. Rosenthal D, Levine K, et al. Femoropopliteal bypass: The preferred site for distal anastomosis. Surgery 93:1, Part 1, 1983.
26. Sonnenfeld T, Cronestrand R. Factors determining outcome of reversed saphenous vein femoropopliteal bypass grafts. Br J Surg 67, 1980.
27. Perdue G, Smith RB, et al. Revascularization for severe limb ischemia. Arch Surg 115, 1980.
28. Turnipseed WD, Detmer DE, et al. Intra-arterial digital angiography: A new diagnostic method for determining limb salvage bypass candidates. Surgery 92:2, 1982.

19
Past and Present Problems in Arterial Grafting

D. Emerick Szilagyi

When in the early 1950s, after the demonstration that arterial allografts were unsuitable for clinical use [1], the search for arterial substitutes began. The concept of the conduit to be achieved was a simple one [2]. The surgeon merely wanted a durable tube that would carry blood consistently for the desired distances.

The basic practical model of this concept was a pipe made of textile fabric. All the variants of this basic model that emerged during the past thirty years were very similar in construction. The fabric proper of the arterial prosthesis is infiltrated by connective tissue, which grows through the pores or crevices between the strands of yarn, eventually reaching the luminal surface. The inner lining is a partially organized layer of blood coagulum, which at intervals is supported by the invading strands of connective tissue. The so-called pseudo-intima has very poor resistance to clotting and does not possess the distinguishing and highly specialized qualities of the true endothelium. The connective tissue in which the prosthesis is embedded forms an outer shell, which may vary greatly in thickness, depending on the reactivity of the prosthesis and on the histologic characteristics of the surrounding tissue.

The early experiments established that porosity, flexibility and durability were the essential qualities desired in this device [3]. From the above description the importance of porosity is obvious. Flexibility in these simple substitutes serves the purpose of accommodation of the prosthesis to anatomic contours. It does not in any way equal the visco-elastic quality of the true arterial wall. Currently, flexibility is usually achieved by crimping, but can also be accomplished by texturing the component fibers, as is done in the so-called Helanca Dacron prosthesis.

Durability is a function partly of the original tensile strength of the component fibers and partly of the chemical reactivity of the synthetic material in the fibers to the surrounding tissues. The ideal synthetic material will have minimal chemical reactivity and will excite just a sufficient amount of histologic reaction to insure incorporation of the synthetic material without excessively thick connective tissue shell and pseudointima. Currently it is universally acknowledged that Dacron is the synthetic material that best combines the qualities favorable to durability.

The problems that arose during the clinical history of this basic model of arterial prosthesis during the past thirty years will be illustrated by a summary of my own clinical and laboratory experience [4,5]. The reason for choosing this approach, aside from the familiarity with the material, is that it contains follow-up studies not available elsewhere.

The experimental work of this prosthesis began in 1955 and was carried out with the McCune preparation [3], which permitted the insertion of prosthetic segments from 20 to 35 centimeters long as bypasses from the proximal thoracic aorta to the distal abdominal aorta. In a group of dogs numbering over 400, gross and microscopic observations of the prosthesis were made for up to 15 years. The prosthesis proved to be well-incorporated in the canine tissues and gave excellent patency rates.

In 1957, after having ascertained that laboratory observations during two years proved the prosthesis to yield satisfactory results and having noted in particular that the tensile strength remained stable, I began the clinical use of this prosthesis.

In 1964, after seven years of clinical use during which the method of fabrication of the prosthesis remained essentially unchanged, a careful survey of the results was conducted [5]. At that time our clinical material consisted of 835 cases, but one should add that experience after 1964 in a total number of 3,500 cases remained in complete accord with the original findings. The evaluation was carried out by three methods: by observing the postoperative angiographic changes; by assessing the gross and microscopic appearances of the recovered grafts; and by calculating the late patency rates.

In the entire clinical material, 561 cases were suitable for angiographic analysis. In 65 percent of these cases, well-preserved and flawless structural qualities were noted. In the remaining 35 percent of the cases, various morphologic changes were observed, almost all of them minor or insignificant. The most common of these was a wavy appearance of the graft, which we call "pleating." This change was mainly the result of the accommodation of the graft to the process of shortening the distance between the arterial anastomoses. With very rare exceptions, grafts with such changes continued to function well. In fact, in less than one percent of the cases the morphologic changes lead to thrombosis.

In femoropopliteal bypass, the most important alteration noted in serial angiograms was the progressive narrowing of the lumen that may have involved isolated segments of all of the prosthesis. Correlation of these roentgen appearances with the gross anatomic findings in the recovered prosthesis proved that the change in contour was due to deposition of layers of mural clo The transit time of the dye from common femoral to popliteal artery may hav n greatly prolonged; from 18 to 48 seconds. The flow was delayed because c the restricted outflow tract brought about by advanced occlusive process in the infrapopliteal arterial branches. This phenomenon was observed in all but 5 of 24 femoropopliteal Dacron prostheses that had been followed by serial angiograms before occlusion. It appears to be the single most important initiating factor in the failures of femoropopliteal prosthesis.

Our angiographic observations were complemented by gross anatomic and microscopic information from the study of the recovered prosthesis. Briefly stated, both the aortoiliac and femoropopliteal grafts that were recovered while still functioning showed good ingrowth of connective tissue and stable but poorly developed neointima.

We classified the results of the gross and microscopic studies of the recovered Helanca Dacron prosthesis according to certain broad categories of qualities, with each category taking into account more minute details. In pure anatomic terms, the results were gratifying. Since the recovered grafts represented a highly selective sample, that is, grafts that were functioning well just before harvesting, these results must not be interpreted as the measure of overall clinical performance. Since 1966 we have added 11 more specimens to the group and the findings have remained consistent. It was especially gratifying that the tensile strength of these grafts remained essentially unchanged for up to 15 years.

The third and perhaps the most impressive proof of performance of prosthetic implants is the late patency rate. During the first seven years of the use of the prosthesis, the most relevant fact was the extremely poor performance of the prosthesis in the femoropopliteal region, where the patency rate dropped to 30 percent in three years. Shortly after this study, the use of this prosthesis in the femoropopliteal region was abandoned.

As regards aortoiliac implants, at five years the postoperative patency rate was 93.1 percent; at ten years 71.0 percent; at 15 years 50.0 percent. We judged these results entirely satisfactory.

The incidence of healing complications was high in the early period of our experience [6], but with the improvement of surgical technique and more recently with the introduction of prophylactic antibiotic medication, their frequency of occurrence rapidly declined. Currently, the rate of incidence of prosthetic graft infection in our practice is 0.2 percent and that of false aneurysm is 1 percent per anastomosis.

If one wishes to summarize the present performance status of synthetic vascular substitutes, all of which in current use behave in a very similar manner, one must say that they represent a synthetic fibrin network around which and into which connective tissue grows, the inner surface of which is covered with a layer of more or less organized blood clot. The body graciously accepts this poor substitute and works well with it as long as the hemodynamic conditions are favorable, that is, as long as the diameter is ample, the length is limited, the flow is fast, and the pressure is high. When the hemodynamic conditions become unfavorable, the conduit gradually stops functioning by a mechanism which is in essence a sequential deposition of mural thrombi on the inner lining or pseudo-intima. The secondary role of the constructional details of the conduit itself is strikingly illustrated by the totally unsatisfactory behavior in the femoro-popliteal regions of the same textile fabrics that give a consistently excellent result in the aortoiliac anatomic area.

Because of the unsatisfactory late results of Dacron prosthesis in the femoropopliteal arterial trunk, by the end of 1956 we had very drastically restricted and during 1957 completely eliminated its use in the treatment of occlusive disease in this anatomic region and turned to the use of the greater saphenous vein as an autogenous implant, first described by Kunlin in 1949 [7], and introduced in this country by Linton. Between January 1, 1963 and December 31, 1967, we performed 597 femoropopliteal operations using saphenous vein for lower limb occlusive arterial disease [8]. Of these, 492 or 82.4 percent left the hospital with open grafts. Among the grafts that left the hospital in a state of patency, in the femoropopliteal grafts there was a yearly attrition of from 3% to 7%, with a patency rate of 50.2 percent in 5 years, 46.0 percent at 10 years, and 27.5 percent in 15 years. The infrapopliteal cases displayed a greater yearly loss, with a patency rate of 37.4 percent at 5 years, and 29.1 percent at 8 years. These results are greatly superior to those we have obtained with any other surgical method.

In 1972, we undertook a study of the problem of the histologic behavior of autogenous vein grafts [9], a problem of obvious importance from the view-point of functional durability. The findings of the review of serial postoperative angiograms and of the microscopic study of vein implants recovered at operation or at autopsy were correlated.

The correlation of histologic findings in 31 cases with the angiographic observations in 260 cases with sequential studies showed six types of morphologic changes: intimal thickening, atherosclerosis, fibrosis of valve, cicatricial stenosis, suture stenosis, and aneurysmal dilatation. Among these, many were preventable by careful surgical technique or remediable by secondary repair. The only lesions that seemed intrinsically unavoidable and usually irreparable were atherosclerosis and intimal thickening, forming about 20 percent of the material under study.

These findings underline the need for extreme care in the harvesting and temporary storing of the venous autografts as well as in the postoperative follow-up of cases bearing such grafts. Careless harvesting undoubtedly increases the probability of later occurrence of degenerative changes. Neglect in the follow-up observation results in failure to detect these lesions early.

While the current needs of the vascular surgeons are satisfactorily met in large-bore arterial replacement, the demand for serviceable small-diameter arterial substitutes, primarily owing to the short supply of autogenous veins, is urgently pressing.

The attempts at the improvement of the performance of the existing arterial substitutes, in particular of small-bore substitutes, have followed three directions: (1) changes in methods of fabrication; (2) introduction of new or modified graft materials, and (3) manipulation of the physicochemical properties of the blood-graft interface.

Research aimed at modifying the blood-graft interactions by a durable or permanent change in the composition of the graft is very active but as yet has produced no clinically applicable advances. The results of the efforts to modify the graft structure by altering the method of fabrication or by introducing new graft materials have, on the other hand, been put to extensive clinical trials. These innovations can be considered under two headings: (1) those with alterations of the basic Dacron construction and (2) those using new graft material.

The so-called velour construction of knitted Dacron prostheses, advocated by Sauvage, has gained wide popularity [10]. This method creates fibriles that stand up on the graft surface, increases the total surface area, and, therefore, is presumed to promote more vigorous connective tissue infiltration. When placed on the outer surface, this construction would be expected to provide a thicker outer shell. On the inner surface it is hoped that this construction encourages tissue ingrowth into the pores and further extension onto the luminal surface, creating a pseudointima that is hoped to be more resistant to clotting.

It is difficult to see the advantage of a thicker outer adventitial connective tissue growth. The connective tissue shell observed about good Dacron prostheses of conventional construction appears to be in every way adequate unless the incorporation has been interfered with by exudate or infection. The claim regarding a better development of the so-called pseudointima leading to superior patency rates has yet to be demonstrated. But in any case, the histologic qualities of the filamentous prosthesis do not show any striking differences from the sections of the Dacron prosthesis discussed earlier.

In the second category of innovations, that of new graft materials, analdehyde-tanned collagen tube of bovine origin was first proposed as a substitute conduit for arteries about 30 years ago and at one time reached rather wide popularity [11]. Histologic studies show that this graft is not incorporated but merely passively accepted. With the passage of time, two great deficiencies became evident, namely, a tendency to aneurysmal change and poor tolerance of the graft to infection.

Specially processed umbilical vein has been more recently offered as an arterial replacement and is in essence another variety of a collagen conduit, but in this instance the tubular structure undergoing the tanning process is the human umbilical cord vein and the tanning agent is glucaraldehyde [12]. Moreover, since the tanned collagen of the umbilical vein has relatively low tensile strength, the entire collagen tube is invested in a highly porous stocking-like Dacron mesh. The histologic behavior of this implant is not significantly different from that of other collagen tubes.

A widely popular current innovation is the use of expanded polytetrafluoroethylene (Teflon) of PTFE for the fabrication of sheets and tubes that are nontextile but appear porous [13]. In spite of the apparent porosity, the incorporation of this prosthesis by connective tissue ingrowth is very limited.

In this respect, however, the fact that the recently introduced nonporous prostheses are capable of sustained function as blood conduits seriously challenges the traditional idea that porosity of the wall is an indispensable quality for function in an artificial artery. The conclusion is inevitable that the degree of thrombogenicity of the inner surface may be an even more important functional determinant.

It is unfortunate that clinical trials with the newer forms of substitute arteries have not been conducted in a statistically rigorous manner, most particularly in their use in the femoropopliteal area. There are no truly convincing data about the relative merits of these new devices, both when one attempts to compare one with another or with the accepted standard, the autogenous vein graft. The only undoubted fact at present seems to be that none can match the performance of the autogenous vein in small-artery replacement.

The ultimate ideal of vascular surgeons is an arterial substitute with a live intima and a permanently compliant wall. One of the most exciting recent advances in this field has been the successful propagation in pure tissue culture of endothelial cells, with the promise that this may be successfully seeded on prosthetic surfaces [14]. The clinical applicability of this concept is, however, still distant.

A fair summary of the current state of the clinical use of arterial substitutes would be to say that while one has only one ideal product—the autogenous vein—all the immediately essential needs of vascular therapeutics are met in a fairly satisfactory though far from ideal manner. For the replacement of large arteries (over 12 mm in diameter) of relatively short length (less than 30 cm) especially in high-flow areas, a number of Dacron and Teflon devices are available that function well in terms of 5-15 years. The requirement for small-bore replacement is splendidly served by the autogenous (greater saphenous) vein graft, but its supply is short of demand. Autogenous vein grafts are applicable to the treatment of all degrees of occlusive disease, but have, of course, serious dimensional limitations. While a search for a man-made artery of qualities equal to or at least closely similar to those of an autogenous vein continues, the use of synthetic small-bore replacement should be limited to far-advanced cases of occlusive involvement. Concurrently, the awareness among the surgical profession of the value of the greater saphenous vein as a limb- and life-saving resource should be emphasized in the hope of avoiding the reckless use of vein-stripping operations, which are very seldom therapeutically justified.

REFERENCES

1. Szilagyi DE, McDonald RT, Smith RF, Whitcomb JG. Biologic fate of human arterial homografts. AMA Arch Surg 75:506–529, 1957.
2. Voorhees AB, Jaretzki A, Blakemore AW. The use of tubes constructed from Vinyon "N" cloth in bridging arterial defects. Ann Surg 135:332–336, 1952.
3. Szilagyi DE, France LC, Smith RF, Whitcomb JG. Clinical use of an elastic Dacron prosthesis. AMA Arch Surg 77:538–551, 1958.
4. Szilagyi DE, Pfeifer JR, DeRusso FJ. Long-term evaluation of plastic arterial substitutes: An experimental study. Surgery 55:165–173, 1964.
5. Szilagyi DE, Smith RF, Elliott JP, Allen HM. The long-term behavior of a Dacron arterial substitute: Clinical roentgenological, and histological correlations. Ann Surg 162:453–456, 1965.
6. Szilagyi DE, Smith RF, Elliott JP, Vrandecic MP. Infection in arterial reconstruction with synthetic grafts. Ann Surg 321–323, 1972.
7. Kunlin J. Le traitement de L'arterite obliterante par le greffe veineuse. Arch Mal Coeur 42:371–374, 1949.
8. Szilagyi DE, Hageman JH, Smith RF, Elliott JP, Brown F, Dietz P. Autogenous vein grafting in femoropopliteal atherosclerosis: The limits of its effectiveness. Surgery 86:836–851, 1979.
9. Szilagyi DE, Elliott JP, Hageman JH, Smith RF, Dall'Olmo CA. Biologic fate of autogenous vein implants as arterial substitutes: Clinical, angiographic and histopathologic observation in femoropopliteal operations for atherosclerosis. Ann Surg 178:232–234, 1973.
10. Sauvage LR, Berger K, Wood SJ, Smith JC, David CC, Hall DG, et al. The USCI-Sauvage filamentous vascular prosthesis: Rationale, clinical results, and healing in man. In PH Sawyer, Martin J Kaplitt (eds.), Vascular Grafts, pp. 185–196. New York, Appleton-Century-Crofts, 1978.
11. Rosenberg N, Gaughran ERL, Henderson J, et al. The use of segmental arterial implants prepared by enzymatic modification of heterologous blood vessels. Surg Forum 6:242–246, 1956.
12. Dardik H, Dardik I. Successful arterial substitution with modified human umbilical vein. Ann Surg 183:252–258, 1976.

13. Campbell CD, Brooks DH, Webster MW, Diamond DL, Peel RL, Bahnson HT. Expanded microporous polytetrafluoroethylene as a vascular substitute: A two year follow-up. Surgery 85:177–183, 1979.
14. Graham LM, Burkel WE, Ford JW, Vinter DW, Kahn RH, Stanley JC. Immediate seeding of enzymatically derived endothelium in Dacron vascular grafts. Early experimental studies with autologous canine cells. Arch Surg 15:1289–1294, 1980.

20
The Diabetic Foot

Moshe Haimov

It is estimated that at present time there are more than ten million diabetics in the United States of whom 70% are currently recognized to have the disease. It is also estimated that 25% of these patients will eventually consult physicians, surgeons or podiatrists for diabetic-related foot or leg problems of various kinds; 200 million dollars are expended yearly in the treatment of diabetic patients and disease-related complications. Two-thirds of limb amputations are done on diabetic patients, who comprise only 5% of the population. More hospital days are spent treating diabetic foot infection than for any other complication of diabetes.

The diabetic patient presents with three primary categories of pathophysiology: infection, neuropathy, and arterial insufficiency. These pathologic processes present as individual problems or a combination of two or all three categories. The problem of infection in diabetic patients is a real one. There is no question that, for reasons not entirely understood, these patients respond with a poor defense mechanism to infection. This poor response to infection may be related to impaired white blood cell function or to the altered metabolism of the diabetic patient. Once infection has occurred, early recognition of the problem is of paramount importance to prevent serious foot destruction or limb loss. To what extent good control of the diabetes in terms of blood sugar levels is important in the prevention of the complications associated with the diabetic foot is not entirely clear and remains controversial. It appears however that the majority of diabetologists agree today that good diabetic control increases the resistance to infection, decreases the likelihood of progressive neuropathy, and decreases the rate of arterial occlusion. Chemically it has been demonstrated that high blood sugars do change the composition of low density lipoproteins of proteins so that fatty deposits in the arterial walls will increase with poorly controlled diabetes. Cigarette smoking is another important factor that has always to be considered. Tobacco increases platelet adhesiveness, which is the precursor of the atherosclerotic plaque. In addition, it increases the concentration of carbon monoxide in the blood which, with its strong affinity to hemoglobin, may decrease the amount of hemoglobin available for oxygen by 30% to 40%. It has been shown experimentally that arterial walls with diminished oxygen supply develop atherosclerosis at a much more rapid rate than would otherwise occur. In addition, nicotine causes vasospasm and increases blood pressure, which further damages the arterial tree.

DIABETIC FOOT INFECTION

Diabetic foot infection as seen by the clinician may manifest various degrees of severity. One sees patients with mild infections consisting of superficial ulcerations without surrounding cellulitis and without involvement of the underlying bone. Other patients present with what is classified as a moderate extent of infection with rather deep ulcerations, with or without bone involvement, with surrounding cellulitis but no systemic toxicity. On the other end of the spectrum we see patients with severe foot infections associated with rather extensive ulceration, abscess formation involving various fascial planes, extensive cellulitis and lymphangitis, and clinical evidence of systemic toxicity. In 90% of these infections one would culture gram-positive cocci; in 50% one would find in addition gram-negative rods, and in 65% anaerobes would play a significant role. In dealing with these infections, it behooves the surgeon to determine the severity of the infection as outlined in the previously mentioned classification. This determination is important since treatment will vary according to the severity of the infection. As much as possible, the accurate extent of tissue destruction will have to be determined as well as the extent of bone or joint involvement. In addition, careful aerobic and anaerobic cultures should be taken and the degree of arterial insufficiency, if any, should be recorded. X-rays of the foot at the acute stage of infection are not very helpful, since only advanced degrees of osteomyelitis would be recognizable. On the other hand if, on probing ulcerations in the foot associated with infection, one can reach bony structures, this in itself would be sufficient evidence for the presence of osteomyelitis. In general, mild foot infections can be treated at home with rest of the injured part, application of local dressings, and the prescription of special appliances aimed at preventing further pressure at the areas of injury. As in all diabetic foot problems, careful follow-up is extremely important. What was mild foot infection 24 or 48 hours previously can rapidly turn into severe foot infection which, in association with diabetic neuropathy, may go unnoticed by the patient. All patients with moderate or severe foot infections have to be treated in the hospital. Again, both require careful diabetic control, cultures and appropriate antibiotic treatment. There are several general principles in the treatment of diabetic foot infections. When surgery is required, all abscesses will have to be opened widely to allow for proper drainage. All sinus tracts should be carefully followed and laid open. All necrotic tissue will have to be debrided. Not infrequently, amputation of one or more toes will be required for proper drainage. If bone appears to be involved, limited amputation would be indicated. In patients in whom arterial insufficiency is present, revascularization will have to be considered once infection has been brought under control. Once local foot amputations have been performed and healing has been achieved, the balance of the foot may be seriously impaired, exposing various areas of the foot to unaccustomed pressure during walking. By using prosthestic appliances, an attempt should be made to rebalance these feet once the patient is fully rehabilitated. Any surgery in the diabetic foot should be carried out in such a way so as to preserve as much tissue as possible. The aim of the surgery is to end up with a functional foot. Once the infection has caused extensive foot damage, primary limb amputation may be the procedure of choice rather than choosing a course of protracted hospitalization and multiple surgical procedures, which eventually culminate with a markedly deformed foot which would be prone to repeated trauma and for which no proper prosthetics are available. In dealing with the diabetic foot, heat or soaking, especially hot soaks, are contraindicated. The diabetic patient would not tolerate undrained pus, and diabetic foot infection is a surgical emergency. Exposed joint capsules or exposed cartilage will not heal. Healing will also not occur if the patient is weight-bearing, and most diabetic foot infections require bed rest to achieve healing. During these sometimes prolonged periods of bed rest, major joint contractures should be avoided with appropriate physiotherapy. Prolonged dependency will cause severe edema in the infected foot and delay healing, and this is also contraindicated. In terms of local care following debridement or limited amputations, there are various solutions that can be used for daily dressing. I have found diluted Betadine solution or Dakin's solution, again diluted to achieve iso-osmolar concentration and prevent wound drying, to be rather inexpensive and practical. Exposed tendons, cartilage or fascia will not heal and will have to be actively debrided. Patients with unusually dry skin are prone to development of cracks which subsequently become infected and may lead to major foot infection. Lanolin has been helpful in preventing this type of complication. As in all problems when dealing with the diabetic foot, preventive measures are equally if not more important than the therapeutic measures. These include early recognition and treatment of infection, trauma prevention, proper diabetic control, control of hypertension, cessation of smoking and weight control.

DIABETIC NEUROPATHY

Diabetic neuropathy is one of the main complications of diabetes mellitus and in 40% of the cases of diabetic foot lesions, it is the primary etiology. The pathology of nerve damage in diabetes is poorly understood. One theory attributes the nerve changes to vascular injuries to the blood supply of the nerves. Another, more popular, suggests the problem is metabolic with the toxic accumulation of sorbitol in Schwann cells. Clinically the symptoms are those of paresthesia, hyperesthesia, hypoesthesia, and radiculopathy and manifested by sharp, stabbing or burning pain in one or both extremities. In contrast to ischemic pain, the aforementioned pain occurs mostly at rest and is often relieved by ambulation. Clinically, in addition to the sensory loss, one finds loss of deep tendon reflexes, loss of vibratory and positional sense, heavy callus formation, trophic ulcer formation and, in more extreme cases, total foot drop and the appearance of Charcot joint with major foot deformities. Muscle paralysis of the small muscles in the foot lead to contractures and hammer toe formation. Plantar ulcer and mal perforant are two of the most important manifestations of diabetic neuropathy. If untreated, these ulcers, which are caused by metatarsal head compression, will eventually lead to major foot infections, which will require partial foot amputations and in more extreme cases lead to major limb loss. Superficial plantar ulcers, which do not extend down to involve the underlying head of the metatarsal bone, can be successfully healed with bed rest and avoiding pressure to the area. Special metatarsal bars can be added to the shoe to avoid ulcer recurrence. Deep ulcerations may require metatarsal head excision to achieve healing. If major infection is not present, this can be done through a separate dorsal foot incision and, following removal of the metatarsal head healing of the ulcer, can be achieved within a matter of weeks. Again, preventive measures are of major importance. The diabetic patient with neuropathic foot should be carefully instructed about foot vulnerability. Both feet should be examined daily by the patient; if any lesion is detected, the attending physician should be consulted immediately. The diabetic patient should be taught to examine his shoes on a daily basis, looking for foreign bodies. Any vascular surgeon with some experience has seen patients who have been walking for weeks with foreign bodies in their shoes without being aware of them. The intradigital spaces should be carefully examined again on a daily basis; if toe deformities are present, cotton or gauze should be applied between the toes to prevent pressure ulcerations. Narrow fashionable shoes should be avoided, since the patient will not be aware of any discomfort caused by excessively narrow shoes. Extensive callus formation can in itself act as a foreign body, causing ulceration and necrosis of the underlying tissue, which is usually followed by infection, which will rapidly involve the underlying bone, requiring limited amputations. If careful follow-up visits are scheduled, these areas of excessive callus formation can be treated on an ongoing basis, thus avoiding the above mentioned complication.

DIABETIC VASCULAR DISEASE

The diabetic patient is more likely to develop early occlusive atherosclerotic disease than his counterpart of similar age and background. A rather useful rule of thumb applied by one of our senior diabetologists states that the true biological age of the diabetic patient can be estimated to be that of his chronological age plus the number of years that the patient has been known to have diabetes mellitus. Thus a 50-year-old diabetic patient who has had diabetes for the last 15 years has the blood vessels of a 65-year-old. In addition, it has been noted that the diabetic patient has a decreased capacity for developing collateral circulation. Also, one finds much more small vessel disease in the diabetic patient than in the nondiabetic. Microscopically there is no typical vascular diabetic lesion in the extremities like the ones found in the kidneys or retina. Some investigators have described thickened capillary basement membrane in the small arterioles in the foot. This lesion, however, is not limited to diabetic patients alone, and its contribution to the overall problems of the diabetic foot are not entirely clear. The diabetic patient with macrovascular disease is not different in terms of diagnostic workup and treatment from his nondiabetic counterpart. The indications for reconstructive surgery in these patients are similar: severe intermittent claudication, rest pain, or gangrene. In some diabetic patients with foot infections, vascular reconstruction may be indicated to allow for limited amputation and healing of various foot lesions. Whenever dealing with any problems associated with the diabetic foot, one should try to conserve as much of the foot as possible. A diabetic patient who looses one extremity has close to a 50% chance of losing the second one within the next five years. Therefore, extreme efforts to preserve the lower extremities in the diabetic patients are in order.

Finally, I would like to stress that in the treatment of the diabetic foot, success is achievable only through a major team effort, the team being the diabetologist, the vascular surgeon, the radiologist, the infectious disease specialist, the podiatrist, and the rehabilitation and prosthetic specialists. It is only through the combined efforts of all these specialists that optimal care can be rendered to this extremely difficult group of patients.

10

Venous Problems

21 Current Management of Varicose Veins

Eric P. Lofgren

The term varicose veins includes all abnormally dilated superficial veins of the lower extremities, ranging in size from minute spider bursts of the skin to large, protruding varicosities in the subcutaneous tissue. Whereas the former do not disrupt the venous physiology, the latter do interfere with the normal venous return because of valvular incompetency. Between these extremes are the more numerous but milder varicosities, which often but not necessarily always enlarge and become of surgical significance. If these smaller veins are included, probably 40% to 50% of adults have varicose veins. However, only 10% to 17% of the adult population have significant varicose veins, meaning that the veins have become dilated, incompetent, and symptomatic because the normal venous hemodynamics have been altered. Because of the protean manifestations of venous disorders of the lower extremities, many options are available for their management, ranging from radical surgery, elastic support, and sclerotherapy to no treatment at all. The severity of the venous problem must be weighed against the patient's overall general medical condition, since the basic objective of treatment is rehabilitation and prophylaxis.

Of the 1,066 primary consultations seen by me in our Section of Peripheral Vein Surgery over one year, 202 patients, or 19%, had problems that were clearly not due to venous disease, such as edema, lymphedema, lipedema, and other conditions. Of the 864 patients, or 81%, who did have venous problems, 244 had deep venous insufficiency, as evidenced by edema, cyanosis, breakdown of cutaneous venules, and skin changes such as stasis dermatitis, pigmentation, cellulitis, and ulceration. Often these patients had secondary varicosities of the saphenous system. The remaining 620 patients had varicosities that appeared to represent primary involvement of the saphenous systems. In 373 patients, the varicosities were considered to be of such severity that surgical removal was recommended. In 247, the venous problems were of lesser magnitude, for which surgical treatment was not indicated; instead, elastic support for symptoms, elevation of the legs, exercise, or sclerotherapy was considered. Some had varicosities so trivial that no treatment seemed necessary. Coon, Willis, and Keller have estimated that the prevalence of significant varicose veins is 24 million among adults in the United States, which is approximately 12% of the adult population. By "significant" is meant that these are incompetent symptomatic veins for which treatment is advisable.

The purposes of treating significant varicose veins are threefold. The first is to relieve the symptoms of venous stasis. Common complaints ascribed to varicose veins are aching, swelling, heaviness, cramping, itching, and burning, in that order of frequency. The second is to remove or to prevent complications of varicose veins such as thrombophlebitis, dermatitis, hemorrhage, and ulcers. The third is to provide long-term control of the venous insufficiency.

It has been our experience that surgical removal of the varicose veins offers the best long-term control and, ideally, this is our treatment of choice. As mentioned, not all venous stasis problems require surgical treatment; nor should all patients undergo the operation, even though their varicose veins are of surgical caliber. Varicose veins should not be operated on in a patient who has uncontrolled malignant or metabolic disease, advanced cardiovascular or peripheral vascular disease, or impaired leg function due to neuromuscular or orthopedic problems. Overall, the treatment should not be more hazardous than the venous disease itself.

Of the 373 patients who were offered vein stripping, only 155 actually underwent the operation. The others may have had more compelling problems.

The diagnosis of varicose veins is established by the history and clinical examination alone. The tortuosity of the veins and the condition of the overlying skin are observed. Palpation may detect induration of the veins if they are thrombosed and may delineate areas of stasis cellulitis. The retrograde filling test, as described originally by Sir Benjamin Brodie in 1846, will demonstrate the function of the valves. This examination will also reveal significant incompetency of the perforating veins. If incompetent perforating veins are noted, there is most likely an underlying chronic deep venous insufficiency, which is often secondary to an ancient deep thrombophlebitis. On occasion, the vascular noninvasive laboratory will be helpful in confirming the clinical diagnosis, but it is not routinely used. In obscure problems involving ligation, venography may be indicated. Conditions such as lymphedema and lipedema, congenital venous anomalies, and chronic deep venous insufficiency must be differentiated in the physical diagnosis. Varicose veins may indeed coexist, but the complaints described may not be due to the varicosities but be caused by degenerative joint disease and referred pain.

If reflux is demonstrated in the main channels of the greater and lesser saphenous systems, these veins have lost their useful function in returning the blood to the heart. Instead, they now interfere with lowering of the ambulatory venous pressure and thus cause the signs and symptoms already described. Therefore, under ideal conditions, they should be removed.

Our technique for the stripping operation had until recent years followed the "all or none" principle, in which all obvious varicosities and those tributaries potentially varicose are removed as thoroughly as possible.

The surgical treatment of varicose veins of the lower extremity has been under reappraisal in recent years by both the patient and the physician. This reassessment is appropriate, since the conventional stripping operation contradicts the surgeon's philosophy of repair and restoration of function and calls for an ablative procedure, destroying the veins, rather than one that restores to normal the deranged venous hemodynamics. Factors that have been responsible for this reappraisal are the usefulness of the saphenous vein for arterial grafting, the increasing concern over cost containment, the search for a better and simpler form of care in an ambulatory setting, and the introduction of new noninvasive laboratory aids for a more precise assessment of venous function such as the use of the Doppler method and photoplethysmography.

Although there has been no decrease in the incidence of varicose veins, which, as mentioned, is estimated to range from 10% to 17% of the adult population, there has been a decrease in the number of vein-stripping operations at the Mayo Clinic. The impact of arterial reconstructive surgery that makes use of the saphenous vein for bypass grafting has without question ushered in an attitude of conservatism in our treatment of varicose veins and has also unquestionably influenced us to be more selective and more discriminating in our technique. We may, on occasion, perform a limited vein-stripping procedure, leaving the thigh segments of the saphenous channel intact; however, a retained saphenous vein is a possible nidus for recurrence of varicosities inasmuch as the pathogenesis of varicose veins is a sequential retrograde breakdown of the valves from the saphenofemoral juncture. It thus compromises a good long-term result from vein stripping, which is based on the premise that a vein removed cannot create a recurring problem. One might speculate whether this retained segment of the saphenous system will escape the progressive degeneration seen in varicose veins and still remain a good arterial graft if it is ever needed. Therefore, if significant varicose veins are removed in one leg and minor varicosities are found in the contralateral leg, the latter may be excised locally through multiple small incisions while the main channels are left intact. A large tributary vein with a clinically competent main channel can be excised without disturbing the saphenous vein. Isolated incompetent perforating veins, which are commonly found on the lateral aspect of the thigh and in the popliteal space, do not communicate with the saphenous system. Ligation of the perforating veins and excision of the overlying tributaries should suffice in these instances. If the varicosities are mild, reevaluation in 1 to 2 years may be the wisest choice.

Sclerotherapy has not been a planned procedure to follow a limited vein-stripping operation, but smaller veins that appear after a thorough vein-stripping operation can be treated with sclerotherapy with a moderate degree of success. Sclerotherapy is also commonly used for cosmetic purpose for venous stars and in the eradication of small venules on the foot and ankle, which may erode through the skin and cause troublesome bleeding. The patient should always be forewarned that a hemosiderin pigment stain may follow the infection.

That varicose veins is a progressive degenerative disorder has been demonstrated by a group of patients whom we have followed for 20 or more years after operation. Veins that were clinically normal at the time of surgery and thus were not removed have shown a gradual, progressive breakdown. Results at the 10-year mark, which have been published, showed 85% good to excellent control, but at 20 years, only 68% were in this category, the remainder having acquired varicosities that became of surgical caliber. The recurrent pattern was nearly always found in the very system that had been operated on.

Some surgeons advocate that both legs should be operated on even though varicosities are present in only one leg, believing that it is merely a matter of time before the other leg veins become varicose. Of the 52 patients who were examined 20 years or more after surgery and in whom only one leg had been operated on, 6 needed subsequent vein surgery in the other leg. In seven additional patients, varicosities had developed in the other leg that were of surgical caliber. Thus, only one in four patients acquired varicosities over the many years in the contralateral leg. This confirms our long-held conviction that there is no place for the prophylactic surgical removal of normal veins in the contralateral leg.

It is not known how many patients with varicose veins eventually require arterial bypass surgery. None of the 140 patients who were examined at 20 years had that need. Of the 440 patients responding to a letter inquiry, 8 had received and 5 had been denied arterial reconstructive surgery. These 13 patients (3% of the respondents) would have benefited from a good saphenous vein if it had been available. This low incidence may be due to the good general health of these patients at the time of surgery, the predominance of female over male patients, and the relatively young age (mean age of 48.7 years) when these patients were operated on.

In summary and conclusion, the long-term control of the inherently progressive and degenerative disease of varicose veins appears to be quite satisfactory with the conventional stripping operation. A limited vein-stripping procedure may be justifiable in selected conditions. Sclerotherapy should not be a cover-up for incomplete surgery but may be indicated for smaller veins after effective surgery. The prophylactic stripping of clinically normal veins in the contralateral leg does not appear to be justified, because the probability of a subsequent breakdown of the veins is slight. To withhold stripping of clinically incompetent varicose veins for possible later need for arterial bypass surgery does not appear justified, for a diseased vein is not an acceptable graft; in any case, from the results of this study, the probability of this event is not significant.

22
Diagnostic Evaluation and Surgical Treatment of Chronic Venous Insufficiency

Harry Schanzer

Chronic venous stasis of the lower extremity remains a devastating health problem. The multiple modalities of therapy advocated for this condition suggest that no single treatment is good for the entire population.

The purpose of this study was to evaluate patients with this condition by ambulatory venous pressure and ascending and retrograde phlebography and, by understanding the specific pathogenetic factor, to be able to rationally prescribe a surgical treatment.

MATERIALS AND METHODS

Fifty-two lower extremities in forty-nine patients suffering from chronic venous stasis were included in this study. Ambulatory venous pressure measurements were performed as described previously [1]. A #18 catheter was placed in a dorsal vein of the foot and the patient was asked to walk in place for 15 seconds. Pressures were measured with a Statham strain gauge transducer and recorded. Determinations were done without tourniquet, and with one or two tourniquets at different levels of the extremity. The percent of pressure drop during exercise and the time of return to standing levels were used to calculate a Venous Sufficiency Index.

Ascending phlebography was done by injecting 50 ml of Hypaque 50% into a dorsal vein of the foot with the patient in a 60° position and a tourniquet applied to his ankle. A femoral retrograde phlebogram was done by making a similar injection into the femoral vein in the same position while performing a Valsalva maneuver.

RESULTS

Four different pathogenetic groups could be distinguished:

1. Incompetence of perforators (59.6%). This group could be divided into two subgroups:
   a. Incompetent perforators alone (20 patients).
   b. Combination of incompetent perforators and those with incompetent saphenous system (11 patients).
2. Incompetence of deep veins (26.8%).
3. Incompetence of saphenous system (5.7%).
4. Deep vein obstruction (7.6%).

Based on these results, the following surgical procedures were performed:

1. Subfascial ligation of perforators (25 cases).
2. Superficial femoral valvuloplasty (3 cases).
3. Ligation of the superficial femoral vein (1 case).
4. Segmental venous transfer (1 case).
5. Saphenous vein cross femoral vein bypass (1 case).
6. High ligation and stripping of the long saphenous vein (3 cases).

The complications of these procedures were as follows: Skin sloughing was seen in three cases of perforator ligation after long posteromedial incisions. One of these cases required a skin graft. A postoperative hematoma occurred in the patient who underwent segmental venous transfer and required surgical evacuation.

The follow-up period in these cases had been between 1 and 37 months (see Table 1). Of the 25 cases that had ligation of perforators, 22 could be followed (88%). Only 2 cases did not show improvement; 1 case had recurrence of ulcer after 8 months. Postoperative ambulatory venous pressure demonstrated significant deep vein incompetence, and this patient underwent ligation of the superficial femoral vein and has been free of recurrence for 5 months. The second case had recurrence of a small ulcer after 34 months and healed quickly with Unna boot treatment. All patients undergoing other procedures have shown improvement in their symptomatology.

Table 1. Follow-Up Surgery, Venous Stasis, March 1981

Type of surgery	Time follow-up (months)	Result
Ligation Perforators[a]	1	improved
	3	improved
	4	improved
	4	improved
	7	improved
	8	improved
	9	improved
	9	improved
	10	improved
	10	improved
	12	improved
	12	improved
	13	improved
	13	improved
	20	improved
	21	improved
	22	improved
	24	improved
	27	recurrence of ulcer
	27	improved
	33	improved
	37	recurrence of ulcer
Segmental venous transfer	9	improved
Valvuloplasty	3	improved
	17	improved
	20	improved
Ligation superficial femoral vein	5	improved
High ligation saphenous vein	17	improved
	22	improved
	22	improved
Cross femoral venous bypass	4	improved

[a]Of 25 cases, 3 cases lost to follow-up.

In an attempt to have a more objective evaluation of these patients, postoperative ambulatory venous pressure studies were performed in 10 patients after perforator ligation, 2 patients after valvuloplasty, 1 patient after segmental venous transfer, and 1 patient after cross-femoral venous bypass (see Table 2). Results show improvement in all cases. Return to normal values nevertheless was seen only in 5 patients after perforator ligation and in 1 case after cross-femoral bypass.

Table 2. Venous Sufficiency Index (VSI) In 10 Patients

Procedure	Preoperative VSI[a]	Postoperative VSI
Ligation Perforators	4.6	8.3
	2.7	6.3
	4	12
	4	14
	4	16
	0.4	17.5
	5	27
	4.6	35
	0.8	38.7
	0.15	54
	1.7	74
Valvuloplasty	2.7	5.7
	4	6
Segmental Venous Transfer	0.6	7
Cross-Femoral Venous Bypass	1	26

[a]Normal Value = 58±30.

DISCUSSION

Chrcnic venous stasis of the lower extremity has been treated over the years by many different methods, both medical and surgical. Medical treatment consists basically in the prevention of stasis by bed rest, leg elevation and different elastic compression stockings. Surgical treatments aimed at treating the ulcer directly by resecting it and covering it with skin grafts [2], ligating incompetent perforators [3], treating incompetent superficial venous systems [4], and, more recently, correcting incompetent deep femoral valves by valvuloplasty [5] or segmental venous transfer [6] or by bypassing obstructive venous systems [7,8].

Previous studies done by us [1] demonstrate that this chronic condition is the result of different alterations in the venous system of the lower extremity. These pathogenetic factors can be identified by the combined use of ambulatory venous pressure with the use of tourniquet and ascending-retrograde phlebography. By understanding the mechanism of disease in each instance, a rational therapy can be prescribed. Clinical results of the present surgical series have been very encouraging in the short follow-up of 1–37 months. The postoperative functional evaluation demonstrates that all cases show improvement. Most of the cases, however, do not return to normal values. If this improvement is enough to shift the balance from an uncompensated to a compensated state, it will ony be determined by long follow-ups.

REFERENCES

1. Schanzer H, Peirce EC II. Pathophysiological evaluation of chronic venous stasis with ambulatory venous pressure studies. Angiology (in press).
2. Homans J. The operative treatment of varicose veins and ulcers based upon a classification of these lesions. Surg Gynecol Obstet 22:143–158, 1916.
3. Linton RR. The communicating veins of the lower leg and the operative technique for their ligation. Ann Surg 107:582, 1938.
4. Recek C. A critical appraisal of the role of ankle perforators for the genesis of venous ulcers in the lower leg. J Cardiovascular Surg 12:45–49, 1971.
5. Kistner RL. Surgical repair of the incompetent femoral vein valve. Arch Surg 110:1336–1342, 1975.
6. Kistner RL, Sparkuhl M. Surgery in acute and chronic venous disease. Surgery 85:31–43, 1979.
7. Husni EA. Clinical experience with femoropopliteal reconstruction. In Bergen JJ, Yao JS (eds.), A New Look at Venous Problems, pp. 485–491. Chicago, Year Book Medical Publishers, 1978.
8. Palma EC, Esperon R. Vein transplants and grafts in the surgical treatment of the post phlebitic syndrome. J Cardiovascular Surg 1:94, 1960.

23
Evaluation of Venography

Alfred R. Ernst

Ascending venography remains a valuable and frequently used method for the objective diagnosis of deep vein thrombosis (DVT) in the legs. In the county of Queens, New York City 13 of 17 hospitals with 50% of the bed capacity do not have noninvasive laboratories and must resort to venography as the only objective means in the diagnosis of DVT. The American Hospital Association does not have figures concerning how many hospitals in America have a noninvasive vascular laboratory.

This report is supported by a retrospective study of 300 consecutive cases of venography at our institution. The technique, as described, requires moderate quantities of contrast material and includes thorough removal of dye from the leg vein, using both elevation and flushing.

The review revealed generally good-quality venograms, of which 39% showed evidence of DVT. The procedure was associated with very low morbidity. The reliability of the negative venogram was again demonstrated. Some difficulties in performance and interpretation of venograms are discussed.

General use of venography is on the wane at university and other teaching hospitals, due to the rapid improvements in noninvasive studies. These are associated with no complications and less discomfort, easier accessibility and patient acceptance as compared to venography, and are almost as accurate. However, since it is most often unacceptable to treat patients with long-term anticoagulants on the basis of clinical diagnosis, well-performed venography will continue to be of great value in those institutions that are not equipped with noninvasive laboratories. A review of the literature of the past 12 years reveals that three changes have occurred in the diagnosis of DVT in the legs.

1. There have been brilliant advances in noninvasive diagnostic methods.
2. Venography has been used with rapidly decreasing frequency at the university and large teaching hospital levels.
3. There have been numerous reports of the problems and complications associated with ascending venography.

We recently tried to determine to what degree these changes had occurred at the community hospital level. The American Hospital Association has no statistics on vascular labs throughout the country. In the county of Queens, New York City, with a population of 2½ million, there are 18 hospitals. Four of these hospitals, with a bed capacity of 2,438, have noninvasive labs. Fourteen hospitals, with a bed capacity of 3,245, do not have vascular labs. Therefore, venography is the only objective test for DVT available to most hospitals in Queens. In 1980, Hull stated, "Venography is the most definitive method currently available to confirm or exclude the diagnosis (of DVT) in patients who have clinically suspected venous thrombosis." Since it became apparent that the use of venography was still common, at least in our area, we felt that a reevaluation of some aspects of the procedure would be in order. We addressed the following questions: (1) When should it be done? (2) How is it to be done? (3) How can problems associated with venography be minimized?

WHEN SHOULD IT BE DONE?

There is universal agreement that the clinical diagnosis of DVT is unreliable. Haeger made two studies in 1965 and 1969 and showed that the venous tree was normal in 45% of the cases that were hospitalized and treated for DVT. In 1976, Cranley presented similar findings in a very careful study. In 1980, Hirsh presented similar findings in 1,000 cases, showing that the clinician is wrong at least 50% of the time on both the positive and negative side in the diagnosis of DVT. This was true whatever the signs and symptoms were, including pain, swelling and tenderness.

Because of these and other similar studies, it is now unacceptable that any patient be subjected to 4 to 6 months of anticoagulant therapy before diagnosis in made by an objective method. Usually, phlegmasia cerulea dolens is one of the few exceptions to the above statement. Therefore, venography should be done:

1. On all patients suspected of having DVT in a hospital without a vascular lab.
2. It is suggested that it be done on all patients with suspicion of DVT in hospitals where vascular labs are not yet well calibrated.
3. In institutions with established labs when noninvasive studies are equivocal.

In institutions that have obtained the degree of accuracy of Doctors Cranley, Strandness, Raines or many other leaders in the fie.d, venograph· can well be restricted to problem cases. However, in newly formed labs, it would seem in order to continue venography on all of the first few hundred cases until specificity and sensitivity have reached a 90% level. This degree of accuracy apparently is not too easy to obtain. I have visited vascular labs that have been functioning for 3 or 4 years. While their arterial evaluations are excellent, the clinicians still have reason to doubt venographic evaluations, which are often only at the 80% accuracy level.

HOW SHOULD VENOGRAPHY BE DONE?

This question is somewhat more difficult to answer. There are numerous techniques used for venography. The most popular of these are those of Rabinov and Paulin, Nicolaides and Kakar, Gallus and Thomas and Albrechtson. Some are done with the patient horizontal, most with a tilt table at 30-60 degrees. Dosages vary from 50 cc to as much as 400 cc of dye. Some use tourniquets at the ankle and above the knee; some use no tourniquets. There is little question that the larger the dose used, the more soleus and gastrocneumius venous sinuses will be visualized. However, it is also probable that the more dye used, the greater the irritation to the venous intima and the greater the possibility of a problem arising therefrom.

We have chosen to use a low-dosage technique. Our management of cases requiring venography is described next. The patient suspected of having DVT is given a bolus of heparin I.V. and venography is done the same day, providing edema has not obliterated the superficial femoral veins. If the vein is not visible, the patient is started on continuous I.V. heparin and the hip Gatch is elevated 10 degrees. Usually within 24 to 48 hours, the edema subsides sufficiently so that the foot veins reappear and venography can be performed. We prefer to avoid cut-downs. This was done on only 2 in our series of 254 cases. Tourniquets are used at the ankle and above or below the knee, 50 cc of Conray 60 is injected into the leg; the injection takes 60 seconds. Two plates are taken of the leg below the knee in the AP and oblique planes, and two plates are taken of the thigh. These are done as quickly as the technician can change the plates and move the tube. For the pelvic view, the cassette is placed at the proper level, the tube is set over the patient's lower abdomen, and the table is corrected to the horizontal position. The surgeon then immediately lifts both legs to 50 to 60 degrees, counts a long one second, and calls "shoot!" In this manner, good visualization is obtained of the iliac veins and the lower vena cava. Pictures are not always suitable as slide material, but certainly are readable. The patient is sent down to his room with an I.V. going into the foot. Four hundred cc of saline or 5% glucose in distilled water is run through the foot vein during the next two hours, while the hip Gatch is elevated to 20 degrees.

Using this technique we have recently reviewed 254 consecutive venograms performed over a six-year period. All x-rays were personally reviewed. The hospital charts on 210 of these patients were reviewed. Subsequent records on all 254 patients were obtained for a 2-month follow-up either by the reviewing of clinic charts or contacting the attending physician who followed the patient in his office. Our criteria for diagnosis of DVT were those usually used:

1. Constant filling defects which are reasonably delineated.
2. Abrupt termination of opaque column noted in two views.
3. Nonfilling of the entire deep venous system.
4. Increased collateral flow.

Regarding the evaluation of constant filling defects, these represent demonstration of the thrombosis and are the best demonstration of venous thrombosis. Most often, one plate is sufficient and leaves little question regarding diagnosis. The next two signs are more of a problem, especially as they occur in the tibial vessels. There are many cases with nonfilling in the tibial vessels. Certainly, these findings require confirmation in two views and probably also require reinjection with and without tourniquets, and assurance that there is no weight bearing by the affected leg and no hyperextension of the knee. We frequently do a venogram of the other leg to have an idea of the normal anatomy of the tibial veins in the patient. Increased collateral flow is, of course, an indirect sign. In itself, it is never used an a diagnostic sign, since, if it is significant, it will always be accompanied by any of the first three signs.

The following are some more pertinent findings in this study of the 254 venograms; 97 were performed unilaterally and 157 bilaterally. Venography was thus performed on a total of 411 extremities. Of the 254 patients suspected of having DVT, 103 showed x-ray evidence of DVT and 151 had negative venograms. This represented a positive finding of 41%. The areas of involvement in the positive grams were as follows:

Tibial veins	33
Tibial popliteal veins	13
Tibial popliteal femoral veins	35
Tibial popliteal femoral iliac veins	11
Femoral vein only	6
Ilio femoral veins	2
Iliac veins	3

The tibial veins, therefore, contained clots in 90% of the cases. There were a few cases in which skip lesions were visable. In other words, clots were present in the tibial and upper femoral veins, with a normal popliteal or lower femoral segment visible. There were no isolated soleus and gastrocnemius vein clots found. This was in distinction to the findings of Nicolaides, in which 20% of his positive grams revealed clots that were localized to either large gastrocnemius or soleus veins.

There has been relatively little written regarding the validity of the negative venogram. This was alluded to in 1970 by Rabinov who stated, "While the possibility that minor clot formations may escape detection cannot be completely excluded, we feel that, for all practical purposes, a negative phlebogram indicates the absence of thrombophlebitis." In 1980, Hull specifically addressed the question of validity of the negative venogram. He followed 150 cases with negative venograms for 3 months. There were 2 cases who developed DVT, which he considered due to the procedure itself. However, he concluded that there were no cases of DVT missed by his negative venograms.

In our two-month follow-up of all 151 patients with negative venograms in our study, there were no cases who developed pulmonary embolism or DVT. Three of these patients died in the two-month follow-up, one of a stroke and two of cardiac failure.

COMPLICATIONS

The complications of the procedure were relatively few and minor in nature. There were some minor cases of local superficial phlebitis, which subsided in a few days. As previously stated, there were no cases of DVT. There were very few patients who complained of local calf discomfort for 12 or 18 hours following the gram. There were occasional mild reactions to the dye, manifested by flushing or mottled rash of the face and neck and several episodes of nausea or vomiting. There were no cases of anaphylaxis or other major complications. No episodes of pulmonary embolism could be attributed to the procedure.

There were, however, some disturbing findings in reviewing all of these x-rays. There were those in which the technique was less than perfect. I found cases in which I considered the technique poor and the plates unreadable. The problem area usually involved suitable demonstration of the tibial veins. Repeat studies with better technique should have been, but were not, done. In these cases, the most common problems involved taking the tibial vessels in only one view. Tibial vessels should be in two views and should include a high KV technique to suppress bone opacity so that the tibial veins become more apparent. There were at least a dozen other tibial vein demonstrations which I considered less than optimal, but they were readable. Nonetheless, it demonstrates that the "gold standard" is only the "gold standard" if it is well done.

Therefore, regarding question three, take tibial pictures in at least 2 planes and give a repeat injection with 3 or 4 shots. If necessary, take the pictures with and without tourniquets, avoid too much weight-bearing of the foot of the leg being examined, and avoid hyperextension of the knee. Also, use KV technique that will burn out the bone to some extent so that the tibial vessels become more apparent. Post x-ray, elevate the limb for a period and wash it out thoroughly with saline. We have no experience with the use of isotonic dye.

CONCLUSIONS

Finally, in our evaluation of venography in 1983, we make the following statements:

1. It is not acceptable to treat DVT without an objective confirmatory test.
2. Venography is still very frequently done and has served us well.
3. The "gold standard" has some problems when not well done.
4. Develop and perfect your noninvasive vascular laboratories.

BIBLIOGRAPHY

Albrechtsson U, Olsen CG. Thrombotic side effects of phlebography. Lancet 1976:723.

Albrectsson U, Olsen CG. Thrombosis after phlebography. Cardiovasc Radiol 2:9, 1979.

Bettmann MA, Paulin S. Leg phlebography incidence, nature and modification of undesirable side effects. Radiology 122:101, 1977.

Cranley JJ. Diagnosis of deep venous thrombosis. Arch Surg 3:34, 1969.

Gallus A, et al. Small subcutaneous doses of heparin in prevention of venous thrombosis. New Engl J Med 288:545, 1973.

Haeger K. Problems of acute deep venous thrombosis. Angiology 20:219–223, 1969.

Health Facilities in Southern New York State. United Hospital Fund, 1982.

Hirsh J. Noninvasive tests for thromboembolic disease. Hospital Practice 1982:77.

Hull R. Current approach to diagnosis of deep venous thrombosis. Modern Concepts of Cardiovascular Disease 51:129–132, 1982.

Hull R, et al. Clinical validity of a negative venogram. Circulation 64(3):622, 1981.

Rabinov K, Pauline S. Roentgen diagnosis of venous thrombosis in the legs. Arch Surg 104:134, 1972.

Thomas ML. Phlebography. Arch Surg 104:145, 1972.

11

Esophageal Varices

24
Emergency Treatment of Bleeding Esophageal Varices

Marshall J. Orloff

Since 1963, *all* patients who have entered our institution with bleeding esophageal varices due to cirrhosis have been treated by emergency portacaval shunt (EPCS) within 8 hours of admission. The results have improved progressively with time, and during the past 6 years the improvement has been highly significant. This report describes our experience from 1977 through 1982 in 84 unselected cirrhotic patients, and compares the recent results with those obtained in 180 similarly unselected, consecutive patients during the first 15 years of our prospective study of EPCS. An extensive diagnostic workup was completed within 3 to 7 hours of admission to the emergency department, and all of the survivors underwent lifelong follow-up at regular intervals, so that the current status of 97% of the patients is known. On admission, 48% had jaundice, 42% had ascites, 42% had severe muscle wasting, 19% had encephalopathy or coma, and 90% had a hyperdynamic state. The incidences of these signs of far-advanced cirrhosis were almost identical in the recent and earlier groups of patients. In every patient, bleeding varices were demonstrated by emergency endoscopy, and cirrhosis was documented by operative liver biopsy. Systemic intravenous vasopressin temporarily controlled varix hemorrhage in 95% of patients, and EPCS permanently controlled varix bleeding in *every* patient by reducing the mean corrected portal pressure from 250 to 16 mm saline. Long-term patency of the PCS has been proven in 100% of patients by yearly angiography and shunt catheterization. Thirty-six percent of patients had a documented history of encephalopathy before EPCS, and 16% of the survivors have had one or more episodes of encephalopathy postoperatively. The operative (30-day) survival rate was 83% in 84 recent patients, compared to 58% in our earlier group of 180 patients. Five-year actuarial survival is 72% in our recent group, compared to 38% in the earlier group. These results of EPCS in *unselected* patients not only reflect a striking improvement in our own experience, but also they are as good as or better than the results of elective PCS in *highly selected patients* reported by other surgeons. Moreover, in comparison with our previous prospective studies, EPCS produced a significantly greater long-term survival rate than either emergency medical therapy or emergency varix ligation followed by elective shunt.

QUESTIONS

1. Encephalopathy occurs in approximately one-third of cirrhotic patients with bleeding varices who have not undergone portacaval shunt.

   a. True
   b. False

   Answer: **a (True)**

2. In recent years, the survival rates following emergency portacaval shunt in unselected cirrhotic patients with bleeding varices have been (choose one):

   a. One year 80+%; five years 70+%
   b. One year 60+%; five years 50+%
   c. One year 40+%; five years 30+%
   d. One year 60+%; five years 30+%

   Answer: a

3. Cirrhotic patients with bleeding varices are characterized by the following *one or more* features:

   a. Hyperdynamic state
   b. High mortality rate
   c. Coagulopathy
   d. Hyperkalemic alkalosis
   e. High incidence of recurrent bleeding

   Answer: **a, b, c, d, e**

4. Which of the following measures provides definitive treatment of bleeding esophageal varices (choose one or more)?

   a. Endoscopic sclerotherapy
   b. Transesophageal varix ligation
   c. Intravenous vasopressin
   d. Esophageal balloon tamponade
   e. Portacaval shunt
   f. All of the above
   g. None of the above

   Answer: **e**

5. It is often difficult to make the diagnosis of bleeding esophageal varices.

   a. True
   b. False

   Answer: **b (False)**

BIBLIOGRAPHY

Orloff MJ, Bell RH, Hyde PV, Skivolocki WP. Long-term results of emergency portacaval shunt for bleeding esophageal varices in unselected patients with alcoholic cirrhosis. Ann Surg 192:325, 1980.

Orloff MJ. Portal hypertension: Portacaval anastomosis. In HAF Dudley, WJ Pories, (eds.), Rod and Smith's Operative Surgery, Abdomen, Fourth ed. London, Butterworths, 1983.

Orloff MJ, Duguay LR, Kosta LD. Criteria for selection of patients for emergency portacaval shunt. Am J Surg 134:146, 1977.

Orloff MJ, Chandler JG, Charters AC, Condon JK, Grambort DE, Modafferi TR, Levin SE. Portacaval shunt as emergency procedure in unselected patients with alcoholic cirrhosis. Surg Gynecol Obstet 141:59. 1975.

Orloff MJ, Chandler JG, Charters AC, Condon JK, Grambort DE, Modafferi TR, Levin SE. Comparison of end-to-side and side-to-side portacaval shunts in dogs and humans with cirrhosis and portal hypertension. Am J Surg 218: 195, 1974.

12

Law and Medicine

25
How to Prevent and Minimize Malpractice Claims

Seymour Boyers

Mention the word "malpractice" to physicians and most every conversation will cease in the ensuing passionate exchange of opinions, experiences and fears. One principle remains constant—good medicine is good law. Good medicine can be and is defended, and will remain defensible in the courtroom.

A malpractice suit is a traumatic event in any doctor's professional career. It projects him into an unfamiliar arena of legal conflict. It is, therefore, important that the doctor be made aware of the nuances and pitfalls so that he can be prepared to proceed.

What do we mean when we talk in terms of medical malpractice? Once a patient visits a doctor for treatment, a physician-patient relationship is established. A physician who undertakes to treat a patient implies that he possesses, and the law places upon him the duty of possessing, that reasonable degree of learning and skill that is ordinarily possessed by physicians and surgeons in the community where he practices. Upon consenting to treat a patient, it becomes the duty of a physician and surgeon to use reasonable care and diligence in the exercise of his skill and the application of his learning to accomplish the purpose for which he was employed, and he is under a further obligation to use his best judgment in exercising his skill and applying his knowledge. The law holds a physician and surgeon liable for any injury to his patient resulting from want of the requisite knowledge and skill, or the failure to exercise reasonable care, or failure to use his best judgment.

What should you do when you receive a letter from an attorney representing your patient, who states that he has a viable claim against a third party physician, and he solicits your opinion as to what caused the condition or injuries to the patient? You should be very careful before you go into great detail as to the causal relationship or proximate cause of the injury complained of by your patient. You should never include words that would indicate what caused a particular condition or incident, because the moment you do that—the moment you give a causal connection—you may well be providing the foundation for a lawsuit against yourself. The better procedure to follow upon receiving such a letter is to communicate immediately with your insurance carrier, emphasizing the fact that you would like to have an attorney advise you how to respond, because you can be sure that a lawsuit has started its course well before you receive the first legal paper. Likewise, if before receiving any written communication you receive a telephone call from a lawyer who represents that he is the attorney for your patient, and solicits your opinion, you would be well advised not to discuss the case on the telephone with anyone, first, because you don't know whether or not the conversation is being recorded, and second, because a doctor who is not trained in legal niceties may unwittingly make statements that can later prove damaging. You can always advise the attorney that if he wishes an opinion, he should: (1) submit to you a written authorization from the patient, and (2) reduce to writing the opinion he seeks.

In the same vein, if you should receive a letter from an attorney together with an authorization signed by your patient requesting a copy of your office records, it is axiomatic that you never send your original records. If I may suggest, at this early request stage, do not send a copy of your records either, but rather, a medical certificate, comprehensively describing, from information culled from your records, what disease or condition the patient was suffering from, what you did for your patient, what prescriptions you wrote, what instructions you gave, the nature of the treatment, and your diagnosis. The certificate, however, should never include words as to what caused the condition. Further, I would again emphasize that upon receipt of a lawyer's letter, the importance of immediately communicating with your insurance carrier to obtain legal advice before responding to it should be paramount in your mind.

Now, if you should be served with a summons and complaint, don't let the papers sit in your office. Time is of the essence! After you make a copy of the pleadings and open your own litigation file, you should contact your insurance company and advise them of the service of papers upon you, and arrange for the immediate delivery of the summons and complaint to their office. They, in turn, will set up a file and the usual practice is to put a claims supervisor in charge of the claim. The claim department will assign a defense lawyer to handle the case for you. Generally, it is essential that the defense lawyer and the doctor arrange for an early face-to-face meeting to discuss the problems of the case in totality. Otherwise, a delay may cause certain facts and positions to be stratified, which could be disastrous for the doctor. To illustrate the need for early investigation and evaluation, one merely has to conjur up what happens in the O.R. when a cardiac arrest occurs. When this catastrophic "code" event takes place, there is naturally some lack of attention to record-keeping procedures, because everyone is intent upon trying to do the best he (or she) can for the patient—precise record-keeping becomes a secondary concern. Unfortunately, however, following resolution of the emergency, the patient's chart is not updated and nothing is often done until an action has been instituted, by which time the events of the incident have become blurred and ambiguous. That is why it is so important that immediately following such an occurrence, within two or three days at most, all the participants in the event should be questioned while recollections are fresh, so that an existing record of what actually occurred can be put together. In that way, you prevent the kind of collusion or misperception that may arise when an alert and eager plaintiff's attorney conducts an early investigation of the occurrence. An immediate on-the-spot record will absolve from blame those who are not at fault, and at the same time, prevent the possible danger of collusion, if there is true negligence. But those who are free from fault should be absolved at the outset.

If a doctor is served with legal papers, how can he protect himself? I think the doctor can protect himself by a level of awareness that he is a client. After the lawyer who has been assigned to represent him by the insurance company communicates with the doctor, he should keep in close touch with that lawyer. The doctor should ask for copies of the pleadings; he should keep abreast of what is going on in the case, what strategy is being developed, what tactics are being used, and I mean, not only as to the merits of the case, but also insofar as settlement is concerned. The lawyer and doctor may conclude, after evaluating the case, that although the case may be defensible, there are certain aspects of the case that are potentially dangerous to the doctor. Under such circumstances, if the case can be settled for a reasonable sum, within the limits of the policy, it might be advisable to consent to a settlement, and thereby avoid the trauma of a protracted trial.

After sending the summons and complaint to the insurance company, the doctor may receive a notice from the carrier to the effect: "Doctor, you are being sued in an amount in excess of your coverage. We therefore suggest that you may want to obtain your own lawyer for your protection on the excess sued upon above your coverage." If such is the case, don't contact a real estate lawyer, or a criminal lawyer, but contact a lawyer who is conversant with the field of medical malpractice litigation, and who can work meaningfully and cooperatively with the lawyer assigned to represent you by your insurance company. Again, I wish to emphasize the importance of an early meeting with the attorney who has been assigned to represent you by the insurance carrier. You can be sure that such attorney will instruct you about not discussing the case with anyone—and that means your relatives, your patients, or any investigators who may come to question you about the action and its attendant events. If you are contacted by anyone at all about the facts of the case, your response should be that the matter is being handled by your attorney, and if the person wants any information, he (or she) can call your attorney. Any discussion on the part of the doctor is usually detrimental to his cause.

In the State of New York, since 1975 the Statute of Limitations for a medical malpractice cause of action is that an action may be instituted within 2½ years of the date of the occurrence of the alleged negligent act (CPLR 214-a). An exception to that rule is when the course of treatment that includes the wrongful acts or omissions has run continuously, and is related to the same original condition or complaint. Where there is continuous treatment, the Statute of Limitations does not begin to run until after the last day of treatment. The concern, of course, is whether there has been continuous treatment, and not merely a continuing relationship between physician and patient.

As a starting point, continuous treatment does not contemplate circumstances where a patient initiates return visits merely to have his or her condition checked. The Statute of Limitations may begin to run "once a hospital or physician considers the patient's treatment to be completed and does not request the patient to return for further examination." This is not to say, however, that a complete discharge by a physician forever bars a finding of continuous treatment. Included within the scope of "continuous treatment" is a timely return visit instigated by the patient to complain about, and seek treatment for, a matter related to the initial treatment. Thus, there will be continuous treatment when a patient, instructed that he or she does not need further attention, soon returns to the doctor because of continued pain in that area for such medical attention was first sought. Continuous treatment serves simply as a toll—the action may be brought at any time, but the patient will not be compelled to initiate judicial proceedings as long as the physician continues to treat the injury. Thus, whenever treatment of a patient is found to have ended, under present New York State law, a 2½ year time period for bringing suit is imposed.

Talking about the Statute of Limitations, I might also advise you that where, during the course of an operation, a foreign object, such as a cottonoid, a pad, or an instrument is left inside the body cavity following surgery and it is not discovered until ten years later, the patient is allowed to commence an action within one year following the discovery of the foreign object.

Even if treatment is undertaken pursuant to an express contract between physician and patient, except in most unusual circumstances, courts do not assume a guarantee or warranty from a physician that he will cure the patient. The only promises the physician is usually held to make are that he has the normal degree of skill, care and knowledge, and that he will use all three in treating the patient. Sometimes, however, a physician does make the mistake of guaranteeing results. If those results are not obtained, he may be liable for breach of warranty, even if he has used the highest skill. The results of any treatment, however, may vary under the best of circumstances, skill and care from excellent to poor. In other words, the physician who accepts a patient for treatment holds himself out as qualified to make a careful diagnosis and plan of treatment, and to use good judgment in carrying out the treatment. He does not hold himself out as a miracle worker, and he is not liable simply because his treatment produces a poor result.

Corollary to an action based upon malpractice is an action for lack of informed consent. Now, there are two distinct and separate entities, i.e., *consent*, which merely requires that you obtain the permission of the patient to operate, or treat him at all. This consent can be expressed in writing, or can be implied from the conduct of the parties. When we talk, however, of the cause of action based on lack of informed consent, we are saying that consent for a particular operation or treatment was obtained, but that the risks and hazards of such operation or treatment, and the alternatives, if any, were not intelligently and sufficiently explained to the patient, to the extent that the patient could make an understanding, independent decision to accept the operation or treatment, choose some available alternative, or decide to undergo *no* operation or treatment at all. Lack of informed consent is part of the legal theory of negligence. For example, with respect to a surgical procedure, the doctor is being charged with being negligent in not informing the patient of the risks and alternatives to the operation, and the consequences, if the operation is not undertaken. The fact that the doctor had the right to treat and operate is not disputed. The foundation underpinning of the lawsuit based on lack of informed consent is that had the physician explained the risks, the patient would not have undergone the operation or treatment. Accordingly, it follows that the injury or harm complained or, whatever it is, would not have come about. That is the distinction between *consent* and *lack of informed consent*.

I want to make it clear, however, that the gravamen of the action for lack of informed consent is not based upon the subjective determination of the patient–that is–following the procedure, the patient says that if he (or she) knew what the dangers or hazards of the operation were, that he (or she) would not have undergone the operation. No, it is not the subjective attitude of the patient, but rather, lack of informed consent is based upon an objective determination, that is, what a reasonably prudent person in the position of your patient would opt for if he (or she) were properly informed of the risks and hazards of the operation.

An example of a situation in which application of the doctrine of lack of informed consent is found is the case of *Fogal* v *Genessee Hospital* (41 AD2d 468). In that case, the patient suffered from an abdominal aortic aneurysm, and the doctor recommended that the patient, Mrs. Fogal, undergo an operative repair procedure. However, he did not inform the patient that this surgery involved stopping the blood supply to portions of the body for extended periods of time, and that recognized surgical practice suggested the use of hypothermia to cool and slow the body's metabolism during the operation. The hypothermia was accomplished by the use of a blanket placed under the patient's body on the operating table. The blanket was cooled or warmed by circulating alcohol through tubes in it at preset temperatures. The temperature of the coolant was regulated by control units, either automatic or manual, monitored by the anesthesiologist. When set on automatic, the action was designed to cool, until the desired body temperature, 89.6° Fahrenheit was reached, and then the automatic adjustment took over and recirculated warm liquid in the tubes in place of the cold, to warm the blanket, so that it maintained the prescribed body temperature. The hot and cold liquids were thus alternating to keep Mrs. Fogal's body temperature constant, as recorded by an esophogeal probe or thermometer. Mrs. Fogal was injured as a result of the use of the hypothermia blanket; her feet, thighs and buttocks became necrotic, necessitating excision of parts of her legs and buttocks and amputation of parts of both feet. It was one of plaintiff's contentions that since the automatic control was subsequently found to be defective, the body never warmed, but was continuously cooling throughout the time the patient was in the operating room from 8:00 A.M. until 1:05 P.M. There was evidence in the case that the doctors recognized cold injury as a risk incident to the use of hypothermia, particularly to a person in the physical condition of Mrs. Fogal. The cardiovascular surgeon in that case testified that he did, in fact, warn Mrs. Fogal of that danger. However, both Mr. and Mrs. Fogal denied that cold injury was ever mentioned or suggested as an inherent danger of the operation. Whether they possessed sufficient knowledge of the risks of cold injury before consenting to the procedure was a question of fact for the jury. Here, as a result of the defective automatic controls of the hypothermia machine, plaintiff suffered frostbite on the heels of both feet and the buttocks. That the hypothermia was appropriate or necessary to the surgery is beside the point. As the court, in *Fogal* observed, the patient may always choose between two apparent dangers, one attendant upon the surgery, the other resulting from the continuation of an existing condition because of the decision not to undergo surgery.

Now as stated previously, the determination as to whether there is lack of informed consent is an objective one. Let us assume, therefore, that the risk of the defective hypothermia machine occurs in 8% of the cases where hypothermia is used, whereas the failure to undergo an operative procedure for an abdominal aortic aneurysm is life-threatening. If the doctor had informed the patient, there is not doubt, if given the choice between a minimal risk of a defective hypothermia machine and that of a life-threatening condition, a reasonably prudent person would likely consent to the operation.

In dealing with the problem of informed consent, one must make a determination as to the mental capacity of a patient. Obviously, someone who is legally adjudicated insane cannot give consent, let alone informed consent. The real problem arises in the borderline cases, where a person has not been adjudicated insane, but there is a question as to the individual's mental capacity. What do you do with that type of person? You try to obtain the patient's consent in writing, and of course, whomever he lives with; or if you know any member of his family, get his (or her) consent. And please—make certain to document your records as to what you did in this regard.

Talking about records, in general, it is essential that you keep complete records of your treatment of the patient; what medications you prescribe, what instructions you give, and if there are any erasures in your records or different-colored inks used by you or your nurse, or information squeezed in between two lines on your records, make certain that you have a reasonable explanation for these changes. Otherwise these changes in your records may come back to haunt you, when you are examined by the plaintiff's attorney with regard to these changes at deposition or trial.

Now, a special problem with consent, and more particularly informed consent, arises with respect to sedated patients. The law is well settled that a sedated patient who is not in possession of his faculties cannot give a valid informed consent. This special problem arises when you have a patient who comes into the hospital in need of an operation. When do you get your surgical consent? The answer must be, if at all possible, prior to the administration of any sedation. You have the added problem as to the time limits of the consent. If a patient comes into the hospital, and you obtain the surgical consent on the first day of admission but don't operate until fifteen days later, the consent is worthless. The timeliness and the care requisite in obtaining a consent is so crucial, that you should never leave it to a nurse. And if you leave it to a resident, please, always check it to see that the patient gave an understanding and informed consent.

Doctors should be aware that the doctrine of informed consent applies also to the administration of drugs. Particularly where a doctor plans to use a clinical investigative drug, the doctor should obtain specific consent from the patient, the risk being that the FDA licenses a drug for prescription sale, but while the drug is being clinically investigated, the drug is not truly approved. It is a sine qua non in the law that if you use a drug that has not been approved by the

FDA, you do so at your own risk. It is therefore imperative that before using such a drug, you carefully explain to the patient the status of the drug, the reason why you feel it is necessary to use the drug, and the contraindications of its use.

From time to time there are special problems of consent that arise due to a patient's religion. It is a well-known fact, for example, that Jehovah's Witnesses will not accept a blood transfusion. A doctor must be very careful to examine the facts and circumstances before deciding to overrule a patient's religious freedom. If the patient is an adult, lucid individual who refuses to give any consent to treatment, the law permits him to exercise that right, and the doctor should abide by the patient's judgment. If, however, the patient is an infant and is suffering, for example, from bone cancer, and the doctor has recommended that the only way the patient's life can be saved is through immediate surgery, and the parent, because of religious principles refuses to permit such treatment, under those circumstances the doctor, or hospital administrator, can apply to the court for an immediate order waiving the parent's consent, and permitting the appointment of a temporary guardian, so that the child's life can be saved by authorizing the necessary treatment. This is so because a child is always a ward of the court, and the court may exercise its parens patrae status, which is in the best interests of the child.

A great Justice once observed, and I wholeheartedly agree, "I stand second to none in my boundless admiration for the medical profession." Doctors, in their dedication to the health of their patients, have contributed enormously to human happiness. In the best of medical hands, a patient may experience a bad result, and the doctor may, nevertheless, be sued, even though he has done nothing wrong. In most instances the doctor has done everything humanly and medically possible to effect a cure. An attorney should, therefore, hesitate before bringing a malpractice action, and carefully weigh all the facts and the medical literature. Charging a doctor with malpractice is a serious matter, and should not be done without careful deliberation. The attorney has a duty not to proceed, unless he is fully satisfied that malpractice has, in fact, occurred.

Index